T0353520

WOMEN AND POSITIVE AGING

WOMEN AND POSITIVE AGING

AN INTERNATIONAL PERSPECTIVE

LISA HOLLIS-SAWYER
AMANDA DYKEMA-ENGBLADE

AMSTERDAM • BOSTON • HEIDELBERG • LONDON
NEW YORK • OXFORD • PARIS • SAN DIEGO
SAN FRANCISCO • SINGAPORE • SYDNEY • TOKYO

Academic Press is an imprint of Elsevier

Academic Press is an imprint of Elsevier
125 London Wall, London EC2Y 5AS, UK
525 B Street, Suite 1800, San Diego, CA 92101-4495, USA
50 Hampshire Street, 5th Floor, Cambridge, MA 02139, USA
The Boulevard, Langford Lane, Kidlington, Oxford OX5 1GB, UK

Notices
Knowledge and best practice in this field are constantly changing. As new research and experience broaden our understanding, changes in research methods, professional practices, or medical treatment may become necessary.

Practitioners and researchers must always rely on their own experience and knowledge in evaluating and using any information, methods, compounds, or experiments described herein. In using such information or methods they should be mindful of their own safety and the safety of others, including parties for whom they have a professional responsibility.

To the fullest extent of the law, neither the Publisher nor the authors, contributors, or editors, assume any liability for any injury and/or damage to persons or property as a matter of products liability, negligence or otherwise, or from any use or operation of any methods, products, instructions, or ideas contained in the material herein.

ISBN: 978-0-12-420136-1

British Library Cataloguing-in-Publication Data
A catalogue record for this book is available from the British Library

Library of Congress Cataloging-in-Publication Data
A catalog record for this book is available from the Library of Congress

For information on all Academic Press publications
visit our website at https://www.elsevier.com/

  Working together
to grow libraries in
developing countries

www.elsevier.com • www.bookaid.org

Publisher: Nikki Levy
Acquisition Editor: Emily Ekle
Editorial Project Manager: Barbara Makinster
Production Project Manager: Julie-Ann Stansfield
Designer: Maria Inês Cruz

Typeset by MPS Limited, Chennai, India

On Aging

"When you see me sitting quietly, like a sack left on a shelf,
Don't think I need your chattering. I'm listening to myself.
Hold! Stop! Don't pity me! Hold! Stop your sympathy!
Understanding if you got it, otherwise I'll do without it!
When my bones are stiff and aching and my feet won't climb the stair,
I will only ask one favor: Don't bring me no rocking chair.
When you see me walking, stumbling, don't study and get it wrong.
'Cause tired don't mean lazy and every goodbye ain't gone.
I'm the same person I was back then, a little less hair, a little less chin,
A lot less lungs and much less wind.
But ain't I lucky I can still breathe in."

–*Maya Angelou, And Still I Rise (1978).*

Contents

Authors   xiii
Preface   xv
Acknowledgments   xvii

I

THE PSYCHOLOGY OF WOMEN'S AGING

1. Older Women and Their Mental Health Needs

Women and Harmonious Aging   4
Aging Women's Resources and Mental Health   5
Women's Later-Life Role Transitions   6
Social Power, Empowerment, and Coping of Older Women   7
"Mind-Body" Connection in Aging Women's Mental Health   8
Factors Determining Aging Women's Mental Health Outcomes   10
Role of Culture in Aging Women's Positive Mental Health   12
Societal "Messages" of Women's Positive Aging   13
Summary   15
Discussion Questions   15
Supplemental Book Readings   16
Supplemental Aging Videos   19
Additional Information Links   21
References   21

2. Women's Resiliency and Psychological Adaptation to Aging

Aging Women's Social Roles and Resiliency   28
The Ecology of Women's Positive Aging   31
Generativity and Personal Growth   33
Positive Resilience as a Learning Process within a Cultural Context   35
Positive Cultural Attitudes and Influences   37
Gerotranscendance and Spirituality   38
Educating about Personal Resiliency Strategies   39
Summary   40
Discussion Questions   40
Supplemental Book Readings   41
Supplemental Aging Videos   43
Additional Information Links   44
References   44

3. Aging Self-Acceptance for Women

Cultural Roles and Aging Self-Acceptance	51
Physical Aging Self-Acceptance	52
Societal Feedback About Women's Aging	53
Personal Adjustment, Self-Forgiveness, and Self-Acceptance	54
Life Role Transitions	56
Positive Psychosocial Adjustment and Self-Actualization	58
Realistic Aging and Sense of Self	60
Summary	63
Discussion Questions	63
Supplemental Book Readings	64
Supplemental Aging Videos	66
Additional Information Links	66
References	67

4. Aging Women and Mental Aerobics

Older Women and Mental Aerobics	71
Self-Regulation Theory and Older Women's Cognitive Engagement	73
Mental Aerobic Interventions with Older Women	74
Mental Aerobics as a Preventative or Rehabilitative Factor for Aging Women	74
Later-Life Health Correlates with Mental Engagement Activities for Women	75
Summary	77
Discussion Questions	77
Supplemental Book Readings	78
Supplemental Aging Videos	79
Additional Information Links	80
References	81

II

PHYSICAL HEALTH IN WOMEN'S AGING

5. Physical Changes and Self-Perceptions in Women's Aging

Aging Women and Their Body Image	87
Psychological Mechanisms and Cognitive Biases That Influence Self-Perceptions	89
The "Culture" of Youth	91
Summary	93
Discussion Questions	94
Supplemental Book Readings	95
Supplemental Aging Videos	96
Additional Information Links	96
References	97

6. Aging Women and Health Longevity

Income   102
Social Support   104
Education   106
Healthy Choices: Smoking and Physical Activity   107
Interventions   109
Summary   111
Discussion Questions   111
Supplemental Book Readings   112
Supplemental Aging Videos   114
Additional Information Links   115
References   115

7. Importance of Daily Physical Activity for Older Women

Being Active Is a Quality-of-Life Issue   121
The Influence of Physical Activity on the Brain   123
The Influence of Physical Activity on the Body   124
Factors That Support Physical Activity   125
Barriers to Working Out   128
Recommendations/Interventions   130
Summary   132
Discussion Questions   132
Supplemental Book Readings   134
Supplemental Aging Videos   134
Additional Information Links   135
References   135

III

WOMEN'S DIVERSE AGING EXPERIENCES

8. Diversity among Older Women

Diversity and Quality-of-Life Perceptions   146
Women's Race, Culture, and Ethnicity Factors in Getting Older 148
Generational Experiences Shaping Women's Aging   149
Societal Status for Older Women   149
Changing Living Situations with Aging   150
Sexuality and Gender Identity in Later Life   151
Education Access   151
Quality-of-Life Factors   152
Summary   156
Discussion Questions   157
Supplemental Book Readings   158
Supplemental Aging Videos   160
Additional Information Links   160
References   160

9. Expansion of Women's Roles in Later Life

Expanded Role Duration   170
Multiple Social Roles in "Balance"   172
Within-Role Task Expansion   175
Summary   177
Discussion Questions   177
Supplemental Book Readings   178
Supplemental Aging Videos   179
Additional Information Links   180
References   180

10. The Role of Social Relationships for Aging Women

The Importance of a Strong Social Support System   185
Theories About Social Relationships in Aging Adults   186
The Quality and Function of Social Support   188
The Importance of Social Support on Physical and Mental/Cognitive Health   189
Social Network Interventions   192
Summary   193
Discussion Questions   193
Supplemental Book Readings   194
Supplemental Aging Videos   196
Additional Information Links   196
References   197

11. Women's Sexuality in Later Life

Older Women and Sexual Engagement   201
Barriers to Older Women's Sexual Activity   203
Biology of Women's Later-Life Sexual Desire   205
Positive Supports for Older Women's Sexuality   208
Summary   210
Discussion Questions   210
Supplemental Book Readings   211
Supplemental Aging Videos   212
Additional Information Links   212
References   213

IV

AGING WOMEN'S ROLES IN SOCIETY

12. Women's Economic Health and Work/Retirement in Later Life

Issues Related to Retirement   219
The Psychological Function of Work   220
Positively Aging at the Workplace   222
Advantages of a Mature Worker   222

Stereotypes of the Mature Worker 223
On-the-Job Factors that Influence the Aging Worker 225
Extending Career Work Life Expectancy 225
Factors to Consider 226
Remaining Updated 228
Summary 229
Discussion Questions 230
Supplemental Book Readings 231
Supplemental Aging Videos 232
Additional Information Links 233
References 233

13. Breaking Stereotypes of Aging Women

Stereotypes Impacting Positive Aging 237
Why Are Stereotypes Harmful? 241
What Can We Do to Combat These Stereotypes? 243
Summary 244
Discussion Questions 245
Supplemental Book Readings 246
Supplemental Aging Videos 247
Additional Information Links 247
References 248

14. Civic Engagement and the Power of Older Women

Benefits of Older Women's Civic Engagement to Aging Women 252
Empowerment of Older Women 260
Summary 260
Discussion Questions 261
Supplemental Book Readings 262
Supplemental Aging Videos 263
Additional Information Links 263
References 264

15. Public Policies and the Next Steps in the Evolution of Women's Aging

Changing Definition of "Quality-of-Life" Standards for Older Women
    Across the World 270
Evolving Definition of "Later Adulthood" as a Public Policy Concept 270
Shifting Social Image of an "Older Woman" in Different Cultures 271
Specific Issues of Public Policy Supports 272
Summary 279
Discussion Questions 279
Supplemental Book Readings 280
Aging Videos 282
Additional Information Links 283
References 283

Appendix A: Aging Knowledge and Attitude Surveys   289
Appendix B: List of National and International Support
   Resources by Topic   301
Index   327

Authors

Dr. Lisa Hollis-Sawyer is an Associate Professor in the Psychology department and Coordinator of the Gerontology program at Northeastern Illinois University. She received her doctorate in Industrial Gerontology from The University of Akron and conducted postdoctoral aging-related training at Boston University. Her research interests range from eldercare to aging workforce issues, especially focusing on aging women's issues within these roles. Dr. Hollis-Sawyer has coauthored three textbooks and authored/coauthored 24 scholarly articles.

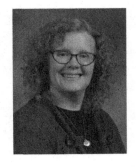

Dr. Amanda Dykema-Engblade is an Associate Professor in the Psychology department and Vice Chair at Northeastern Illinois University. She earned an MA and PhD in Applied Social Psychology from Loyola University (Chicago). Her research interests include small group performance/decision-making, the psychology of food, and women's studies. Dr. Dykema-Engblade has authored/coauthored 10 scholarly articles.

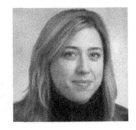

Preface

The focus of this book is about important topics related to women positively aging across many different races, ethnicities, and backgrounds. Related to this aim, the book's sections and chapters cover topics encompassing a "holistic" model of women's aging and will range in focus from the physical and psychological experiences of women's aging to societies' perceptions of older women in many different cultures. All topics related to the focus of contemporary issues with aging women are presented and discussed.

In addition to incorporating timely research on aging women's issues, each chapter provides readers with engaging stories and activities to further reinforce their learning of this content. By design, the content of each book chapter is tailored to offer both theoretical and practical perspectives in how to best support and optimize the aging of women. For example, testimonies and advice from self-identified successfully aging women (Words of Wisdom) are presented in select chapters.

The topics discussed in this book are helpful for both women experiencing aging issues across the life span and/or those involved in their care. Many of the issues examined in this book, of course, have implications toward all individuals who are navigating the complex, sometimes unanticipated "journey" of aging. The aim of this book is to discuss both women's *universal* experiences of aging and their *unique* experiences within specific cultural, historical, and genetic contexts of human development over time.

This book is meant as a helpful guide for all women experiencing the aging process from birth onward, as well as those involved in their lives (eg, significant other, caregiver). The main "message" from the contents of this book is that women should find ways to live their lives to the fullest and to embrace the many different challenges and transitions that aging offers. To effectively adapt in such a way requires a conscious, ongoing self-examination of changing personal capabilities (eg, physical strength), environmental resources (physical, social, and living), and support services, which need to be optimized in combination (ie, best "fit") for women's aging. This book offers advice to achieve positive aging for women, as well as anyone aging across the life span. In addition to the content within the chapters, please review the supplemental attitude scales (Appendix A) and national and international support resources (Appendix B) presented in this book.

Dr. Lisa Hollis-Sawyer
Gerontology Program Coordinator,
Northeastern Illinois University, Chicago, IL, United States

Acknowledgments

The authors would like to give a heartfelt "thank you" to the people who helped and supported them throughout the book writing process. Both authors would like to thank Linda Rada, Marta Bartasiute, and Wendy De Leon for their invaluable help in both conducting and summarizing the interviews of wise older women from many different cultural backgrounds for this book. Lisa Hollis-Sawyer, would also like to thank Tom, Josh, and May for their wonderful support and understanding during this busy time. Amanda Dykema-Engblade, would like to thank David, Zeke, and Evelyn for their equally wonderful support and understanding over the many months of writing and editing this book. Without their help and support, this book would not have been possible!

THE PSYCHOLOGY OF WOMEN'S AGING

Relevant chapters

1   Older Women and Their Mental Health Needs   3
2   Women's Resiliency and Psychological Adaptation
to Aging   27
3   Aging Self-Acceptance for Women   51
4   Aging Women and Mental Aerobics   71

The first section of the book examines issues related to aging women's health on psychological, physical, cognitive, and social bases. In order to ensure positive aging for women from a societal perspective, it is vital to understand the factors that precipitate and impact a woman's aging trajectory over time. The purpose of this section of the book is to introduce many foundational research ideas and practical issues related to women's aging from a diversity perspective. A cross-cultural and individual-differences examination of aging women's issues is important in order to identify both "universal" and unique experiences of aging. Across chapters in this section, person-environment "fit" issues are discussed in different ways as they relate to women's positively aging over time.

Older Women and Their Mental Health Needs

Global Fact: Unipolar depression is projected to be the second leading cause of global disability burden by the year 2020, and aging women are twice as likely to report this condition.

—World Health Organization (n.d.)

Across everyone's life span, people are faced with a variety of life situations which require adaptive coping reactions and a healthy mental attitude. The process of getting older is one of those significant life situations to be positively adapted over an extended time period. An understanding of *realistic* aging processes is a vital factor underlying effective personal adaptation. Before reading this chapter further, please take the *Facts of Aging* quiz in Appendix A to assess your knowledge about aging-related facts and associated adjustment issues. What did you learn? Apply what you learned from taking the quiz to the proceeding discussion of aging women's mental health and psychological adjustment.

What factors underlie positive aging attitudes and adaptation? Myint et al. (2011) suggested that many life events significantly impact an older adult's ability to successfully adapt and achieve positive quality-of-life outcomes. Being both actively engaged in daily activities and open to new experiences (eg, learning new information or skills) are two examples of conducive events promoting positive and adaptive responses to aging-related changes. Aging can be a challenging experience for most people, especially within certain living circumstances (eg, community-dwelling older adults; Akincigil et al., 2011).

Aging research started to turn its attention to issues of positive aging and adjustment from a woman's perspective over 30 years ago (eg, Levy, 1981). Whether older women are truly different than their male counterparts in terms of mental health characteristics, as well as predictive factors, needs further examination (eg, Pachana, McLaughlin, Leung, Byrne, & Dobson, 2012). It is interesting to note that although older men and women are very similar in many ways, their patterns of mental health diagnoses show some differences within different cultures (eg, South Korean culture; Lee & Lee, 2011) and life situations (eg, stressful role responsibilities; Darling, Coccia, & Senatore, 2012).

Is it possible that older women are inherently different in aging-related attitudes or coping reactions? Or, is this perception more an outcome of "double jeopardy" bias regarding stereotyped perceptions of women (eg, emotionality) and their aging (eg, decrement and loss)? This concept of "double jeopardy" (eg, Hollis-Sawyer & Cuevas, 2013) is important to explore because this stereotype may have a significant influence on women's positive aging potential. In certain cultures and societies, older women may be at a social disadvantage in terms of financial viability, social power, and associated support resources. Exploring this idea from a positive aging perspective, women who are empowered and supported in their social roles will be better able to cope and proliferate when faced with aging.

Financial resources are important for women's later-life adaptation and personal growth. The concept of "feminization of poverty" speaks toward this issue (Minkler & Stone, 1985), emphasizing the need for society to better understand lifespan issues of workforce participation, participation interruptions (eg, caregiving role demands), and an associated gender disparity in earned income (eg, wage gap and pension acquisition) significantly impacting women's social status and living situations over a life span.

WOMEN AND HARMONIOUS AGING

Positive aging as applied to mental health is analogous to Liang and Luo's (2012) examination of the concept of "harmonious" aging. Brennan et al. (2012) emphasized the idea that there needs to be an examination of positive mental health perspectives to better understand and identify coping factors that assist in later-life adjustment. Grafova, McGonagle, and Stafford (2006) suggested that there is a very important link between older adults' feelings of positive well-being and their associated functional status in conducting activities of daily living.

The delicate "balance" between mental health and functional status is a vital issue to examine with women who are faced with balancing many roles and responsibilities across a life span (Byles, Gallienne, Blyth, & Banks, 2012). The impact of the caregiver role within a woman's life cannot be understated because of its broad range of role demands and responsibilities within the family system. Further, being a caregiver can have a significant impact upon an aging person's mental and physical health (Hoffman, Lee, & Mendez-Luck, 2012; Neysmith, & Reitsma-Street, 2009; Nordtug, Krokstad, & Holen, 2011). Financial and other support resources may be depleted over time for older women who have been caregivers over many decades of their lives.

AGING WOMEN'S RESOURCES AND MENTAL HEALTH

Lack of resources and lack of support may lead to older women developing feelings of depression. Not surprisingly, there is a linkage between depression and being admitted to nursing homes (eg, Miller, Pinet-Peralta, & Elder, 2012). To combat this possible aging trajectory for women, it is important for societies to offer substantially more programs and services to support and supplement the caregiving needs of women across a life span. Chu, Huynh, and Areán (2012) purported that therapeutic interventions need to be grounded in an understanding of cultural beliefs and values (eg, older adults in China). Tailoring community programs and mental health services for aging women to be culturally relevant would only assist in their effectiveness and long-term benefits for all involved.

QUOTES FROM FAMOUS, POSITIVELY AGING WOMEN

Old age is not a disease – it is strength and survivorship, triumph over all kinds of vicissitudes and disappointments, trials and illnesses.

—*Maggie Kuhn, Activist*

If we are strong, and have faith in life and its richness of surprises, and hold the rudder steadily in our hands. I am sure we will sail into quiet and pleasant waters for our old age.

—*Freya Stark, Writer*

Only through these efforts within communities can positive change for women in terms of mental health adjustment be achieved. For communities to change, there must be broader cultural changes. Cultures which may not have conveyed the social value of women and their roles must consciously shift their focus to consciously value and support aging women's efforts and contributions within family systems in the broader society.

WOMEN'S LATER-LIFE ROLE TRANSITIONS

An important aspect of aging across the life span involves examining role transitions over time. Wink and Jacquelyn (2006) posed the question, is later life the "crown" of life? This is an important question in terms of the culmination of life experiences as women age. Women have many social roles, some that are maintained over life spans and some that change. Some roles are defined by family system dynamics such as being a daughter, a sister, a mother, and other possible roles. Other social roles are defined by society with different societal valuations associated with them (eg, career status). Life circumstances can directly impact aging women's health on a daily basis. For example, Jaussent et al. (2011) examined how women experience stressors that cause interruptions in their sleeping behavior. Disrupted sleeping behavior over time can have effects upon both one's mental and physical health. Stressors that women experience need to be addressed through community-based and aging support services to alleviate such potential negative influences on one's otherwise normative aging trajectory.

TIPS FOR WOMEN'S POSITIVE MENTAL HEALTH

1. Be physically active on a daily basis.
2. Eat healthy and take care of yourself.
3. Take a "break" and enjoy life.
4. Get adequate rest.
5. Write down your accomplishments and make a "wish list" of plans to do.

How older adults perceive their social status within communities, based on social-economic status or other social standards, has a significant influence on older women's internalized feelings of social value and relevancy (Kim, Richardson, Park, & Park, 2013; Ladin, Daniels, & Kawachi, 2010; Pudrovska & Anishkin, 2013). Beyond the family system, women may be faced with different role transitions such as retirement. Changes and loss of social roles over time have an impact upon an aging woman's life and adaptation outcomes. How successfully an older woman adapts to these role-related changes is both a product of her own personal resiliency and coping strategies learned over time and how society supports these role transitions within the aging population.

Cultures and broader societies need to better educate aging women in terms of how to best transition between roles as they move from work to retirement and from caregiver to care recipient (eg, Olesen & Berry, 2011). Certainly there is a cultural valuation of working that translates into cognitive activity and stimulation for aging women; degree to which women can maintain an engaged active role in work can have positive benefits on their later-life adjustment (Van der Elst, Van Boxtel, & Jolles, 2012).

It is important to acknowledge that inequities regarding the social power and resources of women over a life span have implications toward older women's mental health outcomes. From positive aging perspective, societies need to focus on empowering women to optimize their aging progress and potential. If achieved, possible gender differences in reported depression, anxiety, and other mental conditions may be minimized among the normal aging population. What factors support aging women's potential for optimal later-life achievements?

CHECK IT OUT!

Search the Internet to find different websites regarding cultural ideas of aging women and mental health. As you review this online content about aging women and mental health (eg, coping) issues, think about the following questions:

1. What are the cultural images about older women and mental health?
2. Are there gender differences in older adults' mental health portrayals? How so?
3. Is the information presented in terms of positive or negative mental health issues for aging women?
4. In your review, what are the issues related to positive mental health for a growing, aging female population?
5. In examining this online content, are there unique mental health issues related to specific generations of women as they age? If so, why?

SOCIAL POWER, EMPOWERMENT, AND COPING OF OLDER WOMEN

The psychological need for independence and autonomy for women as they age can be a critical quality of life issue. Analyzing an older woman's role within a culture helps us better understand both her needed resources and role-related self-esteem needs. Research suggests a possible curvilinear relationship between age and social power (Schwartz & Bilsky, 1987), impacting aging women's quality of life. If older women experience a declining social status in response to their aging, this certainly can impact their feelings of life satisfaction, self-esteem, and other psychological reactions (Dowd, 1975). Conversely, cultures and communities which value the contributions of older women benefit both society and the mental well-being of older adults in their society. This social valuation may translate into older women's internalized feelings of personal self-worth and their ability to adapt to life's many challenges.

Ryff, Friedman, Morozink, and Tsenkova (2012) argued that a key component to positive later-life adjustment is an individualistic trait of psychological resilience. Even though one might think of this as a trait-related issue, it might be argued that this can also be part of training in community programs for older adults. Understanding the influence of culture on aging women is an important factor for support services offered to older women in different cultures. For example, Thorpe et al. (2011) purported that there are interesting cultural differences between how older Caucasian and African-American women mentally adjusted to experiences of disability and loss due to death, with African-American women utilizing more informal social support resources.

Having a positive life perspective (eg, seeing the "glass as half full") in later life in response to aging can be a key predictor of positive aging outcomes in different living environments (in rural Alaska; Lewis, 2013). Steptoe, Leigh, and Kumari (2011) found that one's mood and associated reactions to daily life activities has a significant impact on older adult functioning. Culturally sensitive education within communities may assist in older women developing effective resiliency responses. Lee and Smith (2011) emphasized the need for education as a factor supporting mental well-being among Korean older adults coping with change in life circumstances as they age. Educational interventions can benefit both the body as well as the mind. Health education initiatives within communities are crucial to promote the overall well-being of an aging population (eg, Perrig-Chiello & Hutchison, 2010).

"MIND-BODY" CONNECTION IN AGING WOMEN'S MENTAL HEALTH

There is certainly a "mind-body" connection (Brower, 2006), when we examine positive aging mental health outcomes for women. One's mental health and associated health perspectives can have an impact on one's physical health (Millán-Calenti, Sánchez, Lorenzo, & Maseda, 2012). Fredriksen-Goldsen et al. (2013) investigated the "mind-body" connection of physical and mental health and associated health risk factors for aging lesbians, among other aging groups. This type of research is an important step in better understanding the many diverse needs of aging women from different perspectives and life trajectories. Too often, interventions and support programs may focus on the "external" needs of aging adults without paying attention to the very important "internal" needs. Darling et al. (2012) emphasized the need to acknowledge older women's experiences of stressors as they relate to the feelings of life satisfaction and health status.

This "mind-body" balance applies to the examination of factors (eg, body weight, physical strength, and balance) underlying why women might live longer across many different cultures in the world (eg, Carroll, Blanck, Serdula, & Brown, 2010; Lakey et al., 2012). Both normative and nonnormative health issues are important to understand for intervention purposes (eg, aging Greek patients with Parkinson's disease; Andreadou et al., 2011). Test yourself with the following positivity scale to understand associated factors.

TEST YOURSELF!

Positivity Scale

Source: Caprara, G.V., Alessandri, G., Eisenberg, N., Kupfer, A., & Steca, P. (2012). The positivity scale. *Psychological Assessment, 24(3),* **701–12.**

Instructions: Please respond to the following items using the response scale and fill in the number from the Likert scale:

1	2	3	4	5
Strongly Disagree	Somewhat Disagree	Neutral	Somewhat Agree	Strongly Agree

1. I have great faith in the future. _____
2. I am satisfied with my life. _____
3. Others are generally here for me when I need them. _____
4. I look forward to the future with hope and enthusiasm. _____
5. On the whole, I am satisfied with myself. _____
6. At times, the future seems unclear to me. _____
7. I feel I have many things to be proud of. _____
8. I generally feel confident in myself. _____

Scoring: Reverse score item #6. Add up the scores. The higher the score, the more resilient you are. Read the article by Caprara, Alessandri, Eisenberg, Kupfer, and Steca to gain more understanding of this brief scale and what it measures.

Subjective perceptions are just as important to understand as objective health indices. An aging woman's self-rated health is shown to be equally important to other factors to adjustment in later life (Hamid, Momtaz, & Rashid, 2010). To have a "positive" and/or realistic attitude about one's physical health influence one's feelings of positive mental health adjustment in later life (Ruthig, Hanson, Pedersen, Weber, & Chipperfield, 2011). There are unique issues related to the experience of women aging which impact their mental health.

Positive mental health is vital to assist in adaptive responses to the many different role transitions as both a woman and older adult in their specific family system, culture, and other social contexts. It is important to acknowledge that there are universal aging adjustment issues for women. These mental health concerns will only be exacerbated as women across the world continue to live longer, living longer even with chronic conditions such as arthritis. Across their life span, women are typically the default caregivers of significant others in their lives. This is vital to understand because it does have implications toward the stressors and potential mental health issues that women accumulate over time. Brody (2004) among other researchers has discussed the concept of "women in the middle," highlighting the idea that there are many societal pressures related to the roles of women in society as they attempt to balance their role of caregivers with their other responsibilities (eg, career).

The "mind-body" connection for aging women should be an integral part of how and why mental health support programs are designed and implemented for this aging subpopulation. It will be discussed throughout this book how women's roles have an impact upon their aging processes. Conversely, a woman's aging positively or negatively affects her social roles and associated role transitions over time. Understanding this dynamic process from a cultural perspective is imperative if effective community-based initiatives are to be offered to aging women in many different societies. In this discussion of understanding "universal" stressors and potential mental health concerns with aging women across the world, it is very important to examine the same issues within a cultural context.

FACTORS DETERMINING AGING WOMEN'S MENTAL HEALTH OUTCOMES

Certainly understanding important individual difference factors of life circumstance and lifestyle is necessary for appropriate interventions to be designed to support aging women's mental health outcomes. Gerstorf et al. (2009) suggested that there are many individual differences which determine the degree to which older adults achieve feelings of positive well-being. For example, what social activities an older woman engages in on a frequent basis can certainly have a positive impact on her mental health status. Berner, Rennemark, Jogréus, and Berglund (2012) examined mental health outcomes related to individualistic traits and the use of the Internet in social activities among older adults in Sweden. The degree to which older adults utilized social networks on the Internet predicted the degree of overall social connectedness for most individuals.

The use of technology and its accessibility for aging women as a resource of social communication and support needs further attention within communities on a global basis. Texting emails and chat rooms may be a very positive social resource for women as caregivers and other roles when they feel the need to share their thoughts and feelings with those who share similar life experiences. The use of technology is one way where aging women may feel a sense of "social belongingness" within (and beyond) her community, a concept suggested by Maslow's hierarchy of needs theory (Maslow, 1999) among other adaptation theories.

The concept of social belongingness may be extended to the role of spirituality in one's life and how it relates to social support from two perspectives: one's religious community and one's supportive relationship with a spiritual being (Vahia et al., 2011). Hill (2010) and McFarland (2010) examined gender differences related to religious involvement and older adults associated feelings of positive mental health and adjustment capabilities. Both research studies emphasized the need for older adults to have some degree of religious involvement as a lifestyle factor to support feelings of social connectedness within one's community and social belongingness within one's social support system.

Social belongingness can be associated with older women's feelings of positive self-determination. Bojorquez-Chapela et al. (2012) studied the impact of older adults' feelings of personal autonomy and perceived "social capital" in Mexico, and the degree to which older women and older men reported feeling empowered and having self-determination in their daily activities was related to positive feelings of aging adjustment and acceptance. The degree to which older adults can engage in and have assistance with self-care activities (eg, "Meals on Wheels" program usage) has a meaningful impact upon their positive mental adjustment in later life (Choi, Teeters, Perez, Farar, & Thompson, 2010; Rodriguez-Blazquez, Forjaz, Prieto-Flores, Rojo-Perez, Fernandez-Mayoralas, & Martinez-Martin, 2012), and may assist in aging women's "aging in place" efforts in the home and broader community.

Globally, women occupy many life roles which, in turn, influence their positive aging trajectories. Grundy, Albala, Allen, Dangour, Elbourne, and Uauy (2012) researched the role of "grandparent" and how it impacted the mental well-being and adaptive capabilities among a sample of older Chilean adults. Findings from the research indicated that active and socially engaged grandparents achieved more positive mental health outcomes over time within functionally able persons. Being socially engaged as a grandmother, among other life roles, translates into positive aging for women but role activities are not just simply associated with caregiving. Work and retirement as roles within aging women's life are important to understand in terms of the impact on their mental health. Nuñez (2010) examined the relationship between mental health and work role capacity in England's labor force. Findings suggested that community interventions which support older adults' role transitions may help promote their feelings of security, autonomy, and general well-being. Globally, culturally based community education and mental health support resources can assist aging women in this aim.

ROLE OF CULTURE IN AGING WOMEN'S POSITIVE MENTAL HEALTH

How a cultural society regards and values the contributions of women over a life span can have an impact upon an aging woman's feelings of self-esteem and self-valuation. In examining culture, there are many specific factors that can support aging women's positive mental health in coping with aging changes. Societies should consciously support aging women's health needs, promote holistic perspective, understanding that older women are experiencing multiple life changes from multiple causal factors. Past research has indicated that social support within a cultural context has definitely a positive influence on aging adults' feelings of optimism and personal adaptation to aging changes (MacDonald, 2007; Tiedt, 2010; Zhang & Li, 2011), as well as avoid suicidal ideations (Yur'yev et al., 2010).

What are some of the cultural issues to explore with aging women and their mental health outcomes? This is a complex question because it involves both understanding the cultural role of a woman within a specific society and, at the same time, the cultural role of an aging person within that society. Combining these two ideas, there must be an examination of the interplay between these two cultural role expectations for an aging woman. Proceeding from a micro to macro perspective of aging women's social roles, cross-cultural research has investigated status and role obligations of women within a family system over time. Certainly, the cultural role of "caregiver" is a pervasive theme for women over time and across cultures, although the experiences of caregiving differ as a function of race and culture (Dilworth-Anderson, Williams, & Gibson, 2002). A better understanding of the cultural-based factors impacting women's positive mental health over a life span is an ethical imperative for societies. Only through this investigation can there be appropriate support programs and laws to assist a woman's positive aging mental health trajectory.

SOCIETAL "MESSAGES" OF WOMEN'S POSITIVE AGING

Another important issue to think about with aging and women is how society conveys societal "messages" through media and other sources regarding aging and attractiveness of women over time as they age. For example, Rozanova (2010) examined how popular publications in London (eg, "London Mail" publication) portrayed biased portrayals of aging which perpetuated stereotypes about later-life mental health adjustment. These social messages can directly impact aging women's personal feelings and perceptions of their own positive aging.

Instead, cultures and broader societies across the world should consciously examine approaches for promoting and supporting older women that acknowledge, support, and promote their active involvement in communities (eg, service usage; Currin, Hayslip, & Temple, 2011). Health service usage and associated social support within communities is a vital issue to be paid attention to to promote aging women's physical and mental well-being (Vasiliadis, Gagné, Jozwiak, & Préville, 2013; Wang, Xiong, Levkoff, & Yu, 2010). Older women are a wealth of knowledge and have skills that may be virtually untapped within a culture that does not acknowledge their intrinsic value in many different areas of societal functioning.

As Activity theory (Havighurst, 1961) suggests, older women who are actively engaged in social activities may have better mental and physical health. The mental health of older women, and their male counterparts, greatly benefit from daily social activities with others and, conversely, society would greatly benefit from older women's social involvement. Greenfield and Russell (2011) and Lin and Wang (2011) both purported that later-life decision-making should take into account optimizing living arrangements which must support social engagement and connectedness with older adults. Litwin (2011) emphasized the need for older women and men to maintain social network connections to optimize mental health outcomes. This social connectedness to others is especially crucial for aging women who might feel isolated within certain social roles (eg, caregiver) (Neri et al., 2012), and culture and community supports are important factors in this outcome.

What are the opportunities and support resources for older women's lives to be enhanced on a psychological basis? How do the ideas and belief systems within the culture promote positive aging for women? Does the culture promote and appreciate older women or does it undermine the self-growth and development of women in later life? These questions have to be examined if there is to be true cultural change in response to aging women. For example, past research has examined where older adults reside as important cultural influence on their feelings of positive mental health ranging from living in a city environment to living in a rural community (Mair, 2010; Montesó et al., 2012; Parikh, Fahs, Shelley, & Yerneni, 2009). Such factors have implications toward designing community programs within different living environments for older women, as well as their male counterparts, and this is the logical next step to support positive aging outcomes for decades to come.

When considering the influence of culture on a woman's aging development, it is appropriate to examine the "micro" social system of families. Blomgren, Breeze, Koskinen, and Martikainen (2012) reported meaningful differences in filial social support for aging individuals' daily functioning tasks between English and Finnish families. Their findings suggest that culture plays a significant role in how families respond to the aging needs of older family members. This is important to understand regarding filial support opportunities for aging women in different cultures across the world.

A potential lack of support within a family system should be consciously supported within communities (eg, senior centers and associated community support groups). By extension, communities and cultures should encourage families to better understand and support aging women's needs on many different levels as a transition across stages in the life span. Only through this heightened understanding of the influence of culture (eg, culturally derived family system dynamics) can we hope to optimize the growth and development of older women over their life spans. Relationship dynamics between adult children and aging women can have a significant impact upon filial support resources (Do & Malhotra, 2012). Widowhood in later life, immigration to a new country, and other life circumstances (eg, job stressors) can create feelings of isolation and stress that can be ameliorated through social support systems (Gammonley, 2009; Gerst, Al-Ghatrif, Beard, Samper-Ternent, & Markides, 2010; Ha & Ingersoll-Dayton, 2011).

The consideration of cultural (and other) influences on a woman's life is complex from a global aging perspective because women, as a group, are quite diverse in their needs and perspectives. At the same time, women may not communicate their mental health needs to promote self-growth because of certain perceived or actual cultural restraints on women's social status and power within a culture. Aging women need to receive consistent messages of cultural social support related to their growth and potential as they age. Existing empirical work on mental health treatment needs to be adapted so that it is culturally competent for ethnic and racial minorities (Whaley & Davis, 2007). As people live longer than in previous generations, it is an ethical responsibility of societies to guide citizenry to live full and happy lives. Because older women may be faced with multiple caregiving roles in addition to coping with aging-related changes or loss, it is morally imperative for communities to offer tailored mental health interventions for this growing aging subpopulation within countries and communities across the world. As previously discussed, women may outlive significant others in their lives and these losses (eg, loss of spouse; Das, 2013) have a significant impact on both women's health and their subsequent sustainability in functional status.

SUMMARY

This chapter examined issues of mental health adjustment for women as they age. Positive mental health is a critical factor in women's positive aging outcomes. Resources, which support ongoing women's ability to cope and possibly adjust to the many challenges of aging should be a major priority within communities across the world. The understanding of factors predicting positive mental health for older women requires continual research and updating as cohorts of women have unique characteristics and experiences as they enter middle adulthood and beyond. Some issues are linked to genetic traits while others are identifiable with cultural, environmental factors. Positive proactive strategies to help older women cope with the many changes and challenges of aging are vital. Women have unique stress issues within traditional "gender specific" roles (eg, caregiver) that necessitate the need for heightened societal consciousness toward better educational programs, community services, and support resources for this growing segment of the global population for decades to come.

DISCUSSION QUESTIONS

1. What can communities do to better support older women's mental health?
2. What is the role of families in the effort to optimize aging women's mental health?
3. Should older women be encouraged to do mental health assessments on a more regular basis across a life span? What would motivate them to do so?
4. Acknowledging that women probably occupy multiple roles in their lives, how can this fact be used in a proactive strategy for positive aging?
5. Are there generational differences in women's mental health reactions and adaptability over time? If so, how?
6. What are factors to consider in a mental health support program for aging women?

7. Would it be beneficial to have intergenerational women support groups in communities? If so, why?
8. What are important therapeutic factors to consider with women from diverse cultural backgrounds? Racial backgrounds?
9. Do you believe that some societies are more conducive to supporting the mental health needs of women across their life spans? Which societies, and why?
10. If you were to design a mental health program for aging women, how would you design it?

TEST YOUR KNOWLEDGE!

Take this quiz about positive aging outcomes and adjustment processes: http://health.howstuffworks.com/wellness/aging/aging-process/aging-quiz.htm

---

SUPPLEMENTAL BOOK READINGS

Over the past decades, there have been many books written on the topic of aging women and their mental health needs within a cultural context. Here are some recommended *additional readings*:

Urbancic, J. C., & Groh, C. (2008). *Women's mental health: A clinical guide for primary care providers.* Philadelphia, IL: LWW.
    The book provides helpful guidelines regarding assessments of mental health, treatments of mental health problems, and associated evaluations of psychosocial functioning. Book contents present assessment and screening tools and resource materials for both aging clients and their service professionals. Website information about different informational sources is also provided.

Malatesta, V. J. (2007). *Mental health issues of older women: A comprehensive review for health care professionals.* New York, NY: Routledge.
    A comprehensive guide for health care professionals, health care trainees, and educators interested in better understanding and assisting with mental health problems of aging women is offered. Issues of dementia, cognitive impairment, alcohol abuse, schizophrenia, depression and anxiety disorders, traumatic and dissociative disorders, sexual and eating disorders, and personality disorders are examined in a thoughtful manner.

Trotman, F., & Brody, C. (2001). *Psychotherapy and counseling with older women: Cross-cultural, family, and end-of-life issues.* New York, NY: Springer Publishing Co.

The book examines the aging experiences of women through a feminist perspective. Issues faced by women regarding family relationships, shifting body image, personal sexuality, eldercare, and other quality of life topics are discussed. How counseling professionals can better understand the aging experiences of women for treatment purposes is one of the main aims of the book.

Cruikshank, M. (2013). *Learning to be old: Gender, culture, and aging.* Lanham, MD: Rowman & Littlefield Publishers.

Learning how to be "old" in society is the primary message of this textbook. The adjustment process within cultural and societal attitudes toward aging is discussed. "Schema" development and shift related to how aging is perceived and treated is reflected in the topics discussed. This adaptation process of learning to become "old" in society relates to positive aging but is not a direct message through the book's content.

Weber, Z., Fawcett, B., & Wilson, S. (2011). *International perspectives on mental health: Critical issues across the lifespan.* London, UK: Palgrave Macmillan.

Global perspectives on mental health functioning across the life span into later life are discussed. Important issues of sexuality, gender roles, and other lifespan issues for women are reviewed by the authors. Suggestions toward "best practices" in policies and practices in treating adults across the life span are proffered.

Segal, D. L., Qualls, S. H., & Smyer, M. A. (2010) *Aging and mental health.* Hoboken, NJ: Wiley-Blackwell.

Practical guidelines regarding clinical research and practices in the treatment of older adult clients are presented. The chapters review models of mental health and mental illness, along with their implications for treatment of older adults. Recommended clinical assessment and treatment approaches are provided, using case studies and other information to illuminate ways to better assist a growing aging population with a myriad of mental health needs.

O'Brien, M. D. (2005). *Successful aging.* Concord, CA: Biomed General.

This book contains great information on how to optimize your aging experiences and process over time: The book covers the following topics: aging well, cultivating a youthful attitude, how to make the most of the body you have got, safeguarding yourself against serious stress, making the most of your mind and memory, celebrating your social life, to firm up your finances, searching for your spirit, and enjoying your life.

Nouwen, H., & Gaffney, W. J. (1976). *Aging: The fulfillment of life.* New York, NY: Random House Publishing.
The authors offer a wonderful message of hope for adults' aging experiences. The "lessons" presented tell the reader how to adopt a much more positive philosophy toward the many challenges that may be faced, creating opportunities for growth out of these multifaceted life changes experienced in aging.

Nuland, S. B. (2008). *The art of aging: A doctor's prescription for well-being.* New York, NY: Random House Publishing.
Dr. Nuland offers a great plan of how to create positive adjustments and to optimize the aging process. From a physician's perspective, Dr. Nuland presents helpful and practical recommendations as how to live a life that positively anticipates and successfully adjusts to physical, mental, and social transitions which might occur across a life span.

Resnick, B., Gwyther, L. P., & Roberto, K. A. (Editors) (2010). *Resilience in aging: Concepts, research, and outcomes.* New York, NY: Springer.
This is a great resource guide for those interested in understanding personal aging adjustment and/or in the assistance of older adults in the aim of becoming more resilient in response to the many changes and transitions associated with getting older. The chapters of the book present theories, case scenarios, clinical guidelines, and interventions. This would be a great resource for both practitioners working with aging clients and laypeople who would like to better understand ways to improve personal resiliency in response to aging.

Rowe, J. W., & Kahn, R. L. (1999). *Successful aging.* New York, NY: Dell.
The content of this book is based on the results of the MacArthur Foundation Study of Aging in America. Findings presented in the book present information regarding how to be strong physically and mentally throughout later life.

Schlossberg, N. K. (2009). *Revitalizing retirement: Reshaping your identity, relationships, and purposes.* Washington, DC: American Psychological Association.
Nancy Schlossberg, a counseling psychologist, presents information regarding how older adults can both financially and psychologically

prepare and adjust to the life-changing experiences of retirement. She presents practical advice regarding coping strategies in adjusting to a new self-identity, social networks and relationships, and/or life purpose. How an older adult can optimize this life-changing experience is the aim of the book.

Wykle, M. L., Whitehouse, P. J., & Morris, D. L. (Editors) (2010). *Successful aging through the life span: Intergenerational issues in health.* New York, NY: Springer.
The authors discuss many different issues underlying productive aging, and emphasize the impact of learning and intergenerational relationships across the life span. The social, educational, and community-based aspects to positive aging processes are emphasized throughout the book's sections.

SUPPLEMENTAL AGING VIDEOS

For learning purposes, the use of videos can be very beneficial for both instructors and readers. Here are some recommended *supplemental videos*:

Menopause—Health Matters (Format: Website)
http://www.ucsd.tv/search-details.aspx?showID=20859&subject=health
This website is a helpful video about menopausal changes in later life.

Women's Health from A to Z—Research on Aging (Format: Website)
http://www.ucsd.tv/search-details.aspx?showID=20489&subject=health
This website is a great video about many different topics related to women's aging.

Integrating Mental Health into Occupational Therapy Practice with Older Adults: Occupational Therapy Training Program—Sage Series (Format: DVD)
The DVD instructs practitioners on how best to assess the mental health status of older adults, how best to disseminate services to older adults who may need to be encouraged to participate, how to make referrals for the mental health care of older adults, and how best to utilize their clinical training skills to assist in helping aging clients achieve positive mental health in response to aging adjustments.

Aging Successfully: The Psychological Aspects of Growing Old (1997)
(Format: DVD)
> The DVD presents a positive aging model of adaptive competence
> by the Baltes. The researchers present a "selection, optimization,
> and compensation" (SOC) model of aging adaptation supported by
> supplemental vignettes of positive aging adults such as the author
> Betty Friedan. Individual difference factors of personality and mental
> functioning are discussed as assessment issues with older adults.

Don't Look Back (2009) (Format: DVD)
> This DVD has a powerful message for older adults. Do not
> struggle with role-related stagnation and loss. Rather, work on
> "reinventing" yourself, be creative, and be productive. The film
> features aging adults who have prospered and thrived in the
> second half of their life. Case examples include Frank McCourt,
> author of Angela's Ashes, Tis, and Teacher Man; Nikki Giovanni,
> author of On My Journey Now and Acolytes; and Larry Gelbart,
> script writer and producer of M*A*S*H and Tootsie.

The Language of Aging (2009) (Format: DVD)
> This DVD examines the "language" of aging (eg, the meaning of the
> word "old" in society). Expert panelists provide an analysis of the
> language of aging. Washington Post columnist Abigail Trafford among
> others dissect the meaning of words related to the aging process (eg,
> "frail") and examine the implications of language toward ways to
> avoid ageist attitudes and potential behavioral age discrimination.

Life Stories: Aging and the Human Spirit (2002) (Format: DVD)
> This DVD documents the efforts of two university professors who
> created a writing group with older adults. The focus of the writing
> was for the older adults to write about their personal experiences
> and accomplishments. This insightful storytelling process yielded
> a transformational experience for all involved. This process of self-
> exploration is a wonderful lesson in how to create self-healing and
> self-appreciation in later life.

Aging in Soviet Georgia: A Toast to Sweet Old (Format: DVD)
> This DVD examines aging in Soviet Georgia, a part of the world
> often called an "epicenter of longevity." The societal lessons from
> this region of the world are profound for the appreciation and
> support of an aging population. Georgian older adults are valued
> for their wisdom and contributions to society. This is a great
> model for how communities and broader societies should regard
> and treat their aging citizens.

ADDITIONAL INFORMATION LINKS

The following are some recommended *supplemental Internet links*:

Administration on Aging website: http://www.aoa.gov/AoARoot/Aging_Statistics/index.aspx

Aging in Action website: http://aginginaction.com/2010/12/gender-and-aging-what-do-we-know/

American Federation for Aging Research website: http://www.afar.org/infoaging/

American Public Health Association website: http://www.apha.org/membergroups/sections/aphasections/a_ph/

Centers for Disease Control and Prevention website: http://www.cdc.gov/mmwr/preview/mmwrhtml/mm5206a2.htm

Everyday Health website: http://www.everydayhealth.com/senior-health/enhancing-your-sexuality.aspx

NIH/NIAging website: http://www.nia.nih.gov/about/minority-aging-and-health-disparities

United Nations website: http://www.un.org/esa/population/publications/Worldageing19502050/

U.S. Census Bureau website: http://www.census.gov/newsroom/releases/archives/aging_population/cb10-72.html

World Health Organization website: http://www.who.int/ageing/gender/en/index.html

References

Akincigil, A., Olfson, M., Walkup, J. T., Siegel, M. J., Kalay, E., Amin, S., et al. (2011). Diagnosis and treatment of depression in older community-dwelling adults: 1992–2005. *Journal of the American Geriatrics Society, 59*(6), 1042–1051. http://dx.doi.org/10.1111/j.1532-5415.2011.03447.x.

Andreadou, E., Anagnostouli, M., Vasdekis, V., Kararizou, E., Rentzos, M., Kontaxis, T., et al. (2011). The impact of comorbidity and other clinical and sociodemographic factors on health-related quality of life in Greek patients with Parkinson's disease. *Aging & Mental Health, 15*(7), 913–921. http://dx.doi.org/10.1080/13607863.2011.569477.

Berner, J., Rennemark, M., Jogréus, C., & Berglund, J. (2012). Distribution of personality, individual characteristics and internet usage in Swedish older adults. *Aging & Mental Health, 16*(1), 119–126. http://dx.doi.org/10.1080/13607863.2011.602958.

Blomgren, J., Breeze, E., Koskinen, S., & Martikainen, P. (2012). Help from spouse and from children among older people with functional limitations: Comparison of England and Finland. *Ageing & Society, 32*(6), 905–933. http://dx.doi.org/10.1017/S0144686X11000729.

Bojorquez-Chapela, I., Manrique-Espinoza, B., Mejía-Arango, S., Solís, M., & Salinas-Rodríguez, A. (2012). Effect of social capital and personal autonomy on the incidence of depressive symptoms in the elderly: Evidence from a longitudinal study in Mexico. *Aging & Mental Health, 16*(4), 462–471. http://dx.doi.org/10.1080/13607863.2011.651432.

Brennan, P. L., Holland, J. M., Schutte, K. K., & Moos, R. H. (2012). Coping trajectories in later life: A 20-year predictive study. *Aging & Mental Health, 16*(3), 305–316. http://dx.doi.org/10.1080/13607863.2011.628975.

Brody, E. (2004). *Women in the middle: Their parent care years.* New York, NY: Springer Publishing Company.

Brower, V. (2006). Mind-body research moves towards the mainstream. *EMBO Reports, 7*(4), 358–361. http://dx.doi.org/10.1038/sj.embor.7400671.

Byles, J. E., Gallienne, L., Blyth, F. M., & Banks, E. (2012). Relationship of age and gender to the prevalence and correlates of psychological distress in later life. *International Psychogeriatrics, 24*(6), 1009–1018. http://dx.doi.org/10.1017/S1041610211002602.

Caprara, G. V., Alessandri, G., Eisenberg, N., Kupfer, A., & Steca, P. (2012). The positivity scale. *Psychological Assessment, 24*(3), 701–712.

Carroll, D. D., Blanck, H. M., Serdula, M. K., & Brown, D. R. (2010). Obesity, physical activity, and depressive symptoms in a cohort of adults aged 51 to 61. *Journal of Aging & Health, 22*(3), 384–398. http://dx.doi.org/10.1177/0898264309359421.

Choi, N. G., Teeters, M., Perez, L., Farar, B., & Thompson, D. (2010). Severity and correlates of depressive symptoms among recipients of Meals on Wheels: Age, gender, and racial/ ethnic difference. *Aging & Mental Health, 14*(2), 145–154. http://dx.doi.org/10.1080/136078609-03421078.

Chu, J. P., Huynh, L., & Areán, P. (2012). Cultural adaptation of evidence-based practice utilizing an iterative stakeholder process and theoretical framework: Problem solving therapy for Chinese older adults. *International Journal of Geriatric Psychiatry, 27*(1), 97–106. http://dx.doi.org/10.1002/gps.2698.

Currin, J. B., Hayslip, B., & Temple, J. R. (2011). The relationship between age, gender, historical change, and adults' perceptions of mental health and mental health services. *International Journal of Aging & Human Development, 72*(4), 317–341. http://dx.doi.org/10.2190/AG.72.4.c.

Darling, C. A., Coccia, C., & Senatore, N. (2012). Women in midlife: Stress, health and life satisfaction. *Stress & Health: Journal of the International Society for the Investigation of Stress, 28*(1), 31–40. http://dx.doi.org/10.1002/smi.1398.

Das, A. (2013). Spousal loss and health in late life: Moving beyond emotional trauma. *Journal of Aging & Health, 25*(2), 221–242. http://dx.doi.org/10.1177/0898264312464498.

Dilworth-Anderson, P., Williams, I. C., & Gibson, B. E. (2002). Issues of race, ethnicity and culture in caregiving research: A 20-year review (1980–2000). *The Gerontologist, 42*(2), 237–272. http://dx.doi.org/10.1093/geront/42.2.237.

Do, Y., & Malhotra, C. (2012). The effect of co-residence with an adult child on depressive symptoms among older widowed women in South Korea: An instrumental variables estimation. *Journals of Gerontology Series B: Psychological Sciences & Social Sciences, 67B*(3), 384–391.

Dowd, J. J. (1975). Aging as exchange: A preface to theory. *Journal of Gerontology, 30*(5), 584–594. http://dx.doi.org/10.1093/geronj/30.5.584.

Fredriksen-Goldsen, K. I., Emlet, C. A., Kim, H., Muraco, A., Erosheva, E. A., Goldsen, J., et al. (2013). The physical and mental health of lesbian, gay male, and bisexual (LGB) older adults: The role of key health indicators and risk and protective factors. *Gerontologist, 53*(4), 664–675.

Gammonley, D. (2009). Psychological well-being and social support among elders employed as lay helpers. *Journal of Gerontological Social Work, 52*(1), 64–80. http://dx.doi.org/10.1080/0163437-0802561976.

Gerst, K., Al-Ghatrif, M., Beard, H. A., Samper-Ternent, R., & Markides, K. S. (2010). High depressive symptomatology among older community-dwelling Mexican Americans: The impact of immigration. *Aging & Mental Health, 14*(3), 347–354. http://dx.doi.org/10.1080/1360786-0903292578.

Gerstorf, D., Ram, N., Fauth, E., Schupp, J., & Wagner, G. G. (2009). Between-person disparities in the progression of late-life well-being. *Annual Review of Gerontology & Geriatrics, 29*(205–232), R12–R13.

Grafova, I., McGonagle, K., & Stafford, F. P. (2006). Functioning and well-being in the third age: 1986–2001. *Annual Review of Gerontology & Geriatrics, 26*(19–38), R10–R11.

Greenfield, E. A., & Russell, D. (2011). Identifying living arrangements that heighten risk for loneliness in later life: Evidence from the U.S. national social life, health, and aging project. *Journal of Applied Gerontology, 30*(4), 524–534. http://dx.doi.org/10.1177/073346481036-4985.

Grundy, E. M., Albala, C., Allen, E., Dangour, A. D., Elbourne, D., & Uauy, R. (2012). Grandparenting and psychosocial health among older Chileans: A longitudinal analysis. *Aging & Mental Health, 16*(8), 1047–1057. http://dx.doi.org/10.1080/13607863.2012.692766z.

Ha, J., & Ingersoll-Dayton, B. (2011). Moderators in the relationship between social contact and psychological distress among widowed adults. *Aging & Mental Health, 15*(3), 354–363. http://dx.doi.org/10.1080/13607863.2010.519325.

Hamid, T., Momtaz, Y., & Rashid, S. (2010). Older women and lower self-rated health. *Educational Gerontology, 36*(6), 521–528. http://dx.doi.org/10.1080/03601270903534606.

Havighurst, R. J. (1961). Successful aging. *The Gerontologist, 1*, 8–13. http://dx.doi.org/10.1093/-geront/1.1.8.

Hill, T. D. (2010). A biopsychosocial model of religious involvement. *Annual Review of Gerontology & Geriatrics, 30*(1), 179–199.

Hoffman, G. J., Lee, J., & Mendez-Luck, C. A. (2012). Health behaviors among baby boomer informal caregivers. *Gerontologist, 52*(2), 219–230.

Hollis-Sawyer, L., & Cuevas, L. (2013). Mirror, mirror on the wall: Ageist and sexist double jeopardy portrayals in children's picture books. *Educational Gerontology, 39*(12), 902–914. http://dx.doi.org/10.1080/03601277.2013.767650.

Jaussent, I., Dauvilliers, Y., Ancelin, M., Dartigues, J., Tavernier, B., Touchon, J., et al. (2011). Insomnia symptoms in older adults: Associated factors and gender differences. *American Journal of Geriatric Psychiatry, 19*(1), 88–97. http://dx.doi.org/10.1097/JGP.-0b013e3181e049b6.

Kim, J., Richardson, V., Park, B., & Park, M. (2013). A multilevel perspective on gender differences in the relationship between poverty status and depression among older adults in the United States. *Journal of Women & Aging, 25*(3), 207–226. http://dx.doi.org/10.1080/08952841.2013.795751.

Ladin, K., Daniels, N., & Kawachi, I. (2010). Exploring the relationship between absolute and relative position and late-life depression: Evidence from 10 European countries. *Gerontologist, 50*(1), 48–59.

Lakey, S. L., LaCroix, A. Z., Gray, S. L., Borson, S., Williams, C. D., Calhoun, D., et al. (2012). Antidepressant use, depressive symptoms, and incident frailty in women aged 65 and older from the women's health initiative observational study. *Journal of the American Geriatrics Society, 60*(5), 854–861. http://dx.doi.org/10.1111/j.1532415.2012.03940.x.

Lee, E., & Lee, J. (2011). Gender differences in predictors of mental health among older adults in South Korea. *International Journal of Aging & Human Development, 72*(3), 207–223. http://dx.doi.org/10.2190/AG.72.3.c.

Lee, J., & Smith, J. P. (2011). Explanations for education gradients in depression: The case of Korea. *Research on Aging, 33*(5), 551–575. http://dx.doi.org/10.1177/0164027511409440.

Levy, S. M. (1981). The aging woman: Developmental issues and mental health needs. *Professional Psychology, 12*, 92–102. http://dx.doi.org/10.1037/0735-7028.12.1.92.

Lewis, J. P. (2013). The importance of optimism in maintaining healthy aging in rural Alaska. *Qualitative Health Research, 23*(11), 1521–1527.

Liang, J., & Luo, B. (2012). Toward a discourse shift in social gerontology: From successful aging to harmonious aging. *Journal of Aging Studies, 26*(3), 327–334.

Lin, P., & Wang, H. (2011). Factors associated with depressive symptoms among elderly living alone: An analysis of sex difference. *Aging & Mental Health, 15*(8), 1038–1044. http://dx.doi.org/10.1080/13607863.2011.583623.

Litwin, H. (2011). The association between social network relationships and depressive symptoms among older Americans: What matters most? *International Psychogeriatrics, 23*(6), 930–940. http://dx.doi.org/10.1017/S1041610211000251.

MacDonald, M. (2007). Social support for centenarians' health, psychological well-being, and longevity. *Annual Review of Gerontology & Geriatrics, 27,* 107.

Mair, C. A. (2010). Social ties and depression: An intersectional examination of Black and White community-dwelling older adults. *Journal of Applied Gerontology, 29*(6), 667–696. http://dx.doi.org/10.1177/0733464809350167.

Maslow, A. H. (1999). *Towards a psychology of being.* New York, NY: John Wiley & Sons.

McFarland, M. J. (2010). Religion and mental health among older adults: Do the effects of religious involvement vary by gender? *Journals of Gerontology Series B: Psychological Sciences & Social Sciences, 65B*(5), 621–630.

Millán-Calenti, J., Sánchez, A., Lorenzo, T., & Maseda, A. (2012). Depressive symptoms and other factors associated with poor self-rated health in the elderly: Gender differences. *Geriatrics & Gerontology International, 12*(2), 198–206. http://dx.doi.org/10.1111/-j.1447-0594.2011.00745.x.

Miller, N. A., Pinet-Peralta, L. M., & Elder, K. T. (2012). A profile of middle-aged and older adults admitted to nursing homes: 2000–2008. *Journal of Aging & Social Policy, 24*(3), 271–290. http://dx.doi.org/10.1080/08959420.2012.684528.

Minkler, M., & Stone, R. (1985). The feminization of poverty and older women. *The Gerontologist, 25*(4), 351–357. http://dx.doi.org/10.1093/geront/25.4.351.

Montesó, P., Ferre, C., Lleixa, M., Albacar, N., Aguilar, C., Sanchez, A., et al. (2012). Depression in the elderly: Study in a rural city in southern Catalonia. *Journal of Psychiatric & Mental Health Nursing, 19*(5), 426–429. http://dx.doi.org/10.1111/j.1365-2850.2011.01798.x.

Myint, P. K., Smith, R. D., Luben, R. N., Surtees, P. G., Wainwright, N. J., Wareham, N. J., et al. (2011). Lifestyle behaviours and quality-adjusted life years in middle and older age. *Age & Ageing, 40*(5), 589–595.

Neri, A., Yassuda, M., Fortes-Burgos, A., Mantovani, E., Arbex, F., de Souza Torres, S., et al. (2012). Relationships between gender, age, family conditions, physical and mental health, and social isolation of older adults' caregivers. *International Psychogeriatrics, 24*(3), 472–483. http://dx.doi.org/10.1017/S1041610211001700.

Neysmith, S. M., & Reitsma-Street, M. (2009). The provisioning responsibilities of older women. *Journal of Aging Studies, 23*(4), 236–244. http://dx.doi.org/10.1016/.j.jaging.2008.-03.001.

Nordtug, B., Krokstad, S., & Holen, A. (2011). Personality features, caring burden and mental health of cohabitants of partners with chronic obstructive pulmonary disease or dementia. *Aging & Mental Health, 15*(3), 318–326. http://dx.doi.org/10.1080/13607863.2010.519319.

Nuñez, I. (2010). The effects of age on health problems that affect the capacity to work: An analysis of United Kingdom labour-force data. *Ageing & Society, 30*(3), 491–510.

Olesen, S. C., & Berry, H. L. (2011). Community participation and mental health during retirement in community sample of Australians. *Aging & Mental Health, 15*(2), 186–197. http://dx.doi.org/10.1080/13607863.2010.501053.

Pachana, N. A., McLaughlin, D., Leung, J., Byrne, G., & Dobson, A. (2012). Anxiety and depression in adults in their eighties: Do gender differences remain? *International Psychogeriatrics, 24*(1), 145–150. http://dx.doi.org/10.1017/S1041610211001372.

Parikh, N. S., Fahs, M. C., Shelley, D., & Yerneni, R. (2009). Health behaviors of older Chinese adults living in New York City. *Journal of Community Health, 34*(1), 6–15. http://dx.doi.org/10.1007/s10900-008-9125-5.

Perrig-Chiello, P., & Hutchison, S. (2010). Health and well-being in old age: The pertinence of a gender mainstreaming approach in research. *Gerontology, 56*(2), 208–213. http://dx.doi.org/10.1159-/000235813.

Pudrovska, T., & Anishkin, A. (2013). Early-life socioeconomic status and physical activity in later life: Evidence from structural equation models. *Journal of Aging &Health, 25*(3), 383–404. http://dx.doi.org/10.1177/0898264312468601.

Rodriguez-Blazquez, C., Forjaz, M., Prieto-Flores, M., Rojo-Perez, F., Fernandez-Mayoralas, G., & Martinez-Martin, P. (2012). Health status and well-being of older adults living in the community and in residential care settings: Are differences influenced by age? *Aging & Mental Health, 16*(7), 884–891. http://dx.doi.org/10.1080/13607863.2012.684664.

Rozanova, J. (2010). Discourse of successful aging in The Globe & Mail: Insights from critical gerontology. *Journal of Aging Studies, 24*(4), 213–222. http://dx.doi.org/10.1016/j.jaging.2010.05.001.

Ruthig, J. C., Hanson, B. L., Pedersen, H., Weber, A., & Chipperfield, J. G. (2011). Later life health optimism, pessimism and realism: Psychosocial contributors and health correlates. *Psychology & Health, 26*(7), 835–853. http://dx.doi.org/10.1080/08870446.2010.506574.

Ryff, C. D., Friedman, E. M., Morozink, J. A., & Tsenkova, V. (2012). Psychological resilience in adulthood and later life: Implications for health. *Annual Review of Gerontology & Geriatrics, 32*, 73–92.

Schwartz, S. H., & Bilsky, W. (1987). Toward a universal structure of human values. *Journal of Personal and Social Psychology, 53*(3), 550–562.

Steptoe, A., Leigh, E. S., & Kumari, M. (2011). Positive affect and distressed affect over the day in older people. *Psychology & Aging, 26*(4), 956–965. http://dx.doi.org/10.1037/a0023303.

Thorpe, R. J., Koster, A., Kritchevsky, S. B., Newman, A. B., Harris, T., Ayonayon, H. N., et al. (2011). Race, socioeconomic resources, and late-life mobility and decline: Findings from the health, aging, and body composition study. *Journals of Gerontology Series A: Biological Sciences & Medical Sciences, 66A*(10), 1114–1123.

Tiedt, A. (2010). The gender gap in depressive symptoms among Japanese elders: Evaluating social support and health as mediating factors. *Journal of Cross-Cultural Gerontology, 25*(3), 239–256. http://dx.doi.org/10.1007/s10823-010-9122-x.

Vahia, I. V., Depp, C. A., Palmer, B. W., Fellows, I., Golshan, S., Thompson, W., et al. (2011). Correlates of spirituality in older women. *Aging & Mental Health, 15*(1), 97–102. http://dx.doi.org/10.1080/13607863.2010.501069.

Van der Elst, W., Van Boxtel, M. J., & Jolles, J. (2012). Occupational activity and cognitive aging: A case-control study based on the Maastricht aging study. *Experimental Aging Research, 38*(3), 315–329. http://dx.doi.org/10.1080/0361073X.2012.672137.

Vasiliadis, H., Gagné, S., Jozwiak, N., & Préville, M. (2013). Gender differences in health service use for mental health reasons in community dwelling older adults with suicidal ideation. *International Psychogeriatrics, 25*(3), 374–381. http://dx.doi.org/10.1017/S10416102-12001895.

Wang, H., Xiong, Q., Levkoff, S., & Yu, X. (2010). Social support, health service use and mental health among caregivers of the elderly in rural China. *Ageing International, 35*(1), 72–84. http://dx.doi.org/10.1007/s12126-009-9049-0.

Whaley, A. L., & Davis, K. E. (2007). Cultural competence and evidence-based practice in mental health services: A complementary perspective. *American Psychologist, 62*(6), 563–574.

Wink, P., & Jacquelyn, B. J. (2006). Conclusion: Is the third age the crown of life? *Annual Review of Gerontology & Geriatrics, 26*(305–325), R7–R8.

World Health Organization (n.d.). Gender disparity and mental health: The facts. Retrieved from: <http://www.who.int/mental_health/prevention/genderwomen/en/>.

Yur'yev, A., Leppik, L., Tooding, L., Sisask, M., Värnik, P., Jing, W., et al. (2010). Social inclusion affects elderly suicide mortality. *International Psychogeriatrics, 22*(8), 1337–1343. http://dx.doi.org/10.1017/S1041610210001614.

Zhang, B., & Li, J. (2011). Gender and marital status differences in depressive symptoms among elderly adults: The roles of family support and friend support. *Aging & Mental Health, 15*(7), 844–854. http://dx.doi.org/10.1080/13607863.2011.569481.

2

Women's Resiliency and Psychological Adaptation to Aging

Global fact: Globally, women age 50 or older currently outnumber aging male peers and this is projected to continue through 2050.
—*United Nations, **Women Coordination Division report (2012)***

By definition, the concept of "resiliency" is the ability to change and grow in response to confronting and resolving problems and broader life situations (Carver, 1998). "Resilience" can be applied to how an adult adapts to a wide range of aging-related physical and/or cognitive functioning (eg, Stine-Morrow & Chui, 2012), overall daily functioning (Butler, 1993; Wink, 2006), and family coping with care (Coon, 2012; Walsh, 2012). Positively aging certainly involves a woman's ability to be resilient in response to the many life changes associated with this developmental process. "Adaptation" is a related concept which involves a person's ability to learn from life experiences in order to alter one's behavior and/or attitudes for better coping outcomes (Lazarus, 1991). With aging women, the ability to be resilient and adaptive to the many changes related to getting older is a necessity for positive aging outcomes. This book chapter will examine different individual-difference factors and situational (eg, cultural) contexts that support older women's resiliency and adaptation to aging over time.

Although aging women's resiliency is a vital concept to understand, there has been relatively little research examining the topic as relates to diverse women's experiences over time. How can women better understand factors which influence their ability to adapt to the many different challenges and changes with personal aging? Across many different countries and cultures in the world, there seems to be a lack of consistent educational opportunities for women to learn how to better cope and grow in response to the many different challenges created through the aging process (Piercy, 2007; Rothrauff, Cooney, & Jeong Shin, 2009). Culture plays a significant role in relation to educating women on how to become resilient and optimally adjust to the many demands of personal aging, as well as to the demands of caring for aging others (Felten, 2000).

To better understand "what works" for older women in terms of positively adapting to and growing from aging experiences will only benefit society, assisting in the design of more effective program interventions and community support programs for women and those that care for them (LaFerriere & Hamel-Bissell, 1994; Sarkisian, Hays, & Mangione, 2002; Seicol, 2005). To better support an aging population and their needs across many societies in the world, it is necessary to understand both cross-culture perspectives impacting aging-related coping and resiliency (Fry, 1997). From an ethical perspective, societies need to introspectively examine how they support and prepare vulnerable older adults, such as women, across a life span to effectively cope and grow within their aging experiences (Grundy, 2006).

AGING WOMEN'S SOCIAL ROLES AND RESILIENCY

To appreciate older women's coping strategies and resilience, it is important to understand how lifespan social environment and lifestyle factors generally influence their positive aging processes and outcomes (eg, Consedine, Magai, & Conway, 2004). The many different gains, losses, and adjustment issues in a woman's life can impact her general quality of life. For fun, take the following scale to gain some insights into your own resilient coping style.

TEST YOURSELF!

Brief Resilient Coping Scale

Source: Sinclair, V. G., & Wallston, K. A. (2004). The development and psychometric evaluation of the brief resilient coping scale. *Assessment,* 11(1), 94–101.

Instructions: Consider how well the following statements describe your behavior and actions on a scale from 1 to 5, where "1" means the statement does not describe you at all and "5" means it describes you very well.

1. I actively look for ways to replace the losses I encounter in life. _____
2. I believe that I can grow in positive ways by dealing with difficult situations. _____

---

3. I look for creative ways to alter difficult situations. _____
4. Regardless of what happens to me, I believe I can control my reaction to it. _____
5. I only set goals which I know I can reach without the help of others. _____
6. When I need help, I don't hesitate to ask a friend to help. _____
7. I hesitate to ask others to help me. _____
8. My friends and family frequently don't live up to my expectations of how they should act. _____
9. I really resent anyone telling me what to do. _____

Scoring: Reverse score items #5, #7, and #8. Add up the scores. The higher the score, the more resilient you are. Read the article by Sinclair and Wallston to gain more understanding of this brief scale and what it measures.

In Westernized cultures, aging women occupy roles of daughter, partner, parent, employee, supervisor, friend, and many others. The potential pressure to maintain and fulfill all of these roles can certainly impact the positive aging outcomes of women. To be resilient and cope with these many pressures of multiple time demands, role conflicts, and other social role dynamics is important to consider for all concerned. Freund and Baltes (1998) suggested that it is optimal for older adults to select certain activities that are most conducive to their area of expertise, and optimize their time and effort. Through the conscious selection of "highly effective" performance activities, an older woman can best optimize her positive aging (ie, concept of selective optimization with compensation; Baltes & Baltes, 1990). For example, this idea can be applied to the reduction of social roles that may overwhelm a woman as she attempts to balance too many social roles within the time constraints and other constraints of her social and environmental situation over a life span. This relates to the realization that the pervasive "superwoman syndrome" (Shaevitz, 1984) for many different women across cultures in the world may not be a conducive long-term lifestyle option for supporting aging women's positive outcomes.

Conversely, one can certainly argue that remaining active in later life can stimulate an older woman's physical and mental activities and maintain a beneficial level of social activity (Knapp, 1977). Perhaps the best way to think about an optimal level of social roles for women is through the examination of a woman's specific interests, capabilities, and cultural norms in order to understand their unique "voice" in society (Gilligan, 1984). This entails a definite shift in perspective, from a woman guided by societal expectations to be guided from personal expectations and motivations. This process of introspection and self-determination should empower aging women to fight stereotypes and be guided by personal standards of achievement (Olney, 1972).

The meaning of these social roles influences an aging woman's positive aging outcomes. For example, most women are caregivers in a family system for most of their life in some manner. Both researchers and clinicians need to understand better the ongoing demands and adjustment issues related to being a multi-generational caregiver within a family system, and broader social system for many women. In investigating this topic, the following questions should be considered: How does being a caregiver for most of the life span impact a woman's aging and her ability to adapt to personal aging? Does the caregiving role of women help them better prepare for their own aging-related role transitions and aging changes? Conversely, could the caregiving role of women interfere with positive coping strategies across the life span?

The degree to which a woman's caregiving role or other later-life role transition (eg, retirement) is a positive factor in her development of effective resiliency behaviors and adaptation skills needs to be better understood from an interventionist societal perspective (Hollis-Sawyer, 2003). From a lifespan perspective, the life experiences of women and related growth opportunities within the roles they occupy are significant learning opportunities to be explored to promote resiliency perspective (Kinsel, 2005). To better understand how women learn to be resilient and optimally cope with the many different challenges of later-life existence, both research and aging services should acknowledge how cohort membership affects the dynamic process of women getting older and their associated psychological experiences of adjustment (eg, Seeman et al., 1994).

QUOTES FROM FAMOUS, POSITIVELY AGING WOMEN

There is a fountain of youth: it is your mind, your talents, the creativity you bring to your life and the lives of people you love. When you learn to tap this source, you will truly have defeated age.

—*Sophia Loren, Actress*

Spring passes and one remembers one's innocence.
Summer passes and one remembers one's exuberance.
Autumn passes and one remembers one's reverence.
Winter passes and one remembers one's perseverance.

—*Yoko Ono, Artist, Musician, and Activist*

A sense of freedom is something that, happily, comes with age and life experience.

—*Diane Keaton, Actress*

For a global society to better care for those aging within it, it is crucial to identify factors affecting how women optimize their existence within a cultural context. Some authors have argued that aging women are "invisible" entities in some cultures (Woodward, 1999), who need to be valued and recognized as contributing members. This lack of societal recognition as a person with a range of social roles may significantly undermine women's feelings of personal empowerment and their resultant resilience reactions (Facio, 1995).

In a positive sense, a woman caregiver may learn to be more resilient through facing the multiple challenges of caring for someone else. Within different cultures, women's learning how to age successfully is an extension of Bandura's social learning theory (Bandura, 1969) in which there can be influential social role modeling between generations of women in terms of developing "shared" positive aging schemas. From a positive aging perspective, older women have to utilize effective ways to cope and become resilient through exposure to positive aging models of women in their lives (ie, family, peers, educators, and public figures).

There are certainly stressors related to being an elder caregiver but one might argue that this is unique learning opportunity for women, creating situations for self-insights and personal growth. In different cultures, supporting the efforts of aging women (and men) as caregivers would assist in optimizing learning and self-growth into later life. Education about realistic later-life capabilities, adaptive responses, and positive self-evaluations to aging should be offered to all women across the life span (Kwan, Love, Ryff, & Essex, 2003).

THE ECOLOGY OF WOMEN'S POSITIVE AGING

Resiliency is a vital aspect of human development and has been applied to positive aging (eg, Aldwin & Igarashi, 2012; Fulle-Iglesias, Smith, & Antonucci, 2009). Aldwin and colleagues presented an ecological model of resilience in aging from a positive aging perspective, arguing that adaptation to aging is based on both external issues of available social and cultural resources and internal processes of self-transcendence and mindfulness of one's needs into later life. Dorfman, Mendez, and Osterhaus (2009) examined the themes of coping and resiliency in the personal stories of older women living in rural communities and their adjustment experiences to getting older in this type of living environment. The older women dealing well with daily stresses of aging and other adjustment issues (eg, cost of living into later life) were able to do this through adaptive responses of relying more upon others (eg, social support resources), controlling one's spending (eg, self-control), and acceptance of one's life circumstance. Dorfman and colleagues (2009) suggested that communities should offer intervention education and support services for older women in these life situations to optimize their adaptation to aging in a rural setting. Stark-Wroblewski, Edelbaum, and Bello (2008) investigated the positive attitudes and coping behavior of rural older women in the Midwest. Stark-Wroblweski and colleagues found that rural older women were less likely to report health conditions as "barriers" to daily functioning, although they had as many health-related issues as their male peers in the region. The researchers suggested that the older women studied were more adaptive to the aging process possibly because they exhibited more of an "other focused" rather than "self-focused" orientation in response to aging changes.

To adapt to "aging in place" in a community setting is reality faced by a growing number of aging women living longer with chronic conditions experiencing many life transitions (Brock et al., 2011). Brock and colleagues found that women with chronic health conditions (eg, knee difficulty in mobility) reported more feelings of worry in comparison to female peers with either acute health conditions or were healthy. Functional status and the ability to meet the task demands in activities of daily living is a critical part of women's adjustment to aging. As an extension of this research, it is important to understand how community outreach programs can alleviate older women's concerns about aging in different community settings, be it urban or rural. A better understanding of older adults' health needs, perceptions of health, and how they both relate to their resiliency reactions in accomplishing daily activities (eg, Whitson et al., 2011) needs to be further investigated for intervention program development targeting older women in global communities.

TIPS FOR WOMEN TO ADAPT TO PERSONAL AGING

1. Appreciate the "face" you see in the mirror.
2. Stay active on a physical and cognitive basis every day.
3. Be social and maintain positive relationships over time.
4. View life circumstances in a positive manner ("glass as half full").

Resiliency, among other factors, relates to how well older adults cope and thrive in different living situations (Reker, 2001). Chin and Quine (2012) suggested that resiliency, among other factors, relates to a woman's ability to achieve quality-of-life outcomes.

Chin and Quine examined the quality of life desires and attitudes between women living at home or in care facilities. The researchers found that the women living in formal care settings desired to maintain aspects of living at home in their new living situation. This is a crucial support issue in supporting older women's resiliency reactions to changing care situations and living circumstances, especially as women (and their male counterparts) can expect to live longer with chronic health conditions compared to previous cohorts.

GENERATIVITY AND PERSONAL GROWTH

Resiliency does not simply have to focus on how well an aging woman can overcome difficulties but rather how she can optimize her ego "self" development (ie, file resolution of psychosocial crises) in later life. Cheng, Chan, and Chan (2008) examined the opportunities for older adults in Hong Kong to engage in generativity activities in a society that is experiencing cultural shifts in transitions. Cheng and colleagues discovered a real concern among older adults that the younger generation needed moral guidance to avoid possible "evils" but were criticized in adopting this mentoring role. In order to satisfy this ego-development need, it is interesting to note that older women and men within this culture adopted more of a passive role of advisement within the family system. Applying this idea to aging women and resiliency, it might be argued that education and social support services should help women achieve this feeling of generativity within the context of cultural expectations and norms.

Changing life circumstances can impact an older woman's feelings of stress and associated resiliency capabilities. Unanticipated changes in one's aging trajectory due to living longer than expected (eg, becoming a "Centenarian" or being 100 years old or older; Chun, 2007). Past research suggests the idea that women and men can exhibit different social emotional functioning levels, and this is associated with coping issues in response to physical aging changes (eg, Consedine, Magai, & Krivoshekova, 2005). For example, Dasgupta and Ray (2013) examined the dynamic "mind-body" connection related to older women's reactions to menopausal changes in coping with aging in West Bengal. Ability to control one's body changes in response to menopausal onset (eg, incontinence), feelings of irritability, age onset of menopause, and financial status were some of the significant factors affecting older women's resiliency reactions. Education, health care, and support services need to be focused on how these socio-emotional reactions and life situational factors affect aging women's resiliency capabilities.

Changes in life circumstance can relate to how well aging women adjust to the loss of a spouse and associated coping issues (Hahn, Cichy,

Almeida, & Haley, 2011; Holtslander & Duggleby, 2010; O'Rourke, 2004; Williams, Sawyer, & Allman, 2012). For example, Hahn and colleagues found that older widows can exhibit similar levels of well-being as married women due to key individual-difference attributes of coping ability. This is important to realize, and emphasizes the role of education in helping older women who may be widows to better understand their own unique ways to cope in later life in response to such losses. Losses which older women can experience in later life need appropriate community support resources (Janssen, Abma, & Van Regenmortel, 2012), such as social support groups for sustained friendship networks (eg, Red Hat Society; Hutchinson, Yarnal, Staffordson, & Kerstetter, 2008).

Becoming a caregiver within a family system can certainly test a woman's resiliency in adapting to the many different role demands and decision-making tasks. Because most women across different cultures are the default caregivers and families, it is important to understand how community programs, support services, and educational workshops can be supportive and optimize aging women's psychological and physical resiliency response to these daily tasks. Conversely, the role transition of becoming a care recipient can equally be an issue of resiliency and adjustment for aging women across her life span, and it is imperative that this transition is supported through a contextual care approach which takes into account the context and characteristics of the aging women (and men) involved in this process (Dilworth-Anderson, Hilliard, Williams, & Palmer, 2011).

To understand diverse older women's unique resiliency reactions and needs is an imperative in order for appropriate interventions to be designed properly (Crawley & Lynch, 2012). Crawley and Lynch analyzed older women's interviews regarding feelings of well-being, and found that some women reported experiencing social injustices of being devalued, misunderstood, and excluded in society. Interventions need to be based on such research to best address the needs of aging women and help them to optimize their aging experience.

Overall stress related to getting older and the many health-related issues of risk in later adulthood for women can be mentally rated by appropriate resiliency factors in the person's personality and behavior (Diehl, Hay, & Chui, 2012). Beyond counteracting stress reactions, resilience can promote feelings of general well-being in later life adaption and quality of death outcomes but it is important to acknowledge the complexity of factors interacting together to create well-being outcomes (Gerstorf, Ram, Fauth, Schupp, & Wagner, 2009; Gu & Zeng, 2012; Helson & Cate, 2006). Gerstorf and colleagues suggested that there are many between-person disparities and contextual factors (eg, community and society level) that impact older adults' well-being perceptions and coping reactions. To avoid depression and other negative mental health outcomes, aging women need sufficient support resources and education to assist in this adjustment process as they undergo aging-related changes and losses (Laganá, Spellman, Wakefield, & Oliver, 2011; Lerner et al., 2012; Moe, Ekker, & Enmarker, 2013).

Work and retirement are life transitions for women that are impacted by personal aging trajectories and involve women's ability to positively adapt to these many different role-related changes in addition to perceived inequities as one transitions from work to retirement (Rayman, Allen, Pifer, & Allshouse, 1993). Older women's sustained workforce participation into later life for women necessitates the understanding of personal resiliency response patterns. Personal patterns of resilience are important to identify in order to best optimize adjustment responses to the many changes inherent in later-life workforce involvement, ranging from changing work demands to changing functional ability (eg, relational "fit" issues in the workplace and job demands) (Sterns & Dawson, 2012).

POSITIVE RESILIENCE AS A LEARNING PROCESS WITHIN A CULTURAL CONTEXT

One might argue that resilience is both a trait and a learned coping skill. Older women can have accumulated experiences overcoming adversity and obstacles across their life span in different cultures. One resilience issue for diverse groups of women is related to overcoming possible experiences of prejudice and discrimination in being both a woman and an older adult (ie, "double jeopardy" bias; Chappell & Havens, 1980). Given specific values and beliefs of the culture, an older women can experience different levels of opportunities and support as they age. This is important to acknowledge as we think about the needs and support interventions related to older women in different societies across the world. Further, there could even be "triple jeopardy" issues in response to an aging woman's race, ethnicity, functional status, sexual orientation, or other individual difference issues that impact her quality-of-life outcomes (eg, Averett, Yoon, & Jenkins, 2011).

How aging females respond to potential prejudice and discrimination in a social context can be qualitatively different than their male peers (García & Troyano, 2013). García and Troyano (2013) compared younger and older adults on experiences and behaviors related to age discrimination. The investigators surmised, among other findings, that older women tended to exhibit less ageist beliefs and associated age discrimination in behavior. The logical assumption is that knowledge about aging counteracts age discrimination, and this argues for more education in communities about realistic aging information to reduce the prevalence of stereotypes in cultures and societies. Further, a better understanding of the social reactions to aging women can have useful implications toward community programs and educational interventions for both training older adults and the broader society to avoid biased behavior and decision-making processes.

Resiliency of a woman can be in response to later-life changes and, in turn, affects a woman's health-related stress level and functional status (Jacobs & Kane, 2011; Lavretsky, 2012; Rybarczyk, Emery, Guequierre, Shamaskin, & Behel, 2012). A woman's experiences in overcoming loss and surviving traumatic life events (eg, psychological and/or physical trauma related to an accident) may impact her resiliency reactions to later-age-related changes in crises (Bonanno, Westphal, & Mancini, 2012). For example, being diagnosed with a life-changing disease (eg, AIDS/HIV) can elicit individual different reactions among older women with some evincing a strong resiliency and will to survive a response to this physical and mental adjustment challenge (Emlet, Tozay, & Raveis, 2011; Henry & Jones, 2011). Rybarczyk and colleagues suggested that older adults may actually develop a heightened resiliency reaction after resolving stressful life events over the course of a life span. Conversely, an aging woman's health outcomes can be affected by her level of resiliency in coping with situations and changes over a life span (Ryff, Friedman, Morozink, & Tsenkova, 2012). If it is possible to train resiliency skills through posed simulations of aging-related changes and challenges, this could assist in both the psychological and physical health of aging women through community education programs.

Culture has a significant influence on older women's willingness to seek out testing and support resources or can be a long-term chronic health condition (eg, Craig, Beaulaurier, Newman, La Rosa, & Brennan, 2012). Craig and colleagues concluded that community support of health-care resources (ie, provider endorsement, healthcare services) was a vital determinant of women's resiliency and coping responses in seeking HIV testing in the Latina culture.

Traumatic life events and associated role demands for aging women can be on the family system level. Grandmothers may be faced with the unanticipated "second parenthood" due to family members being lost to drugs and/or disease (eg, Casale, 2011). Women as default caregivers (eg, dementia care) across many cultures/societies would necessitate the ability to utilize resiliency responses to optimize their positive aging as well as those for whom they are caring (Harris, 2008).

For aging women to optimize their coping and resiliency responses to the many challenges of getting older, it is important for communities to offer educational interventions and support services that promote positive coping skills across a life span into later life (Bode, de Ridder, Kuijer, & Bensing, 2007; Smith & Hayslip, 2012). Utilizing Proactive Coping

Theory, Bode and researchers (2007) concluded that education is key to helping older adults develop proactive coping, especially if it assists in them developing concrete personal goals to guide resiliency responses. "Community" in a broader sense is important to understand as it impacts older women's feelings of resiliency. Having social ties and daily activities can bolster older women's (and men's) feelings of mastery in their coping ability in later life (eg, Pachana, McLaughlin, Leung, McKenzie, & Dobson, 2011). Volunteerism and community engagement can also be a productive aspect of community interventions that can enhance older women's feelings of self-efficacy and resilience (eg, Resnick, Klinedinst, Dorsey, Holtzman, & Abuelhiga, 2013; Sougleris & Ranzijn, 2011).

POSITIVE CULTURAL ATTITUDES AND INFLUENCES

How society responds to an aging woman is an important issue to reflect upon. Are aging women treated differently than aging men in society? The degree to which there may be different social supports and resources allocated to aging women may suggest a serious misunderstanding and bias within a given culture toward women's roles in later life (Canetto, Kaminski, & Felicio, 1995). If women experience attitudinal bias and discrimination as they get older, their social learning about ways to adapt and cope may be negative and limited in scope. In the extreme, some aging men and women may internalize these negative attitudes and develop a sense of "learned helplessness" (Peterson & Bossio, 1989).

Instead, cultures and broader societies need to promote the capabilities and positive contributions of older women in order to better enhance their feelings of resiliency, self-esteem and focus on both their mental and physical health. Exercise programs designed for aging women can have the effect of alleviating feelings of depression, raising self-esteem, and improving general well-being (Khalil, Callaghan, Carter, & Morres, 2012). Psychological resilience has been suggested to be linked to exhaustion recovery among other health conditions (Whitson et al., 2011). Interestingly, personal expectancies about positive aging can be a "self-fulfilling" prophecy related to the degree to which the older women (or men) may seek healthcare support and be resilient in response to healthcare needs (Sarkisian et al., 2002).

The need for personal control at a time in life when there are many changes and losses experienced by an older adult may lead to feeling out-of-control and is crucial to understand when designing interventions for older women (Ross & Mirowsky, 2002). Community education and support programs should attempt to incorporate as best as possible the unique beliefs, values, and self-care issues in activities of daily living to best address the personal control needs of older women. Encountering diverse health issues may be able to assist older women in improving their resiliency reactions and help them function better on a daily basis (eg, Leach & Schoenberg, 2008).

CHECK IT OUT!

Search the Internet to find different cultural ideas regarding women and adaptation to aging. Examine the ideas about women's positive aging adjustment and resiliency reactions. Are there factors to be considered according to what you found? In considering these factors, ask yourself the following questions:

1. What are the cultural "images" about women successfully aging? Are these predominantly positive or negative images?
2. Within and across cultures, are there basic ideas about resiliency and aging that apply to women's gender roles?
3. What advice seems to be conveyed about positive ways for women to adjust to aging changes?
4. As the nature of aging changes with a growing aging population within many different countries, what are some anticipated issues of resiliency and adaptation to aging facing women in the coming decades?

GEROTRANSCENDANCE AND SPIRITUALITY

Positive feelings of "gerotranscendance" (Wadensten, 2007) and women finding proactive ways to cope with aging-related changes are relatable concepts in their coping with the accomplishment of daily activities utilizing functional abilities (physical, mental). Interventions with older women can assist in helping them achieve a clearer purpose/meaning in life that rises above age-related client and loss issues (Nygren et al., 2005). This process of introspection and self-examination through training with older women could assist possibly generations of women across many different cultures in achieving positive resiliency coping skills and positive aging outcomes (Wiggs, 2010; Winter, Torges, Stewart, Henderson-King, & Henderson-King, 2006).

Personal spirituality is a meaningful, culturally derived social support factor to consider (Seicol, 2005). Across different parts of the world, many aging women may utilize personal spiritual beliefs as a navigational "tool" to traverse the many challenges of getting older (eg, life trauma survival; Bowland, Biswas, Kyriakakis, & Edmond, 2011). Crowther and colleagues argued that spirituality is often overlooked as a critical determinant of positive aging outcomes (Crowther, Parker, Achenbaum, Larimore, & Koenig, 2002). Ramsey (2012) purported that personal spirituality is an important life factor to examine from many different perspectives (ie, affective, situational, and cognitive) in order to best understand older adults' resiliency reactions which may be guided by spiritual beliefs.

EDUCATING ABOUT PERSONAL RESILIENCY STRATEGIES

Education is an important variable to consider when different cultures across the world think about ways to better help aging women become more resilient. Education can be in many forms, from informal to formal venues of instruction. Starting in early education, children should be taught about the positive aspects of aging and how women and men can achieve positive aging over time (eg, children's books; Hollis-Sawyer & Cuevas, 2013). Within family systems, older women can model positive aging adaptation styles to younger generations of girls. Aging education needs to start early in development in order to avoid negative aging stereotypes that may be learned and internalized before reaching adulthood. Across a life span, all ages of women should be exposed to positive messages about growing older and how they can optimize each stage of this development. Instead of thinking about aging as "decline," it is important for different cultures to promote the concept of aging as simply a new phase of existence that has challenges but equally has opportunities for learning and growth. Education in the community may be especially important for women in order to ensure the development of effective adaptive skills across their life span and into later life.

The value of education can also be extended to all members of society who need to better understand the aging experiences of women in their lives. Significant others, family, peers, and friends all need education about women's aging issues in order to best support their efforts in optimizing their unique aging experiences. Conversely, this broad-based educational effort in communities will help all more positively aging in response to the many different changes of aging. Through this effort, there is also hope that there'll be less aging stereotypes and bias in response to this growing segment of the aging population.

Resiliency responses to biological changes as a woman ages are important to examine. How well a woman may feel about her changing appearance and associated attractiveness is very much grounded in one's culture and societal learning. The interplay between aging women's biological changes and their adaptive responses to this changing sense of "self" is complex and rooted in social and cultural belief systems. How a woman feels about her aging and the degree to which she is resilient in response to aging changes may be reflection of the social models she has been exposed to within her family system and or culture. For example, unconsciously or consciously a woman may be following the same motion reactions that she witnessed with her mother and grandmother. The degree to which relevant social models exhibit positive resiliency and effective adaptation to aging changes can significantly impact how well the resultant aging woman copes and grows in later life. Bandura (1969) suggested that much of the feelings of "enactive mastery" people develop over time in response to certain contexts and tasks is learned through observational learning, especially in childhood. We mimic the social messages and behaviors received from relevant social "others" in our lives. Instead of judging aging women as having losses (eg, loss of youthful appearance), people's cultural attitudes should empower older women and value them for their contributions.

SUMMARY

There are many changes and losses that may occur as we age, and it is important for aging women and the larger community to be aware of these issues in order to assist in older women's resiliency reactions. From a psychological perspective, identifying individual difference factors for women across their life span, which help achieve strong and adaptive resiliency reactions would be critical for therapeutic and/or educational community-based programs.

Personal growth for aging women can only be better supported when we, as a society, more closely examine specific aging issues with older women. Once understood, it is vital to assess how communities and associated cultures respond to older women's later-life needs. Only through this process of "self" analysis within communities and broader societies can better, more supportive programs be developed for aging women faced with multiple transitions in later life. The interventions to help aging woman better cope with the many changes of later-life changes and transitions will benefit all involved. It is an ethical responsibility for communities to better support the growth potential of women across their life spans.

DISCUSSION QUESTIONS

1. Is an older woman's resiliency primarily learned through life experiences, or is it primarily an innate personality trait that can be used to adapt to later-life situations?

2. What are the common situations that require women's coping responses in later life?
3. Can educational programs within communities (eg, senior centers) assist women in learning better coping strategies?
4. What is the role of culture in women's development of coping skills?
5. Do you think communities adequately support older women's adaptation needs?
6. Do women and men cope differently, and does that impact their general aging trajectories?
7. What are the factors to consider in a coping support program for aging women?
8. Would it be beneficial to have an intergenerational women support group in communities? If so, why?
9. What are the important factors to consider in developing a community-based coping education program for women from diverse cultural backgrounds? Racial backgrounds?
10. Do you believe that community-based educational programs can assist in promoting resiliency responses of women across their life spans? Why or why not?

TEST YOUR KNOWLEDGE!

Take this quiz to test your personal resiliency and coping ability:

http://www.webmd.com/balance/stress-management/resilience-quiz

---

SUPPLEMENTAL BOOK READINGS

Over the past decades, there have been many books written related to aging women's coping and resiliency. Here are some recommended *additional readings*:

Sellers, R. (Editor) (2013). *70 things to do when you turn 70*. South Portland, ME: Sellers Publishing, Inc.
> *70 Things to Do When You Turn 70* presents wonderful life stories regarding ways to live a meaningful, fulfilling existence into later life. Seventy essays from diverse contributors communicate inspiring examples of ways to be resilient and succeed in response to the many challenges faced through the aging process.

Ramsey, J. L., & Blieszner, R. M. (1999). *Spiritual resiliency in older women: Models of strength for challenges through the life span.* Thousand Oaks, CA: Sage Publications, Inc.

The book offers an interesting collection of narratives about aging and resiliency by older women from Germany and America. The authors purport that positive coping in later life is assisted by an aging woman's dependence upon faith and maintenance of social support networks.

Henderson, M. C. (2014). *Optimistic aging: From midlife to the good life, an action plan.* Boise, ID: Resilient Publications.

Making a positive choice about aging processes is suggested by the present text. The author of the book suggests that the "key" to positive aging is to make a concise plan of activities that support positive aging outcomes. Being active and socially engaged in daily activities are encouraged through the topics presented.

Orel, N. A., & Fruhauf, C. A. (2014). *The lives of LGBT older adults: Understanding challenges and resilience.* Washington, DC: American Psychological Association.

The authors discuss important aging issues with the lesbian, gay, bisexual, and transgendered (LGBT) population who may have unique personal factors contributing to the aging trajectories; utilizing a life course perspective to investigate how LGBT older adults may be affected by systematic discrimination and stigma within society. Importantly, the book examines the resiliency of aging LGBT individuals in response to their life experiences and needs.

Thomas, A. (1996). *The women we become: Myths, folktales, and stories about growing older.* Denmark: Prima Lifestyles.

The Women We Become book explores the journey of aging women in many different cultures. Further, the book compares the social treatment and regard for women in Western and non-Western cultures. The author presents folktales, stories, and myths from various cultures in the world to help aging women approaching mid-life and beyond to successfully navigate their aging path with resiliency and empowerment.

Fry, P. S., & Keyes, C. L. M. (2013). *New frontiers in resilient aging: Life-strengths and well-being in late life.* New York, NY: Cambridge University Press.

This book offers a strong message of hope and support for aging women facing the many challenges of getting older. The authors argue that older adults must actively utilize psychological resources of personal engagement, social support, sustained mental activity, and physical activeness to create resilient aging outcomes. Older adults can better cope with the many losses and changes associated with aging through their on-going focus on skill utilization, compensatory strategies, positivity in attitudes, and growth-oriented development.

Loe, M. (2011). *Aging our way: Lessons for living from 85 and beyond.* New York, NY: Oxford University Press.
The author presents real stories about the everyday lives of a set of older adults coping with activities of daily living. This is an empowering book of stories about adults from diverse backgrounds and circumstances dealing with a myriad of challenges and achieving many different life successes in the process.

Greenstein, M., & Holland, J. (2014). *Lighter as we go: Virtues, character strengths, and aging.* London, UK: Oxford University.
The book examines the strength of aging attitudes, sometimes negative in nature due to worries related to aging, upon one's quality of life, health, and aging resiliency reactions. Ultimately, an older adult can achieve a positive sense of well-being and wisdom through the development and maintenance of positive aging attitudes across the life span.

SUPPLEMENTAL AGING VIDEOS

For learning purposes, the use of videos can be very beneficial for both instructors and readers. Here are recommended *supplemental videos*:

Healthy Body/Health Mind: http://www.itvisus.com/programs/hbhm/ (Format: Website)
This is a great website offering different videos about healthy aging.

I Know a Song: A Journey with Alzheimer's Disease (Format: DVD)
This film is a heartfelt depiction of the filmmaker's mother as she developed and then died from Alzheimer's disease. This positive depiction of the experience for both the patient and the family who took care of her exemplifies the coping strategies and resiliency factors underlying needed in such a life-changing aging situation for all involved.

ADDITIONAL INFORMATION LINKS

The following are some recommended *supplemental Internet links*:

Aging in Action website: http://aginginaction.com/2010/12/gender-and-aging-what-do-we-know/

Everyday Health website: http://www.everydayhealth.com/senior-health/enhancing-your-sexuality.aspx

NIH/NIAging website: http://www.nia.nih.gov/about/minority-aging-and-health-disparities

WebMD website: http://www.webmd.com/healthy-aging/guide/sex-aging

World Health Organization website: http://www.who.int/ageing/gender/en/index.html

References

Aldwin, C., & Igarashi, H. (2012). An ecological model of resilience in late life. *Annual Review of Gerontology & Geriatrics, 32*, 115–130.

Averett, P., Yoon, I., & Jenkins, C. L. (2011). Older lesbians: Experiences of aging, discrimination and resilience. *Journal of Women & Aging, 23*(3), 216–232. http://dx.doi.org/10.1080/08952841.2011.587742.

Baltes, P. B., & Baltes, M. M. (1990). Psychological perspectives on successful aging. The model of selective optimization with compensation. In P. B. Baltes & M. M. Baltes (Eds.), *Successful aging: Perspectives from the behavioral sciences* (pp. 1–34). Cambridge, MA: Cambridge University Press.

Bandura, A. (1969). Social-learning theory of identificatory processes. In D. A. Goslin (Ed.), *Handbook of socialization theory and research*. New York, NY: Rand McNally.

Bode, C., de Ridder, D. D., Kuijer, R. G., & Bensing, J. M. (2007). Effects of an intervention promoting proactive coping competencies in middle and late adulthood. *Gerontologist, 47*(1), 42–51.

Bonanno, G. A., Westphal, M., & Mancini, A. D. (2012). Loss, trauma, and resilience in adulthood. *Annual Review of Gerontology & Geriatrics, 32*, 189–210.

Bowland, S., Biswas, B., Kyriakakis, S., & Edmond, T. (2011). Transcending the negative: Spiritual struggles and resilience in older female trauma survivors. *Journal of Religion, Spirituality & Aging, 23*(4), 318–337. http://dx.doi.org/10.1080/15528030.2011.592121.

Brock, K., Clemson, L., Cant, R., Ke, L., Cumming, R. G., Kendig, H., et al. (2011). Worry in older community-residing adults. *International Journal of Aging & Human Development, 72*(4), 289–301. http://dx.doi.org/10.2190/AG.72.4.a.

Butler, S. S. (1993). Older rural women: Understanding their conceptions of health and illness. *Topics in Geriatric Rehabilitation, 9*(1), 56–68.

Canetto, S. S., Kaminski, P. L., & Felicio, D. M. (1995). Typical and optimal aging in women and men: Is there a double standard? *International Journal of Aging and Human Development, 40*(3), 187–207.

Carver, C. S. (1998). Resilience and thriving: Issues, models, and link-ages. *Journal of Social Issue, 54*, 245–266.

Casale, M. (2011). 'I am living a peaceful life with my grandchildren. Nothing else.' Stories of adversity and 'resilience' of older women caring for children in the context of HIV/AIDS and other stressors. *Ageing & Society, 31*(8), 1265–1288. http://dx.doi.org/10.1017/S0144686X-10001303.

Chappell, N. L., & Havens, B. (1980). Old and female: Testing the double jeopardy hypothesis. *The Sociological Quarterly, 21*, 157–171.

Cheng, S., Chan, W., & Chan, A. C. M. (2008). Older people's realisation of generativity in a changing society: The case of Hong Kong. *Ageing and Society, 28*, 609–627. http://dx.doi.org/10.1017/S0144686X07006903.

Chin, L., & Quine, S. (2012). Common factors that enhance the quality of life for women living in their own homes or in aged care facilities. *Journal of Women & Aging, 24*(4), 269–279. http://dx.doi.org/10.1080/08952841.2012.650605.

Chun, K. (2007). Living past 100 years: Perspectives from anthropology of longevity. *Annual Review of Gerontology & Geriatrics, 27*, 173–204.

Consedine, N. S., Magai, C., & Conway, F. (2004). Predicting ethnic variation in adaptation to later life: Styles of socioemotional functioning and constrained heterotypy. *Journal of Cross-Cultural Gerontology, 19*(2), 97–131.

Consedine, N. S., Magai, C., & Krivoshekova, Y. S. (2005). Sex and age cohort differences in patterns of socioemotional functioning in older adults and their links to physical resilience. *Ageing International, 30*(3), 209–244.

Coon, D. W. (2012). Resilience and family caregiving. *Annual Review of Gerontology & Geriatrics, 32*, 231–249.

Craig, S. L., Beaulaurier, R. L., Newman, F. L., La Rosa, M. D., & Brennan, D. J. (2012). Health and cultural determinants of voluntary HIV testing and counseling among middle-aged and older Latina women. *Journal of Women & Aging, 24*(2), 97–112. http://dx.doi.org/10.1080/08952841.2012.639650.

Crawley, L., & Lynch, K. (2012). The emotional significance of affective inequalities and why they are important to women in old age. *Journal of Women & Aging, 24*(4), 313–328. http://dx.doi.org/10.1080/08952841.2012.708584.

Crowther, M. R., Parker, M. W., Achenbaum, W. A., Larimore, W. L., & Koenig, H. G. (2002). Rowe and Kahn's model of successful aging revisited: Positive spirituality—The forgotten factor. *The Gerontologist, 42*(5), 613–620.

Dasgupta, D., & Ray, S. (2013). Attitude toward menopause and aging: A study on postmenopausal women of West Bengal. *Journal of Women & Aging, 25*(1), 66–79. http://dx.doi.org/10.1080/08952841.2012.720203.

Diehl, M., Hay, E. L., & Chui, H. (2012). Personal risk and resilience factors in the context of daily stress. *Annual Review of Gerontology & Geriatrics, 32*, 251–274.

Dilworth-Anderson, P., Hilliard, T. S., Williams, S., & Palmer, M. H. (2011). A contextual conceptualization on transitions of care for older persons: Shaping the direction of care. *Annual Review of Gerontology & Geriatrics, 31*, 1–14.

Dorfman, L. T., Mendez, E. C., & Osterhaus, J. K. (2009). Stress and resilience in the oral histories of rural older women. *Journal of Women & Aging, 21*(4), 303–316. http://dx.doi.org/10.1080/08952840903285237.

Emlet, C. A., Tozay, S., & Raveis, V. H. (2011). "I'm not going to die from the AIDS": Resilience in aging with HIV disease. *Gerontologist, 51*(1), 101–111.

Facio, E. (1995). Being an older woman means being more than just a grandma: *Understanding the older chicanas: Sociological and policy perspectives.* New York, NY: Sage.9099

Felten, B. S. (2000). Resilience in a multicultural sample of community dwelling women older than age 85. *Clinical Nursing Research, 9*(2), 102–124.

Freund, A. M., & Baltes, P. B. (1998). Selection, optimization, and compensation as strategies of life management: Correlations with subjective indicators of successful aging. *Psychology and Aging, 13*(4), 531–543.

Fry, C. (1997). Cross-cultural perspectives on aging. In K. Ferraro (Ed.), *Gerontology: Perspectives and issues* (pp. 138–152). New York, NY: Springer.

Fulle-Iglesias, H., Smith, J., & Antonucci, T. C. (2009). Theories of aging from a life-course and life-span perspective: An overview. *Annual Review of Gerontology & Geriatrics, 29*(3–25), R12–R13.

García, A. J., & Troyano, Y. (2013). Different ways of perceiving the aging process: Social behaviors of women and men in relation to age discrimination. *Psychology, 4*(3A), 279–282. http://dx.doi.org/10.4236/2013.43A041.

Gerstorf, D., Ram, N., Fauth, E., Schupp, J., & Wagner, G. G. (2009). Between-person disparities in the progression of late-life well-being. *Annual Review of Gerontology & Geriatrics, 29*(205–232), R12–R13.

Gilligan, C. (1984). *In a different voice: Psychological theory and women's development.* Cambridge, MA: Harvard University Press.

Grundy, E. (2006). Aging and vulnerable elderly: European perspectives. *Aging and Society, 26,* 105–129. http://dx.doi.org/10.107/s104468X05004484.

Gu, D., & Zeng, Y. (2012). Healthiness of survival and quality of death among oldest old in China using fuzzy sets. *Journal of Aging & Health, 24*(7), 1091–1130. http://dx.doi.org/10.1177/-0898264312453069.

Hahn, E. A., Cichy, K. E., Almeida, D. M., & Haley, W. E. (2011). Time use and well-being in older widows: Adaptation and resilience. *Journal of Women & Aging, 23*(2), 149–159. http://dx.doi.org/10.1080/08952841.2011.561139.

Harris, P. B. (2008). Another wrinkle in the debate about successful aging: The undervalued concept of resilience and the lived experience of dementia. *International Journal Aging and Human Development, 67*(1), 43–61.

Helson, R., & Cate, R. A. (2006). Late middle age: Transition to the third age. *Annual Review of Gerontology & Geriatrics, 26*(83-101), R9–R10.

Henry, E., & Jones, S. H. (2011). Experiences of older adult women diagnosed with attention deficit hyperactivity disorder. *Journal of Women & Aging, 23*(3), 246–262. http://dx.doi.org/10.1080/-08952841.2011.589285.

Hollis-Sawyer, L., & Cuevas, L. (2013). Mirror, mirror on the wall: Ageist and sexist double jeopardy portrayals in children's picture books. *Educational Gerontology, 39*(12), 902–914. http://dx.doi.org/10.1080/03601277.2013.767650.

Hollis-Sawyer, L. A. (2003). A path-analytic investigation of factors underlying positive, adaptive mother-daughter eldercare relationships. *Journal of Adult Development, 10*(1), 41–52.

Holtslander, L., & Duggleby, W. (2010). The psychosocial context of bereavement for older women who were caregivers for a spouse with advanced cancer. *Journal of Women & Aging, 22*(2), 109–124. http://dx.doi.org/10.1080/08952841003716147.

Hutchinson, S. L., Yarnal, C. M., Staffordson, J., & Kerstetter, D. L. (2008). Beyond fun and friendship: The red hat society as a coping resource for older women. *Ageing and Society, 28*(7), 979–999. http://dx.doi.org/10.1017/S0144686X08007058.

Jacobs, R. J., & Kane, M. N. (2011). Psychosocial predictors of self-esteem in a multiethnic sample of women over 50 at risk for HIV. *Journal of Women & Aging, 23*(1), 23–39. http://dx.doi.org/10.1080/08952841.2011.540484.

Janssen, B. M., Abma, T. A., & Van Regenmortel, T. (2012). Maintaining mastery despite age related losses. The resilience narratives of two older women in need of long-term community care. *Journal of Aging Studies, 26*(3), 343–354. http://dx.doi.org/10.1016/j.jaging.2012.-03.003.

Khalil, E., Callaghan, P., Carter, T., & Morres, J. (2012). Pragmatic randomised controlled trial of an exercise programme to improve well-being outcomes in women with depression: Findings from the qualitative component. *Psychology, 3*(11), 979–986. http://dx.doi.org/10.4236/psych.2012.311147.

Kinsel, B. (2005). Resilience as adaptation in older women. *Journal of Women & Aging, 17*(3), 23–39.

Knapp, M. R. (1977). The activity theory of aging: An examination in the English context. *The Gerontologist, 17*(6), 553–559.

Kwan, C. M. L. K., Love, G. D., Ryff, C. D., & Essex, M. J. (2003). The role of self-enhancing self-evaluations in a successful life transition. *Psychology and Aging, 18*, 3–12.

LaFerriere, R. H., & Hamel-Bissell, B. P. (1994). Successful aging of oldest-old women in the Northeast kingdom of Vermont. *IMAGE: Journal of Nursing Scholarship, 26*, 319–323.

Laganá, L., Spellman, T., Wakefield, J., & Oliver, T. (2011). Ethnic minority status, depression, and cognitive failures in relation to marital adjustment in ethnically diverse older women. *Clinical Gerontologist, 34*(3), 173–189. http://dx.doi.org/10.1080/07317115.2011.554627.

Lavretsky, H. (2012). Resilience, stress, and mood disorders in old age. *Annual Review of Gerontology & Geriatrics, 32*, 49–72.

Lazarus, R. S. (1991). *Emotion and adaptation.* New York, NY: Oxford University Press.

Leach, C., & Schoenberg, N. (2008). Striving for control: Cognitive, self-care, and faith strategies employed by vulnerable Black and White older adults with multiple chronic conditions. *Journal of Cross-Cultural Gerontology, 23*(4), 377–399. http://dx.doi.org/10.1007/s10823-008-9086-2.

Lerner, R. M., Weiner, M. B., Arbeit, M. R., Chase, P. A., Agans, J. P., Schmid, K. L., et al. (2012). Resilience across the life span. *Annual Review of Gerontology & Geriatrics, 32*, 275–299.

Moe, A., Ekker, K., & Enmarker, I. (2013). A description of resilience for Norwegian home-living chronically ill oldest older persons. *Open Journal of Nursing, 3*, 241–248. http://dx.doi.org/10.4236/ojn.2013.32033.

Nygren, B. B., Aléx, L. L., Jonsén, E. E., Gustafson, Y. Y., Norberg, A. A., & Lundman, B. B. (2005). Resilience, sense of coherence, purpose in life and self-transcendence in relation to perceived physical and mental health among the oldest old. *Aging & Mental Health, 9*(4), 354–362. http://dx.doi.org/10.1080/1360500114415.

Olney, J. (1972). *Metaphors of the self: The meaning of autobiography.* Princeton, NJ: Princeton University Press.

O'Rourke, N. (2004). Psychological resilience and the well-being of widowed women. *Ageing International, 29*(3), 267–280.

Pachana, N. A., McLaughlin, D., Leung, J., McKenzie, S. J., & Dobson, A. (2011). The effect of having a partner on activities of daily living in men and women aged 82–87 years. *Maturitas, 68*(3), 286–290. http://dx.doi.org/10.1016/j.maturitas.2010.11.009.

Peterson, C., & Bossio, L. M. (1989). Learned helplessness. In R. Curtis (Ed.), *Self-defeating behaviors: Experimental research, clinical impressions, and practical implications* (pp. 235–257). New York, NY: Plenum Press.

Piercy, K. W. (2007). Characteristics intergenerational of strong commitments to family care of older adults. *Journals of Gerontology Series B: Psychological Sciences & Social Sciences, 62B*(6), S381–S387.

Ramsey, J. L. (2012). Spirituality and aging: Cognitive, affective, and relational pathways to resiliency. *Annual Review of Gerontology & Geriatrics, 32*, 131–150.

Rayman, P., Allen, J., Pifer, A., & Allshouse, K. (1993). Resiliency amidst inequity: Older women workers in an aging United States: *Women on the front lines: Meeting the challenge of an aging America.* Washington, DC: Urban Institute Press.133166

Reker, G. T. (2001). Prospective predictors of successful aging in community-residing and institutionalized Canadian elderly. *Ageing International, 27*(1), 42–64.

Resnick, B., Klinedinst, J., Dorsey, S., Holtzman, L., & Abuelhiga, L. S. (2013). Volunteer behavior and factors that influence volunteering among residents in continuing care retirement communities. *Journal of Housing for the Elderly, 27*(1/2), 161–176. http://dx.doi.org/10.1080/02763893.2012.751820.

Ross, C. E., & Mirowsky, J. (2002). Age and the gender gap in the sense of personal control. *Social Psychology Quarterly, 65*(2), 125–145.

Rothrauff, T. C., Cooney, T. M., & Jeong Shin, A. (2009). Remembered parenting styles and adjustment in middle and late adulthood. *Journals of Gerontology Series B: Psychological Sciences & Social Sciences, 64B*(1), 137–146.

Rybarczyk, B., Emery, E. E., Guequierre, L. L., Shamaskin, A., & Behel, J. (2012). The role of resilience in chronic illness and disability in older adults. *Annual Review of Gerontology & Geriatrics, 32*, 173–187.

Ryff, C. D., Friedman, E. M., Morozink, J. A., & Tsenkova, V. (2012). Psychological resilience in adulthood and later life: Implications for health. *Annual Review of Gerontology & Geriatrics, 32*, 73–92.

Sarkisian, C. A., Hays, R. D., & Mangione, C. M. (2002). Do older adults expect to age successfully? The association between expectations regarding aging and beliefs regarding healthcare seeking among older adults. *Journal of Applied Gerontology, 50*, 1837–1843. 0002-8614/02.

Seeman, T. E., Charpentier, P. A., Berkman, L. F., Tenetti, M. E., Guralnik, J. M., Albert, M., et al. (1994). Predicting changes in physical performance in a high- functioning elderly cohort: MacArthur studies of successful aging. *Journal of Gerontology, 49*(3), M97–M108. http://dx.doi.org/10.1093/geronj/49.3.M97.

Seicol, S. R. (2005). A pastoral understanding of positive aging. *Journal of Gerontological Social Work, 45*(3), 293–300. http://dx.doi.org/10.1300/J083v45n03_03.

Shaevitz, M. H. (1984). *The superwoman syndrome*. New York, NY: Warner Books.612

Sinclair, V. G., & Wallston, K. A. (2004). The development and psychometric evaluation of the brief resilient coping scale. *Assessment, 11*(1), 94–101. http://dx.doi.org/10.1177/1073191103258144.

Smith, G. C., & Hayslip, B., Jr. (2012). Resilience in adulthood and later life: What does it mean and where are we heading? *Annual Review of Gerontology & Geriatrics, 32*(1), 1–28.

Sougleris, C., & Ranzijn, R. (2011). Proactive coping in community-dwelling older Australians. *International Journal of Aging and Human Development, 72*(2), 155–168. http://dx.doi.org/10.2190/AG.72.2.d.

Stark-Wroblewski, K., Edelbaum, J. K., & Bello, T. O. (2008). Perceptions of aging among rural, Midwestern senior citizens: Signs of women's resiliency. *Journal of Women & Aging, 20*(3/4), 361–373.

Sterns, H. L., & Dawson, N. T. (2012). Emerging perspectives on resilience in adulthood and later life: Work, retirement, and resilience. *Annual Review of Gerontology & Geriatrics, 32*(1), 211–230.

Stine-Morrow, E., & Chui, H. (2012). Cognitive resilience in adulthood. *Annual Review of Gerontology & Geriatrics, 32*(1), 93–114.

United Nations, Women Coordination Division. (2012). Between gender and ageing: The status of the world's older women and progress since the Madrid International Plan of Action on Ageing. Retrieved from: <http://www.un.org/womenwatch/osagi/ianwge2012/-Between-Gender-Ageing-Report-Executive-Summary-2012.pdf>.

Wadensten, B. (2007). The theory of gerotranscendence as applied to gerontological nursing. *International Journal of Older People Nursing, 2*(4), 289–294.

Walsh, F. (2012). Successful aging and family resilience. *Annual Review of Gerontology & Geriatrics, 32*(1), 151–172.

Whitson, H. E., Thielke, S., Diehr, P., O'Hare, A. M., Chaves, P. M., Zakai, N. A., et al. (2011). Patterns and predictors of recovery from exhaustion in older adults: The cardiovascular health study. *Journal of the American Geriatrics Society, 59*(2), 207–213. http://dx.doi.org/10.1111/j.1532-5415.2010.03238.x.

Wiggs, C. M. (2010). Creating the self: Exploring the life journey of late-midlife women. *Journal of Women & Aging, 22,* 218–233. http://dx.doi.org/10.1080/08952841.2010.495 574.

Williams, B. R., Sawyer, P., & Allman, R. M. (2012). Wearing the garment of widowhood: Variations in time since spousal loss among community-dwelling older adults. *Journal of Women & Aging, 24*(2), 126–139. http://dx.doi.org/10.1080/08952841.2012.639660.

Wink, P. (2006). Everyday life in the third age. *Annual Review of Gerontology & Geriatrics, 26*(243-261), R7–R8.

Winter, D. G., Torges, C. M., Stewart, A. J., Henderson-King, D., & Henderson-King, E. (2006). Pathways toward the third age: Studying a cohort from the "golden age.". *Annual Review of Gerontology & Geriatrics, 26*(103–129), R10–R11.

Woodward, K. (Ed.). (1999). *Figuring age: Women, bodies, generations.* Bloomington, IN: Indiana University Press.

3

Aging Self-Acceptance for Women

Global fact: Mass media, the machine of image-making, is also a link in the globalization chain, and can have profound effects on the developing world, and particularly on the older women who live there.

—Global Aging (2001)

Positive aging self-perceptions are related to positive aging outcomes (eg, longevity; Levy, Slade, Kunkel, & Kasl, 2002). What does it mean to accept one's aging? Aging self-acceptance is a healthy and adaptive response to later-life human development (eg, changing body image), and is an important individual-difference factor to better understand diverse positive aging outcomes of women (Reichstadt, Sengupta, Depp, Palinkas, & Jeste, 2010; Rossen, Knafi, & Flood, 2008). Perceived and actual health status, functional status, and effectiveness in accomplishing activities of daily living in different living contacts (eg, rural settings) have a significant impact on older women's, as well as their male counterparts' feelings of aging acceptance and personal self-identity (Butler, 1993). The proceeding will examine personal and contextual factors significantly impacting women's feelings of self-esteem and self-acceptance in later adulthood.

CULTURAL ROLES AND AGING SELF-ACCEPTANCE

Culture plays a significant role in the development of positive aging self-perceptions (Karasawa et al., 2011). Expectations of society, in terms of what adults are expected to do in everyday life, relate to how well a woman may feel about how she is aging (Ault, 2007; Wink, 2006). Conversely, a woman's perceptions of her "ideal" self may impact her actual aging outcomes and associated personal aging self-acceptance (Ryff, 1991). This idea of "self" is a key aspect of this evaluation process. Ryff and Singer (2008) suggested that it is most important to embrace who you are, in order to

51

achieve feelings of personal self-satisfaction and well-being. Applying this concept to the experiences of aging women across many different cultures, a woman's inner exploration and self-understanding which lead to self-acceptance and other positive aging outcomes are important to explore from a developmental perspective. The interplay of a positive sense of self and one's ability to operate effectively in a physical and social environment is an important quality of life issue for many.

PHYSICAL AGING SELF-ACCEPTANCE

Body image is an important factor to consider when examining women's feelings of positive self-acceptance across their life span (Hurd, 2000). Changes in skin elasticity and other aging-related changes in appearance can significantly influence an aging woman's self-identity and associated aging self-acceptance (Pearlman, 1993). Heuberger, Domina, and MacGillivray (2010) conducted a study and concluded that older women had different identity reactions to being placed in a 3-D body scanner than younger women. The majority of older women had issues with appearance that affected emotional and psychological reactions for their personal aging trajectory. This finding has significant support for a strong linkage between a woman's body image and aging self-acceptance. An important extension of this idea is to examine if body image restricts older women's social and behavioral activities that may negatively impact health in positive aging outcomes (eg, going to the gym). How an older woman perceives her aging body can be a significant variable in the determination of aging-related self-esteem.

QUOTES FROM FAMOUS, POSITIVELY AGING WOMEN

Old age is like a plane flying through a storm.
Once you're aboard, there's nothing you can do.
            —*Golda Meir, Israeli Prime Minister from 1969–1974*

We are always the same age inside.
                        —*Gertrude Stein, Author*

"Age" is the acceptance of a term of years.
But maturity is the glory of years.
            —*Martha Graham, Dancer and Choreographer*

Be eccentric now. Don't wait for old age to wear purple.
                    —*Regina Brett, Journalist*

Leichty (2012) raised an important point that older women's feelings of self-acceptance may be lower or higher in level within certain contexts and aspects of self-image evaluation (eg, body weight) but this self-evaluation may not affect their general feelings of contentment. Beyond simply "body image," it is important to acknowledge that a woman's feelings of self-acceptance can impact critical health-related functioning that is important for both quality and quality-of-life outcomes. Phelan, Love, Ryff, Brown, and Heidrich (2010) found a meaningful association between feelings of self-acceptance and sleep patterns among older women. Agitated sleep was more associated with women who struggle with feelings of self-esteem and self-acceptance. This is the logical idea because stress can certainly be a factor impacting women's inability to rest and avoid interrupting thoughts. Feelings of positive self-acceptance appear to impact a woman's physical health on a daily basis, from physical activities to peaceful sleep.

SOCIETAL FEEDBACK ABOUT WOMEN'S AGING

It is important to understand how society expresses aging attitudes (eg, public humor; Davies, 1977), and its potential impact on older women's feelings of self-acceptance. Perceived and actual women's biological changes across a life span (eg, menopausal changes) may meaningfully impact diverse women's global quality of aging and health-related attitudes within a social context (Ama & Ngome, 2013; Avis, Assmann, Kravitz, Ganz, & Ory, 2004). How an aging woman is regarded (or disregarded) based upon her age-related appearance within diverse cultures across the world is a significant issue to undertake (Porcino, 1986). For example, communication patterns, both verbal and nonverbal, between generations can certainly indicate social valuation of diverse older adults within a cultural context (Nussbaum & Coupland, 2004).

An aging woman's physical appearance, and the social message to "defy aging" in response to her appearance and/or social roles, might have a strong psychological influence on her internalized self-image (Sawchuk, 2009). In order to better understand women's reactions to aging-related body changes, one must understand the cultural context that a woman lives within as she ages. Reel, SooHoo, Summerhays, and Gill (2008) reported a meaningful difference in personal satisfaction and adjustment issues to aging between Caucasian and African-American women. Older African-American women were not as concerned about their changing body image. In examining the African-American culture, on-going social support and positive social feedback related to being an older woman create positive standards of support for positive aging self-acceptance and growth. Schuler and colleagues investigated body image and associated body mass index (BMI) levels between older European and African-American women (Schuler et al. (2008). There was a significant cultural difference, with older African-American women being significantly less concerned about changing body image. Clarke and Bundon (2009) conducted research on the symbolic meaning of women using lipstick as a way to maintain a youthful self-image. Specifically, the researchers suggested that the meaning behind the action may actually undermine a woman's positive aging self-acceptance if the motivation is to obscure age-related changes. The psychological concept of hiding or disguising one's true age may certainly create a negative aging trajectory for aging women.

To deny or inhibit aging-related changes may create internal psychological conflicts for women who wish to maintain a positive sense of self that are conflicted with the wish of maintaining an increasingly unrealistic external aging persona. In order to successfully age, diverse older women need to examine these feelings of potential negative reactions to personal aging and consciously create strategies for embracing the many age-related changes that can occur without embarrassment or self-consciousness within their cultural context.

PERSONAL ADJUSTMENT, SELF-FORGIVENESS, AND SELF-ACCEPTANCE

Life decision-making and feelings of "self-forgiveness" in light of choices made over time are also important to understand from a positive aging perspective (Ingersoll-Dayton & Krause, 2005). The emotional reaction of getting older, having less energy to maintain earlier life activities (number, degree of activities), and changes in general appearance may lead to feelings of depression and even self-hatred (Ingersoll-Dayton & Krause, 2005). Education and other types of mental health interventions may assist older women in achieving more positive feelings of forgiveness of others, self-forgiveness, and self-acceptance in response to the many physical and social transitions they may experience in later life (Sells & Hargrave, 2002). Spafford, Rudman, Leipert, Klinger, and Huot (2010) speculated that older adults who do not accept aging changes, such as aging-related vision change, may hide their needs and avoid using needed health-related services. This implication toward quality-of-life of aging women is quite serious in nature and needs to be addressed within society so that their aging trajectories are not negatively impacted by this feeling of self-denial regarding aging-related needs.

TIPS FOR WOMEN'S AGING SELF-ACCEPTANCE

1. Appreciate the aging-related changes you see and love the "new you."
2. Engage in volunteer activities to show your social value.
3. Be around other positively aging women and exchange ideas.
4. Mentor a younger woman about positive aging acceptance.

WORDS OF WISDOM

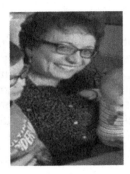

Teresa was a teacher for more than 30 years; she taught in Peru and the United States. Retired for a couple of years now she devotes her time to family and friends. She always keeps herself busy and engages in various activities. When asked how to embrace aging she said that it is important to take care of yourself—eat well, sleep well, and not overdo anything; regardless of age every woman is beautiful, and every woman should love and accept herself. Physical appearances change with age, but it is important to accept those changes, and take care of your physical, mental, and emotional health. "Today is a very important day—I have to be happy; I always dress up": Teresa says that if she looks good she feels good and everything else will be okay.

Women should not try and fit into a "standard" but, on the contrary, women should be themselves and embrace who they are: for example, a woman should always wear what makes her feel good, not what is expected of her.

Women should always accept themselves for who they are: and it is especially true when women age: getting older means your personality is not going to change anymore—you are who you are and you need to be happy with yourself. Keeping a positive self-image, believing in yourself, and doing what makes you content and happy are the most important things.

What advice would Teresa give to younger women? First of all, be yourself! Do not pay attention to others, especially when you are young it is easy to give in to outside pressures and try to live up to expectations, accept yourself the way you are and listen to yourself. Do what makes you happy. Stay connected and share with people who matter in your life. Believe in yourself. "Always be nice to everybody regardless of who they are—life is too short to be cranky!"

Sexuality is a key part of one's identity over time and does not simply extinguish as one gets older, although this is a pervasive biased assumption within general aging stereotypes (Hinchliff & Gott, 2008). Sexual needs are a part of basic human needs, and aging women as well as the societies they live within, should recognize this as a vital aspect of their positive aging. How a culture defines beauty and attractiveness should be reexamined and acknowledged as a lifelong issue for women.

LIFE ROLE TRANSITIONS

In addition to the many internal transitions that a woman can experience as she ages, there are also important contextual and environmental transitions that can be experienced over time. Life transitions for older women may involve migrating to a new location and/or culture. This potentially major life transition can certainly impact women's aging trajectory. The degree to which the older woman adjusts to this life transition depends upon, among other factors, the acceptance of the older woman within the new social context. This adaptation process requires both parties involved to have an open mind and positive attitude about the aging woman's role within the community and her value in the community. The impact of such a life change can be a positive experience that their social support resources and the new culture are accepting of the older woman's culture and beliefs (Binfa, Robertson, & Ransjö-Arvidson, 2010).

An increasingly normative life transition for aging women will be the need to move from independent living to residential care. This is a common and increasingly normative reality for aging women as they live longer than previous generations, long-term chronic conditions. Being open to this experience of adjusting to role dependency in later adulthood underlies feelings of positive self-acceptance for women. Positive adaption to daily life circumstance can directly impact one's feelings about personal performance and capabilities, as well as feelings of self-acceptance under the new life circumstances (eg, eldercare circumstances as a care recipient) (Schanowitz & Nicassio, 2006). The role of caregiver is a significant part of self-identity for many women across different cultures. To lose this significant lifespan role and transition to the role of care recipient can be challenging for many women, but is a necessary issue of adjustment that needs to be better understood through community education and filial social support. Life "transitions" and associated feelings of self-acceptance for aging women may be influenced by cultural traditions and beliefs. Lvgren (2013) examined how traditions within the Swedish Tant culture, and the associated cultural meaning toward women's aging in this culture (eg, a "coming-of-age" in later life), have significant implications toward older women's feelings of competency and efficacy in their daily circumstances. There is a significant cultural and personal benefit in the explicit recognition and valuation of women's developmental transition into later adulthood.

Social support associated with widowhood is an especially relevant issue for women who typically outlive their spouses or romantic partners due to gender-related viability differences (Bennett, 2010). This loss of a romantic partner definitely affects a woman's self-identity, and may affect an older woman's subsequent aging adjustment, potentially exacerbated by a lack of other social support resources. In addition to a loss of social support due to the loss of a romantic partner, some older women may have unique challenges due to never being married (O'Brien, 1991) and/or being childless (Abma & Martinez, 2006). Never-married and/or childless women may require supplemental social support resources within the family system (eg, siblings, extended family) and/or within nonfilial relationships, such as friendships, coworkers at work, and other societal network opportunities (Rubinstein, Alexander, Goodman, & Luborsky, 1991).

It has been said that "it takes a village to raise child," but one might argue that it equally takes the community to support a growing aging female population across countries in the world who will need social, financial, and other resources to achieve and maintain positive aging. For example, there will be a financial support crisis for diverse groups of aging women known as the "feminization of poverty" (Minkler & Stone, 1985). In many countries across the world, better social support and financial support programs will be needed to assist women in achieving financial stability into later adulthood.

POSITIVE PSYCHOSOCIAL ADJUSTMENT AND SELF-ACTUALIZATION

A relevant theory to apply to older women's feelings of self-acceptance would be Erikson's psychosocial stages of development (Erikson, Paul, Heider, & Gardner, 1959), focusing on women's experiences in the last three (or "adult") stages of psychosocial adjustment. Specifically, aging women's achievement of intimate and long-lasting relationship "bonds" within both platonic and nonplatonic relationships (ie, positive resolution of the "relationship intimacy" psychosocial stage), feelings of meaningful contribution to others in society (ie, positive resolution of the "generativity" psychosocial stage), and, ultimately, achieving feelings of personal achievement on a personal, societal, and other relevant criteria of success (ie, positive resolution of the "ego integrity" psychosocial stage).

Issues of establishing and maintaining social support networks are dynamically related to women's roles and the associated costs/benefits for them into later adulthood, such as eldercare and role-related demands as well as the social reciprocity of care among family members/friends. Further, the degree to which older women can contribute to society relies partly on societies' valuation of middle-aged and older women's knowledge and skills to be offered to others. This social feedback contributes to women's feelings of enactive mastery (Bandura, 1977) in their social environment.

In addition to Erikson's theory and Bandura's concept of enactive mastery, applying Maslow's hierarchy of needs theory to aging self-acceptance for older women (see Fig. 3.1) addresses the many needs of aging women.

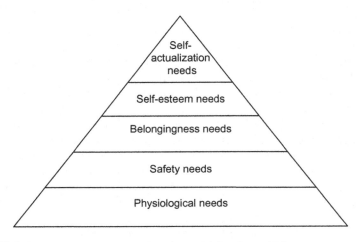

FIGURE 3.1   Maslow's hierarchy of needs model (Maslow, 1971).

Maslow's theory suggested needed foci for educational programs and services offered to aging women in communities. Maslow (1971) spoke about the importance of satisfying the need of "social belongingness" for most individuals. Moving beyond the need to achieve a sense of belongingness for women, Maslow (1954) purported in his theoretical model that "self-esteem" is a next progressive higher-level need important for all human beings to achieve and maintain. For aging women, this concept of self-esteem as a quality of life need relates well to the previous discussions within this chapter related to aging and self-acceptance. The "path" toward this self-acceptance and associated higher-level need for a personal self-esteem is a personal balance of aging identity, and societal acceptance of aging women.

CHECK IT OUT!

Search the Internet to find different cultural ideas of older women and feelings of self-acceptance. What are some of the factors that relate to how women can achieve personal acceptance of aging for further growth and development? As you are examining these factors about aging women and acceptance, think about the following questions:

1. What are the cultural images about women and aging acceptance?
2. Are there gender differences in older adults' portrayals of aging acceptance?
3. What social factors seem to contribute to older women's self-acceptance?
4. Are there stereotypes associate with aging presented within different cultures across the world?
5. How would you convey a positive message about aging women and self-acceptance?

The degree to which women's aging acceptance is achieved is strongly influenced and embedded within one's culture and community (Keith, 2003; Keith et al., 1994). How family, peers, coworkers, and the larger society view aging can negatively or positively impact women's attitudes about personal aging (Kaufman, 1981, 1986). This influence cannot be understated. The "social messages" sent on a frequent basis to women as they age can potentially have a significant influence on their feelings of aging acceptance.

Communities within and across cultures should make efforts to utilize and empower older women utilizing their expertise, knowledge, and skills. Older women, as with their male counterparts, are an invaluable resource in a society. As aging female "baby boomers" redefine work and retirement, the workplace in many countries need to redefine their employment policies accordingly (Pruchno, 2012). It is imperative that women across a life span engage in lifelong training and societal engagement in order to optimize positive aging outcomes and maintain financial security. In turn, communities need to better support the work life extension efforts of aging women and how they can best transition to retirement (Ainsworth, 2002).

Beyond the workplace, aging women need to be better supported through community programs and services and the many different role-related transitions they will undergo in later life. Family members, peers, and other societal members must better communicate the social value of older women in their lives. Aging women should be better supported in their desire to be actively engaged in social activities which will benefit all involved and assist in the process of self-acceptance during aging-related transitions and changes.

Aging women must regard themselves as ever-evolving, developing individuals capable of many later-life achievements, ranging from career to personal goals. Too often, older adults believe the stereotype that "old dogs cannot learn new tricks" but that is a stereotype that should never be a consideration in decision-making. Aging women need to surpass the expectations of society, breaking stereotypes of being both a woman and an aging adult within a culture.

REALISTIC AGING AND SENSE OF SELF

It is easy for individuals to believe the many stereotypes about aging that exist across the world. To be realistic about personal aging requires more attention, more effort, and more self-examination than might be anticipated. This process also reflects forgiving others and oneself about outcomes from lifespan experiences (eg, Sells & Hargrave, 1998). It is vital for women to achieve feelings of positive self-acceptance. To be realistic about your capabilities and your motivations is an important aspect of this decision-making process when choosing which opportunities to pursue. To "know thyself" in the context of personal aging necessitates a review of one's past experiences and respective self-learning outcomes. It is potentially harmful for any individual to internalize and act on stereotypes, whether negative or positive in nature because either type of stereotype is not realistic in perspective.

TEST YOURSELF!

Brief Aging Perceptions Questionnaire

Source: Sexton, King-Kallimanis, Morgan, and McGee (2014).

Please Tick One Box Per Line Which Shows How You Feel About Each Statement	Strongly Disagree	Disagree	Neither Agree Nor Disagree	Agree	Strongly Agree
1. I always classify myself as old.					
2. I am always aware of the fact that I am getting older.					
3. I feel my age in everything that I do.					
4. As I get older, I get wiser.					
5. As I get older I continue to grow as a person.					
6. As I get older I appreciate things more.					
7. I get depressed when I think about how ageing might affect the things that I can do.					
8. The quality of my social life in later years depends on me.					
9. The quality of my relationships with others in later life depends on me.					
10. Whether I continue to live life to the fullest depends on me.					

continued

Please Tick One Box Per Line Which Shows How You Feel About Each Statement	Strongly Disagree	Disagree	Neither Agree Nor Disagree	Agree	Strongly Agree
11. Getting older makes me less independent.					
12. As I get older I can take part in less activities.					
13. As I get older I cannot cope as well with problems that arise.					
14. Slowing down with aging is not something I can control.					
15. I have no control over the effects which getting older has on my social life.					
16. I worry about the effect that getting older may have on my relationships with others.					
17. I feel angry when I think about getting older.					

Sub-dimensions for Scoring:
Timeline-Chronic: Items 1, 2, and 3
Consequences-Positive: Items 4, 5, and 6
Emotional Representations: Items 7, 16, and 17
Consequences and Control Negative: Items 11, 12, 13, 14, and 15
Control-Positive: Items 8, 9, and 10

Having a positive sense of oneself, especially in response to the many life-changing events that can occur in response to aging, is important for positive aging adjustment. One predictor of aging self-acceptance is rooted within the culture of the woman. The societal messages about the value of aging and the social power related to being an older woman in society are important to understand. Community education related to positive while realistic perception of aging abilities is a vital aspect of supporting women's acceptance of aging processes. Only through such interventions can the quality of life in aging be supported for older women in society.

Optimizing self-acceptance among women during the aging process is important within global communities. Aging adults are faced with many challenges and changes in life roles and self-image understanding and supporting positive aging acceptance outcomes is a moral imperative for society (Hogan & Warren, 2012). Different cultures regard quality of aging in many different ways, but the importance of feelings of self-worth and self-acceptance cannot be understated. Having a realistic assessment of personal capabilities and personal motivations in aging is important to this decision-making process about later-life opportunities.

SUMMARY

There is an on-going need to better understand underlying factors in order to optimize aging women's feelings of self-acceptance in light of the many changes that occur within the aging experience. In attempting to support the aging-related self-acceptance of women, it is a necessity to understand the many different factors which shape and influence this outcome. Both researchers and practitioners working with this population of older adults must acknowledge the significant impact of gender role as women age across a life span.

Culture, physical environment, life experiences, and education are just some of the factors which need to be further explored in order to support women's feelings of positive aging for their quality of life and those that care for them. Getting older should not be perceived as being a deterrent to fully optimizing one's self-growth and self-identity into later life. The cultural "messages" that are presented to women early in their development onward should be scrutinized in order to eradicate negative messages and promote positive messages to achieve positive self-acceptance for women across their life spans into later life.

DISCUSSION QUESTIONS

1. Is an older woman's feelings of aging self-acceptance primarily guided by "internal" (ie, personal self-esteem), "external" (eg, community reactions), or both factors combined?
2. In what ways can society convey supportive "messages" to aging women about aging acceptance? Do you see the messages in today's society and in what ways?
3. What is the role of social support systems in how women achieve positive aging self-acceptance?

4. One might argue that self-acceptance is a lifelong process. How early should education begin in women's lives to teach this positive process of self-acceptance?
5. Intergenerational learning between cohorts of women would be a beneficial strategy to assist in achieving women's developmental feelings of positive adjustment to personal aging. What programs could be developed to offer these opportunities for women across their life span?
6. What would be the key factors to be considered in assisting with women's aging self-acceptance over time?
7. Do aging men have similar issues of concern or are there gender-specific concerns with aging women?
8. Are there cohort (generational) differences to consider in creating support programs and educational programs for women across the world?
9. Are there "universal" or culture-specific factors to consider in developing support programs?
10. If you were to develop a community-based intervention program for women, what topics would you cover? Why?

TEST YOUR KNOWLEDGE!

Take this quiz to assess your personal feelings of self-acceptance:
http://www.beauty-and-the-bath.com/womens-aging-quiz.html

SUPPLEMENTAL BOOK READINGS

Over the past decades, there have been many books written on the topic of aging women and feelings of self-acceptance. Here are some recommended *additional readings* for both course instructors and readers of this book:

Shinoda, J., & Bolen, M. D. (2014). *Goddesses in older women: Archetypes in women over fifty.* New York, NY: HarperCollins Publishers.
> The authors focus on the growth opportunity during the "third age" of life for women after they enter their fifties and beyond. Referred to as "goddesses," the book presents wonderful ideas about the wisdom, strength, and beauty of older women.

Alloway, J. R. (2013). *A quiet strength: Inspirational stories of older American women*. Frederick, MD: America Star Books.
The book presents interviews with 15 inspiring women who lived through the Great Depression and/or a World War and were faced with the very tough task of balancing multiple family and social roles during these challenging historical times. Reflections on their past experiences and how they impact their current aging as women are examined in the book.

Blackmer, J., & Greiner, L. (2004). *Where women walked*. Carol Stream, IL: Tyndale House Publishers, Inc.
Where Women Walked book presents 28 inspiring stories about aging women and their diverse life experiences, struggles, and achievements. The stories show the strength and perseverance of generations of women. The book covers many different topics that resonate with all generations of women across their life span.

Rycraft, R.A., & What, L. (2012). *Winter tales II: Women on the art of aging*. Florham Park, NJ: Serving House Books.
This book is a beautiful tribute to aging through the works of 29 women artists and writers. Contributors explore the portrayals of aging through poetry, essays, pictures, art, and comics. Their reflections on aging also offer interesting insights into the personal meaning of aging as a woman in society from diverse perspectives.

Golden, C. J. (2007). *Tao of the defiant woman: Five brazen ways to accept what you must and rebel against the rest*. Naperville, IL: Sourcebooks.
The author presents a "tao" of positive aging for women that will help with both self-acceptance and the mentoring of other young women to also achieve positive aging outcomes: Principle 1—make the most of relationships, Principle 2—value and depend upon your "community" of women, Principle 3—acquire and become a positive role model of women aging, Principle 4—be yourself, and Principle 5—reimagine your life and take it into exciting new directions.

Zackheim, V. (Editor) (2007). *For keeps: Women tell the truth about their bodies, growing older, and acceptance*. Berkeley, CA: Seal Press.
The book is an empowering resource for women potentially struggling with the many different changes to their appearance and body as they get older. This book challenges women to face these changes with an accepting perspective of self-growth and self-transformation. The lesson from this text is a wonderful resource for all generations of women who wish to reach self-acceptance and can be positive aging role models for others.

SUPPLEMENTAL AGING VIDEOS

For learning purposes, the use of videos can be very beneficial for both instructors and readers. Here are some recommended *supplemental videos* for more information on *aging self-acceptance*:

Let's Face It: Women Explore Their Aging Faces (Format: DVD)
The DVD examines cultural attitudes about youth and associated ideas of what is the standard of "beauty" for women. The film argues that a youth-obsessed culture puts unnecessary pressure on women to remain "young" when they are experiencing realistically aging and should not feel the need to "halt" or "fight" these natural, developmental changes.

Grow Old along with Me: The Poetry of Aging (Format: DVD)
Acceptance of one's life experiences and coming to terms with the past, both with personal achievements and missed opportunities, is the message of this video for aging adults. The film acknowledges that there can be many challenges with getting older, from aging bodies to losses in relationships. Embracing these inevitable aging processes and outcomes is the message from this interesting film.

ADDITIONAL INFORMATION LINKS

The following are some recommended *supplemental Internet links* for more information on the topic:

Aging in Action website: http://aginginaction.com/2010/12/gender-and-aging-what-do-we-*know*/

American Public Health Association website: http://www.apha.org/membergroups/sections/*aphasections/a_ph*/

Everyday Health website: http://www.everydayhealth.com/senior-health/enhancing-your-sexuality.aspx

NIH/NIAging website: http://www.nia.nih.gov/*about*/*minority-aging-and-health-disparities*

WebMD website: http://www.webmd.com/healthy-aging/guide/sex-aging

World Health Organization website: http://www.who.int/ageing/gender/en/index.html

References

Abma, J. C., & Martinez, G. M. (2006). Childlessness among older women in the United States: Trends and profiles. *Journal of Marriage and Family, 68*, 1045–1056. http://dx.doi.org/10.1111/-j.1741-3737.2006.00312.x.

Ainsworth, S. (2002). The "feminine advantage:" A discursive analysis of the invisibility of older women workers. *Gender, Work, and Organization, 9*(5), 579–601.

Ama, N. O., & Ngome, E. (2013). Menopausal perceptions and experiences of older women from selected sites in Botswana. *Advances in Sexual Medicine, 3*, 47–59. http://dx.doi.org/10.4236/asm.2013.33009.

Ault, A. (2007). Aging. In S. Brzuzy & A. Lind (Eds.), *Battleground: Women, gender, and sexuality* (pp. 16–22). Santa Barbara, CA: ABC-CLIO/Greenwood Press.

Avis, N. E., Assmann, S. F., Kravitz, H. M., Ganz, P. A., & Ory, M. (2004). Quality of life in diverse groups of midlife women: Assessing the influence of menopause, health status and psychosocial and demographic factors. *Quality of Life Research, 13*(5), 933–946.

Bandura, A. (1977). *Social learning theory.* Englewood Cliffs, NJ: Prentice Hall.

Bennett, K. M. (2010). "You can't spend years with someone and just cast them aside": Augmented identity in older British widows. *Journal of Women & Aging, 22*(3), 204–217. http://dx.doi.org/10.1080/08952841.2010.495571.

Binfa, L., Robertson, E., & Ransjö-Arvidson, A. (2010). "We are always asked; 'where are you from?'": Chilean women's reflections in midlife about their health and influence of migration to Sweden. *Scandinavian Journal of Caring Sciences, 24*(3), 445–453. http://dx.doi.org/10.1111/j.1471-6712.2009.00734.x.

Butler, S. S. (1993). Older rural women: Understanding their conceptions of health and illness. *Topics in Geriatric Rehabilitation, 9*(1), 56–68.

Clarke, L., & Bundon, A. (2009). From 'the thing to do' to 'defying the ravages of age:' Older women reflect on the use of lipstick. *Journal of Women & Aging, 21*(3), 198–212. http://dx.doi.org/10.1080/08952840903054757.

Davies, L. J. (1977). Attitudes toward old age and aging as shown by humor. *The Gerontologist, 17*(3), 220–226.

Erikson, E. H., Paul, I. H., Heider, F., & Gardner, R. W. (1959). *Psychological issues.* Madison, CT: International Universities Press.

Global Aging. (2001). The ageing of the world's population. Retrieved from: <http://www.globalaging.org/waa2/documents/theagingoftheworld.htm>.

Heuberger, R., Domina, T., & MacGillivray, M. (2010). Older women's comfort with 3-D body scanning technology as compared with younger women. *Journal of Women & Aging, 22*(3), 171–183. http://dx.doi.org/10.1080/08952841.2010.495556.

Hinchliff, S., & Gott, M. (2008). Challenging social myths and stereotypes of women and aging: Heterosexual women talk about sex. *Journal of Women & Aging, 20*, 65–81.

Hogan, S., & Warren, L. (2012). Dealing with complexity in research processes and findings: How do older women negotiate and challenge images of aging? *Journal of Women & Aging, 24*(4), 329–350. http://dx.doi.org/10.1080/08952841.2012.708589.

Hurd, L. C. (2000). Older women's body image and embodied experience: An exploration. *Journal of Women & Aging, 12*(3–4), 77–97.

Ingersoll-Dayton, B., & Krause, N. (2005). Self-forgiveness. *Research on Aging, 27*(3), 267–289. http://dx.doi.org/10.1177/0164027504274122.

Karasawa, M., Curhan, K. B., Markus, H. R., Kitayama, S. S., Love, G. D., Radler, B. T., et al. (2011). Cultural perspectives on aging and well-being: A comparison of Japan and the U.S. *International Journal of Aging & Human Development, 73*(1), 73–98.

Kaufman, S. (1981). Cultural components of identity in old age: A case study. *Ethos, 9*, 51–87. http://dx.doi.org/10.1525/eth.1981.9.1.02a00050.

Kaufman, S. (1986). *The ageless self: Sources of meaning in late life*. Madison, WI: University of Wisconsin Press.

Keith, J., Fry, C. L., Glascock, A., Ikels, C., Dickerson-Putman, J., Harpending, H., et al. (1994). *The aging experience: Diversity and commonality across cultures*. Thousand Oaks, CA: Sage.

Keith, P. (2003). Resources, family ties, and well-being of never-married men and women. *Journal of Gerontological Social Work, 42*(2), 51–75.

Leichty, T. (2012). "Yes, I worry about my weight ... but for the most part I'm content with my body": Older women's body dissatisfaction alongside contentment. *Journal of Women & Aging, 24*(1), 70–88. http://dx.doi.org/10.1080/08952841.2012.638873.

Levy, B. R., Slade, M. D., Kunkel, S. R., & Kasl, S. V. (2002). Longevity increased by positive self-perceptions of aging. *Journal of Personality and Social Psychology, 83*(2), 261–270.

Lvgren, K. (2013). The Swedish tant: A marker of female aging. *Journal of Women & Aging, 25*(2), 119–137. http://dx.doi.org/10.1080/08952841.2013.732826.

Maslow, A. (1954). *Motivation and personality*. New York, NY: Harper.

Maslow, A. (1971). *The farther reaches of human nature*. New York, NY: The Viking Press.

Minkler, M., & Stone, R. (1985). The feminization of poverty and older women. *The Gerontologist, 25*(4), 351–357. http://dx.doi.org/10.1093/geront/25.4.351.

Montemurro, B., & Gillen, M. M. (2013). Wrinkles and sagging flesh: Exploring transformations in women's sexual body image. *Journal of Women & Aging, 25*(1), 3–23. http://dx.doi.org/10.1080/08952841.2012.720179.

Nussbaum, J. F., & Coupland, J. (Eds.). (2004). *Handbook of communication and aging research*. New York, NY: Routledge.

O'Brien, M. (1991). Never married older women: The life experience. *Social Indicators Research, 24*(3), 301–315.

Pearlman, S. F. (1993). Late mid-life astonishment: Disruptions to identity and self-esteem. *Women & Therapy, 14*(1–2), 1–12.

Phelan, C. H., Love, G. D., Ryff, C. D., Brown, R. L., & Heidrich, S. M. (2010). Psychosocial predictors of changing sleep patterns in aging women: A multiple pathway approach. *Psychology & Aging, 25*(4), 858–866. http://dx.doi.org/10.1037/a0019622.

Porcino, J. (1986). Psychological aspects of aging in women. *Women & Health, 10*(2–3), 115–122.

Pruchno, R. (2012). Not your mother's old age: Baby Boomers at age 65. *The Gerontologist, 52*(2), 149–152. http://dx.doi.org/10.1093/geront/gns038.

Reel, J. J., SooHoo, S., Summerhays, J., & Gill, D. L. (2008). Age before beauty: An exploration of body image in African-American and Caucasian adult women. *Journal of Gender Studies, 17*(4), 321–330. http://dx.doi.org/10.1080/09589230802419963.

Reichstadt, J., Sengupta, G., Depp, C. A., Palinkas, L. A., & Jeste, D. V. (2010). Older adults' perspectives on successful aging: Qualitative interviews. *American Journal of Geriatric Psychiatry, 18*(7), 567–575.

Rossen, E. K., Knafl, K. A., & Flood, M. (2008). Older women's perceptions of successful aging. *Activities, Adaptation & Aging, 32*(2), 73–88. http://dx.doi.org/10.1080/01924780802142644.

Rubinstein, R. L., Alexander, B. B., Goodman, M., & Luborsky, M. (1991). Key relationships of never married, childless older women: A cultural analysis. *Journal of Gerontology, 46*(5), S270–S277.

Ryff, C. D. (1991). Possible selves in adulthood and old age: A tale of shifting horizons. *Psychology and Aging, 6*(2), 286–295. http://dx.doi.org/10.1037/0882-7974.6.2.286.

Ryff, C. D., & Singer, B. H. (2008). Know thyself and become what you are: A eudemonic approach to psychological well-being. *Journal of Happiness Studies, 9*(1), 13–39. http://dx.doi.org/10.1007/s10902-006-9019-0.

Sawchuk, D. (2009). The raging grannies: Defying stereotypes and embracing aging through activism. *Journal of Women & Aging, 21*(3), 171–185.

Schanowitz, J. Y., & Nicassio, P. (2006). Predictors of positive psychosocial functioning of older adults in residential care facilities. *Journal of Behavioral Medicine, 29*(2), 191–201. http://dx.doi.org/10.1007/s10865-005-9034-3.

Schuler, P., Vinci, D., Isosaari, R., Philipp, S., Todorovich, J., Roy, J., et al. (2008). Body-shape perceptions and body mass index of older African American and European American women. *Journal of Cross-Cultural Gerontology, 23*(3), 255–264. http://dx.doi.org/10.1007/s10823-008-9061-y.

Sells, J. N., & Hargrave, T. D. (1998). Forgiveness: A review of the theoretical and empirical literature. *Journal of Family Therapy, 20*, 21–36. http://dx.doi.org/10.1111/1467-6427.00066.

Sexton, E., King-Kallimanis, B. L., Morgan, K., & McGee, H. (2014). Development of the brief ageing perceptions questionnaire (B-APQ): A confirmatory factor analysis approach to item reduction. *BMC Geriatrics, 14*(44), 1–11. http://dx.doi.org/10.1186/1471-2318-14-44.

Spafford, M. M., Rudman, D., Leipert, B. D., Klinger, L., & Huot, S. (2010). When self-presentation trumps access: Why older adults with low vision go without low-vision services. *Journal of Applied Gerontology, 29*(5), 579–602. http://dx.doi.org/10.1177/0733464809345494.

Wink, P. (2006). Everyday life in the third age. *Annual Review of Gerontology & Geriatrics, 26*, 243–261.

4

Aging Women and Mental Aerobics

Global fact: *Average levels of illiteracy for women aged 65 or over are as high as 78% in Africa and 53% in Asia, compared to 58% and 29% respectively for men in these regions.*

—**United Nations, Women Coordination Division report (2012)**

Exercising in later life promotes positive aging adjustment and growth (Kramer, Erickson, & Colcombe, 2006; McAuley & Rudolph, 1995). When we think about exercise, most people typically think about the "physical" aspects of exercise. But in actuality the concept of "mental aerobics" is equally if not more important as we get older in later life. What is this concept? To put it simply, it is the process of exercising your mental capabilities to maintain and optimize cognitive functioning over time (eg, memory functioning) (Jak, 2012). Past research has suggested that positive aging is associated with being mentally and physically active with one's daily activities (Flood & Scharer, 2006; Lee & Hung, 2011).

This "mind-body connection" to being active and fully engaged in life is not a new concept, but simply one that requires more crucial application as a number of older adults are living longer than ever before (Gergen & Gergen, 2006; Schaefer & Schumacher, 2011; Swartzberg, 2004). Hogan (2005) purported the idea that there's an integral "mind-body" connection that can be supported through proper design in the quality of the exercise activities and associated proper "fit" with the older adults' needs and capabilities. This mind and body connection is a key component for positive aging and later-life health outcomes (Bashore, 1989; Kramer, Sowon, & McAuley, 2000; Rice, Katzel, & Waldstein, 2010; Verbrugge, 1990).

OLDER WOMEN AND MENTAL AEROBICS

Factors underlying "positive aging" design in living environments for aging women, whether in the home, workplace, or living environments are

71

important to examine (Chin & Quine, 2012). Everyday lifestyle activities for aging Americans may not optimally support mental aerobic activities (Mirowsky, 2011). This important point can be applied to many different living situations for aging women in countries across the world.

Maintaining one's mental functioning is possible through a range of both cognitive and physical activities, on a frequent basis (Kramer, Colcombe, McAuley, Scalf, & Erikson, 2005). Feelings of mental well-being have been associated with on-going physical and mental activity extended into later life (McAuley & Rudolph, 2005). For aging women, the benefits of such activities for both general cognitive performance and specific aspects of memory functioning (eg, episodic memory; Evers, Klusmann, Schwarzer, & Heuser, 2011; 2012) are important to explore through applied interventions in different "living" environments (eg, workplace) (Seligman, Steen, Park, & Peterson, 2005).

Mental exercise interventions may assist in maintaining and improving cognitive functioning (eg, mental processing speed; Bashore, Goddard, & Cerella, 1993). Paggi and Hayslip (1999) were some of the first proponents of daily mental exercises to improve one's general quality of life, and Weaver and Kosan (1992) suggested the mental aerobic activities offer multiple benefits and are enjoyable to do. The "use it or lose it" principle can be used as a key concept underlying the positive mental health of aging women (eg, Ackerman, Kanfer, & Calderwood, 2010; Millington, 2012).

On-going daily physical activity has multiple positive influences on aging women's cognitive functioning across many different performance domains (eg, decision-making; Netz, Dwolatzky, Zinker, Argov, & Agmon, 2011; Swoap, Norvelt, Graves, & Pollock, 1994), as well as feelings of psychological well-being (Netz, Meng-Jia, Becker, & Tenenbaum, 2005). In a Swedish study with normatively aging adults, Lindwall, Rennemark, and Berggren (2008) reported meaningful benefits from physical exercise on mental functioning. This mind-body connection was also shown in the mental concentration of older athletes who were experiencing aging-related declines in physical balance (eg, Vaillant et al., 2006), attentional capacity over time (Pesce, Cereatti, Forte, Crova, & Casella, 2011), or mild Alzheimer's disease (Teixeira et al., 2012; Valenzuela & Sachdev, 2009; Vidovich, Shaw, Flicker, & Almeida, 2011). The same idea of maintaining functioning capability can be applied to the rate of physical and mental decline within a continuing care facility. The degree to which older women can and do engage in mentally and physically challenging activities on a regular basis is a quality-of-life issue that communities and broader societies across the world should address through programs and policies supporting such activities (Gureje, Ogunniyi, Kola, & Abiona, 2011; Huggett, Connelly, & Overend, 2005; Resnick, 2001; Tsantali, Tsolaki, Economides, & Paraskeuaidis, 2008; Yamamoto, Izumi, & Aso, 2012).

SELF-REGULATION THEORY AND OLDER WOMEN'S COGNITIVE ENGAGEMENT

One associated theory to this idea of continual cognitive engagement is self-regulation theory (Kuyper, Van, & Lubbers, 2000). Self-regulation theory suggests that there is a process of anchoring and adjusting our performance, both mental and physical in nature, in response to corrective feedback within our social and physical environment.

QUOTES FROM FAMOUS, POSITIVELY AGING WOMEN

At 81, I don't feel guilty about anything ... There's nothing inside that's 81.
It's just the changes in the body. And the memory.
I don't remember where the keys are. Or as my son says,
'Ma, it's not that you don't remember where you put the keys,
It's when you pick up your keys and you don't know what they're for'.
—*Toni Morrison, Author*

In youth we learn;
in age we understand.
—*Marie von Ebner-Eschenbach, Novelist*

What could be more beautiful than a dear old lady growing wise with age?
Every age can be enchanting, provided you live within it.
—*Brigitte Bardot, Actress*

Training in effective mental and/or physical self-regulation may assist women in their positive aging processes. Positive, effective self-regulation is an important concept to explore under the topics of "aging in place," driving behavior, and other quality-of-life factors (eg, Rudman, Friedland, Chipman, & Sciortino, 2006; Vohs & Baumeister, 2011) which are important positive aging concerns for women as they age. A real-world application of this idea would be specific community-based programs that teach older women how to better identify age-related changes in their daily capabilities and health status (Clark et al., 2000). Further, instructive strategies on how to optimize both mental and physical performance in women's activities of daily living would be highly beneficial for older women, regardless of cultural and environmental locations across the world. Applications can range from web- to exercise-based learning environments tailored to the needs and motivations of aging women.

MENTAL AEROBIC INTERVENTIONS WITH OLDER WOMEN

Computer-based mental activities can be beneficial and flexible in design for older learners (Bozoki, Radovanovic, Winn, Heeter, & Anthony, 2013). Any well-designed mental aerobics activity can have a significant positive impact on an older woman's cognitive memory, physical, and executive functioning (Carlson et al., 2008; Mouton & Cloes, 2013).

Companies such as *Happy Neuron* have created creative approaches to mental aerobics activities through online games that test one's mental problem-solving capabilities and certainly could be a part of an aging woman's daily activities (Dunning, 2007). Relatedly, Van Schaik, Blake, Pernet, Spears, and Fencott (2008) suggested the benefits of using virtual exercise games to motivate mental aerobics activities with older adults. Senior centers within communities across the world can utilize activities that involve exercising both older women's bodies and minds that have direct implications for improving their quality of overall health, such as programs examined in regions of Canada (Fitzpatrick, 2010). For example, community-based health services which coach older women in different aspects of body and mind functioning can have many positive health outcomes, improving their quality of life and personal autonomy in daily activities (eg, Holland et al., 2005).

TIPS FOR WOMEN'S MENTAL AEROBICS ACTIVITIES

1. Learn a new knowledge fact every day (eg, "word of the day").
2. Do a puzzle or read a mystery book.
3. Engage in a social "debate" with friends.
4. Learn a new skill that you always wanted to do (eg, a language).
5. Create a "blog" or a web page.

MENTAL AEROBICS AS A PREVENTATIVE OR REHABILITATIVE FACTOR FOR AGING WOMEN

Engaging in stimulating cognitive exercises can help reduce risk factors toward the development of dementia or help normatively aging older adults recover some cognitive functioning due to mild memory impairment (Hayslip, Paggi, Poole, & Pinson, 2009).

Perceptions about the effectiveness of such interventions to slow cognitive decline can differ by cohort and age level (Horhota, Ositelu, Hertzog, Lineweaver, & Summers, 2012). Early education interventions should be put into place that extol the benefits of cognitive and physical exercise for positive aging and the maintenance of cognitive competencies in later life. Attitudes about the meaning of "aging well" underlie the motivation to engage in such mental health activities, and this has implications toward the education of women across their life span about the benefits of remaining mentally and physically engaged in life activities (Laditka et al., 2009). Maintenance of one's personal autonomy in decision-making and completion of activities of daily living (ADLs) offer opportunities for cognitive engagement and have long-term quality of life results for women adjusting to later-life functioning (Matthews et al., 2011).

LATER-LIFE HEALTH CORRELATES WITH MENTAL ENGAGEMENT ACTIVITIES FOR WOMEN

There are two main aging theories that could be applied to explain the value of such activities for older women. Activity theory (Cummings & Henry, 1961) purports that the more "active" we are, the better the quality of aging. Extending this theory to the daily lives of aging women, a woman needs to focus on daily activities that exercise her brain as well as engage in activities that exercise her body (eg, exercise intensity; Swoap et al., 1994). Older women should select learning activities that challenge the mind across many contexts, in the classroom, workplace, or on the Internet. Social engagement is an important part of these active cognitive processes, supporting cognitive stimulation and social involvement for aging women who may otherwise not be engaged to their full capacity (Fratiglioni, Paillord-Borg, & Winblad, 2004; Parisi, Greene, Morrow, & Stine-Morrow, 2007). Even though social engagement is very beneficial to aging women, solitary activities (eg, completing a crossword puzzle) are equally beneficial to maintain cognitive activities in daily life (LaRue, 2010). Ultimately, the benefit of engaging in various levels of social activities for women from diverse backgrounds and cultures is that older women should be conscious of maintaining desired social roles (eg, volunteerism) and/or relationship activities (eg, maintaining friendships).

Continuity theory (Atchley, 1989) is another relevant concept regarding positive aging that could be applied to mental aerobics for older adults. Continuity theory suggests that activities that an individual engages in should be reflective of past activities, learning, and associated tasks. Applying this idea, women from many different cultures and life situations should engage in culturally relevant, meaningful lifelong activities reflecting what they like to do and what motivates them (eg, constructing a "personal narrative," Chapman, 2005).

CHECK IT OUT!

Search the Internet to find different community activities targeting older women to engage in sociocultural cognitive activities (eg, intergenerational learning exchange program activities). As you are examining these factors, think about the following questions:

1. What are some "mental aerobic" activities that aging women can participate in on a daily basis?
2. What role does culture have in the design of cognitive exercise programs?
3. What technologies could be applied to the design of learning activities for older women?
4. What are the cultural "messages" about women and later-life learning?
5. Are there motivational factors to consider when creating cognitive exercises with older women learners?

The more the daily activities are intrinsically interesting and motivating for older women, the less likely the stressors and strains associated with later-life activities (eg, being an elder caregiver) will significantly impact their mental health (eg, Jin, 1992; Long & Haney, 1989). To understand what is intrinsically motivating for different older women requires a thoughtful analysis of what "fits" with an individual's task preferences. The tailoring of activity programs designed for diverse groups of aging women might be time intensive, but the benefits to both the older adult and the broader community outweigh the effort needed. Promoting active mental engagement could be as simple as providing specific reading material (eg, "pleasure reading" books), puzzles, web-based resources, or games to reduce feelings of loneliness or stagnation (eg, Rane-Szostak & Herth, 1995). In order to best sustain older women's participation in such cognitive activities, the design of the tasks must be understood on a deeper level which entails understanding the unique needs, capabilities, and interests of the old adult (ie, personal competencies; Zhou & Oldham, 2001). Further, having the older woman learner involved in the task development process may better ensure appropriate learner motivation and engagement in the mental exercises (Boulton-Lewis, Buys, & Lovie-Kitchin, 2006).

Within communities, possible ageist attitudes can become internalized within a woman's aging self-image and potentially curtail their activities on a daily basis (Klusmann, Evers, Schwarzer, & Heuser, 2012). Extending this idea to the concept of "self-fulfilling prophecy," older women in certain cultures might internalize a negative viewpoint about their personal cognitive aging and believe that engaging in mental aerobics would not be useful (Levy, Slade, & Kasl, 2002; Wurm, Warner, Ziegelmann, Wolff, & Schüz, 2013). This of course is not true, but reflects a possible "decrement" perspective that may be pervasive in some cultures and broader societies in the world. To combat this possible ageism, older women learners have to break traditions and consciously pursue activities that engage their minds and bodies for positive aging.

SUMMARY

This book chapter focused on proactive strategies for aging women to remain cognitively competent and actively engaged in their social environment. This active engagement assists in many domains of positive aging, from the physical to the psychological for women. As aging populations continue to grow in number and live longer than previous cohorts, it is vital for societies to turn their attention to how older adults can remain actively engaged in community and social activities. Older women have much to offer to younger generations through mentoring, and communicating their experiences to others needing advice and guidance.

This intergenerational sharing of ideas and experiences will serve to enrich the lives and development of all involved. Further, the empowerment of the older woman in society is the larger issue in this discussion. Aging women must actively request needed community programs and services in order to sustain equality of aging existence, for themselves and for those who care for them. To be active mentally and physically within one's capabilities belies the achievement and sustainability of quality-of-life outcomes for all aging populations.

DISCUSSION QUESTIONS

1. How can an older woman engage in mental aerobics on a daily basis?
2. What is the role of community education programs to assist in helping older women engage in cognitive exercises?
3. Is there a "mind-body" connection idea from the chapter that could be applied to beneficial daily activities for aging women?
4. What role does culture and society play in the choice and use of mental exercises?

5. Are there gender-specific activities that best support women's mental competency?
6. Are there cultural considerations in the design of such mental tasks for women?
7. How early should education emphasize the use of mental aerobic tasks for women?
8. Should mental activities be tailored to diverse women's specific interests and motivations? Why or why not?
9. Is technology the "key" to keeping older women mentally active? Give examples.
10. If you were to design a mental aerobics program, what would you include as activities?

TEST YOUR KNOWLEDGE!

Take the following brain teasers and quiz about mental aerobics activities:

http://www.clevelandseniors.com/forever/quiz.htm

SUPPLEMENTAL BOOK READINGS

Over the past decades, there have been many books written on the topic of mental activity and positive aging. Here are some recommended *additional readings*:

Lee, I., & Jones, J. (2008). *In full bloom: A brain education guide for successful aging*. Sedona, AZ: BEST Life Media.
This book empowers older adults to be much more active in their utilization of mental activities to both strengthen and maintain their cognitive functioning into later life. This book is a wonderful resource for both aging women as well as for those for whom they are caring. The content has great suggestions for daily exercises to support older adults' healthy brain functioning. This book will help adults in improving their mental concentration, attentional capacity, creative thinking, and retention of cognitive competency in a normative aging population.

Powell, D. H. (2011). *The aging intellect*. New York, NY: Routledge.
The author focuses on how older adults can change their habits to achieve a positively aging mind when he refers to a positive cognitive vigor. Dr Powell presents a very specific

recommendation regarding characteristics of people who can maintain cognitive vigor over time in a normative age. His suggestions can be integrated easily into daily life activities for people of all ages who wish to increase their mental vigor and maintain positive mental capacity into later life. Dr Powell's recommendations are very "user-friendly" and are easily understandable for laypeople. His recommendations could also be utilized by practitioners working with aging clients who might be experiencing normative changes in intellectual functioning and who would benefit from such interventions.

Depp, C. A., & Jeste, D. V. (2009). *Successful cognitive and emotional aging.* Arlington, VA: American Psychiatric Publishing, Inc.
This book offers helpful scientific evidence regarding ways to support healthy aging brain functioning through strategies to maintain cognitive functioning and well-being into later life. Topics of nutrition, physical exercise, wisdom, and even spirituality are discussed as issues related to lifestyle positively impacting cognitive functioning and positive aging outcomes. Written in an understandable language, this book would be a wonderful resource for students and laypeople interested in how to improve their lives and cognitive functioning in effective and scientifically proven ways.

Nussbaum, J. F., Federowicz, M., & Nussbaum, P.D. (2010). *Brain health and optimal engagement for older adults.* Girona, Spain: Editorial Aresta.
Nussbaum, Federowicz and Nussbaum make a very important linkage between healthy brain functioning and healthy social relationship network within one's life over time. Older adults would greatly benefit from social interactions on a daily basis which both challenge and enhance cognitive functioning. Achieving positive cognitive brain health and supporting an interactive and balanced social network are imperative for all aging women as they engage in multiple life roles and associated cognitive challenges into their later years.

SUPPLEMENTAL AGING VIDEOS

For learning purposes, the use of videos can be very beneficial for both instructors and readers. Here are some recommended *supplemental videos*:

Different video links on aging health: http://www.healthvideo.com/sitemap.php (Format: Website)

This is a great website that offers short videos on different aging-related health.

Different videos on human development: http://www.learner.org (Format: Website)
Supported by the Annenberg Foundation, this website offers several video series on human development and aging. Videos are approximately 60 min in length.

The More We Get Together—Educational Version with Public Performance Rights (Format: DVD)
The More We Get Together gives insights into working with the "oldest-old," cognitively incompetent residents. Ms Feil promotes the need to restore both social engagement and dignity in the lives of these long-term care residents who might otherwise feel lost and be ignored.

Brain Fitness (Format: DVD)
This DVD suggests innovative and engaging brain fitness exercises to promote and maintain brain vitality and agility for women across their life span.

ADDITIONAL INFORMATION LINKS

The following are some recommended *supplemental Internet links*:

Administration on Aging website: http://www.aoa.gov/AoARoot/Aging_Statistics/index.aspx

Aging in Action website: http://aginginaction.com/2010/12/gender-and-aging-what-do-we-know/

American Federation for Aging Research website: http://www.afar.org/infoaging/

American Public Health Association website: http://www.apha.org/membergroups/sections/aphasections/a_ph/

Centers for Disease Control and Prevention website: http://www.cdc.gov/mmwr/preview/mmwrhtml/mm5206a2.htm

NIA Demography Center website: http://agingcenters.org/

NIH/NIAging website: http://www.nia.nih.gov/about/minority-aging-and-health-disparities

United Nations website: http://www.un.org/esa/population/publications/Worldageing19502050/

U.S. Census Bureau website: http://www.census.gov/newsroom/releases/archives/aging_population/cb10-72.html

U.S. Census Bureau website: http://www.census.gov/newsroom/releases/archives/2010_census/cb12-239.html

World Health Organization website: http://www.who.int/ageing/gender/en/index.html

References

Ackerman, P. L., Kanfer, R., & Calderwood, C. (2010). Use it or lose it? Wii brain exercise practice and reading for domain knowledge. *Psychology & Aging, 25*(4), 753–766. http://dx.doi.org/10.1037/a0019277.

Atchley, R. C. (1989). A continuity theory of normal aging. *The Gerontologist, 29*(2), 183–190. http://dx.doi.org/10.1093/geront/29.2.183.

Bashore, T. R. (1989). Age, physical fitness, and mental processing speed. *Annual Review of Gerontology & Geriatrics, 9*, 120–144.

Bashore, T. R., Goddard, P. H., & Cerella, J. (1993). Preservative and restorative effects of aerobic fitness on the age-related slowing of mental processing speed: *Adult information processing: Limits on loss*. San Diego, CA: Academic Press.205228

Boulton-Lewis, G. M., Buys, L., & Lovie-Kitchin, J. (2006). Learning and active aging. *Educational Gerontology, 32*(4), 271–282.

Bozoki, A., Radovanovic, M., Winn, B., Heeter, C., & Anthony, J. C. (2013). Effects of a computer-based cognitive exercise program on age-related cognitive decline. *Archives of Gerontology & Geriatrics, 57*(1), 1–7. http://dx.doi.org/10.1016/j.archger.2013.02.009.

Carlson, M. C., Saczynski, J. S., Rebok, G. W., Seeman, T., Glass, T. A., McGill, S., et al. (2008). Exploring the effects of an "everyday" activity program on executive function and memory in older adults: Experience corps. *Gerontologist, 48*(6), 793–801.

Chapman, S. A. (2005). Theorizing about aging well: Constructing a narrative. *Canadian Journal on Aging/La Revue Canadienne Du Vieillissement, 24*(01), 9–18.

Chin, L., & Quine, S. (2012). Common factors that enhance the quality of life for women living in their own homes or in aged care facilities. *Journal of Women & Aging, 24*(4), 269–279. http://dx.doi.org/10.1080/08952841.2012.650605.

Clark, N. M., Janz, N. K., Dodge, J. A., Schork, M. A., Fingerlin, T. E., Wheeler, J. R., et al. (2000). Changes in functional health status of older women with heart disease evaluation of a program based on self-regulation. *The Journals of Gerontology Series B: Psychological Sciences and Social Sciences, 55*(2), S117–S126.

Cumming, E., & Henry, W. E. (1961). *Growing old: The process of disengagement*. New York, NY: Basic Books, Inc.

Dunning, T. (2007). Happy Neuron launches online brain games. *Activities, Adaptation & Aging, 31*(4), 59–60. http://dx.doi.org/10.1300/J016v31n04_05.

Evers, A., Klusmann, V., Schwarzer, R., & Heuser, I. (2011). Improving cognition by adherence to physical or mental exercise: A moderated mediation analysis. *Aging & Mental Health, 15*(4), 446–455.

Evers, A., Klusmann, V., Schwarzer, R., & Heuser, I. (2012). Does adherence moderate the effect of physical or mental training on episodic memory in older women? *Advances in Physical Education, 2*(2), 68–72. http://dx.doi.org/10.4236/ape.2012.22012.

Fitzpatrick, T. R. (2010). Brain fitness activities and health among older female senior center participants in Montreal, Quebec. *Activities, Adaptation & Aging, 34*(1), 30–47. http://dx.doi.org/10.1080/01924780903552287.

Flood, M., & Scharer, K. (2006). Creativity enhancement: Possibilities for successful aging. *Issues in Mental Health Nursing, 27,* 939–959. http://dx.doi.org/10.1080/01612840600899832.

Fratiglioni, L., Paillard-Borg, S., & Winblad, B. (2004). An active and socially integrated lifestyle in late life might protect against dementia. *The Lancet Neurology, 3*(6), 343–353.

Gergen, M., & Gergen, K. (2006). Positive aging: Reconstructing the life course: *Handbook of girls' and women's psychological health: Gender and well-being across the life span.* New York, NY: Oxford University Press.416426

Gureje, O., Ogunniyi, A., Kola, L., & Abiona, T. (2011). Incidence of and risk factors for dementia in the Ibadan study of aging. *Journal of Applied Gerontology, 59,* 869–874. http://dx.doi.org/10.1111/j.1532-5415.2011.03374.x.

Hayslip, B., Jr., Paggi, K., Poole, M., & Pinson, M. (2009). The impact of mental aerobics training on memory impaired older adults. *Clinical Gerontologist, 32*(4), 389–394. http://dx.doi.org/10.1080/07317110903112233.

Hogan, M. (2005). Physical and cognitive activity and exercise for older adults: A review. *International Journal of Aging and Human Development, 60*(2), 95–126.

Holland, S. K., Greenberg, J., Tidwell, L., Malone, J., Mullan, J., & Newcomer, R. (2005). Community-based health coaching, exercise, and health service utilization. *Journal of Aging & Health, 17*(6), 697–716. http://dx.doi.org/10.1177/0898264305277959.

Horhota, M., Ositelu, M., Hertzog, C., Lineweaver, T., & Summers, K. (2012). Young and older adults' beliefs about effective ways to mitigate age-related memory decline. *Psychology & Aging, 27*(2), 293–304. http://dx.doi.org/10.1037/a0026088.

Huggett, D. L., Connelly, D. M., & Overend, T. J. (2005). Maximal aerobic capacity testing of older adults: A critical review. *Journal of Gerontology: Medical Sciences, 60A*(1), 57–66.

Jak, A. J. (2012). The impact of physical and mental activity on cognitive aging: *Behavioral neurobiology of aging.* Berlin, Germany: Springer.273291

Jin, P. (1992). Efficacy of Tai Chi, brisk walking, meditation, and reading in reducing mental and emotional stress. *Journal of Psychosomatic Research, 36*(4), 361–370.

Klusmann, V., Evers, A., Schwarzer, R., & Heuser, I. (2012). Views on aging and emotional benefits of physical activity: Effects of an exercise intervention in older women. *Psychology of Sport and Exercise, 13*(2), 236–242.

Kramer, A. F., Colcombe, S. J., McAuley, E., Scalf, P. E., & Erickson, K. I. (2005). Fitness, aging and neurocognitive function. *Neurobiology of Aging, 26*(1), 124–127.

Kramer, A. F., Erickson, K. I., & Colcombe, S. J. (2006). Exercise, cognition, and the aging brain. *Journal of Applied Physiology, 101*(4), 1237–1242.

Kramer, A. F., Sowon, H., & McAuley, E. (2000). Influence of aerobic fitness on the neurocognitive function of older adults. *Journal of Aging & Physical Activity, 8*(4), 379.

Kuyper, H., Van, W. M. P. C., & Lubbers, M. J. (2000). Motivation, meta-cognition, and self-regulation as predictors of long-term educational attainment. *Educational Research and Evaluation: An International Journal on Theory and Practice, 6*(3), 181–205.

Laditka, S. B., Corwin, S. J., Laditka, J. N., Liu, R., Tseng, W., Wu, B., et al. (2009). Attitudes about aging well among a diverse group of older Americans: Implications for promoting cognitive health. *The Gerontologist, 49*(S1), S30–S39. http://dx.doi.org/10.1093/geront/gnp084.

LaRue, A. (2010). Healthy brain aging: Role of cognitive reserve, cognitive stimulation, and cognitive exercises. *Clinics in Geriatric Medicine, 26*(1), 99–111.

Lee, Y., & Hung, W. (2011). The relationship between exercise participation and well-being of the retired elderly. *Aging & Mental Health, 15*(7), 873–881. http://dx.doi.org/10.1080/13607863.-2011.569486.

Levy, B. R., Slade, M. D., & Kasl, S. V. (2002). Longitudinal benefit of positive self-perceptions of aging on functional health. *The Journals of Gerontology Series B: Psychological Sciences and Social Sciences*, 57(5), P409–P417.

Lindwall, M., Rennemark, M., & Berggren, T. (2008). Movement in mind: The relationship of exercise with cognitive status for older adults in the Swedish National Study on Aging and Care (SNAC). *Aging & Mental Health*, 12(2), 212–220.

Long, B. C., & Haney, C. J. (1989). Coping strategies for working women: Aerobic exercise and relaxation interventions. *Behavior Therapy*, 19(1), 75–83.

Matthews, M. M., Hsu, F., Walkup, M. P., Barry, L. C., Patel, K. V., & Blair, S. N. (2011). Depressive symptoms and physical performance in the lifestyle interventions and independence for elders pilot study. *Journal of the American Geriatrics Society*, 59(3), 495–500. http://dx.doi.org/10.1111/j.1532-5415.2011.03319.x.

McAuley, E., & Rudolph, D. (1995). Physical activity, aging, and psychological well-being. *Journal of Aging & Physical Activity*, 3(1), 67–96.

Millington, B. (2012). Use it or lose it: Ageing and the politics of brain training. *Leisure Studies*, 31(4), 429–446. http://dx.doi.org/10.1080/02614367.2011.589865.

Mirowsky, J. (2011). Cognitive decline and the default American lifestyle. *Journals of Gerontology Series B: Psychological Sciences & Social Sciences*, 66B(supp_1), i50–i58.

Mouton, A., & Cloes, M. (2013). Web-based interventions to promote physical activity by older adults: Promising perspectives for a public health challenge. *Archives of Public Health*, 71(1), 16.http://dx.doi.org/10.1186/0778-7367-71-16.

Netz, Y., Dwolatzky, T., Zinker, Y., Argov, E., & Agmon, R. (2011). Aerobic fitness and multi-domain cognitive function in advanced age. *International Psychogeriatrics*, 23(1), 114–124. http://dx.doi.org/10.1017/S1041610210000797.

Netz, Y., Meng-Jia, W., Becker, B., & Tenenbaum, G. (2005). Physical activity and psychological well-being in advanced age: A meta-analysis of intervention studies. *Psychology & Aging*, 20(2), 272–284. http://dx.doi.org/10.1037/0882-7974.20.2.272.

Paggi, K., & Hayslip, B. (1999). Mental aerobics: Exercises for the mind in later life. *Educational Gerontology*, 25(1), 1–12. http://dx.doi.org/10.1080/036012799267972.

Parisi, J. M., Greene, J. C., Morrow, D. G., & Stine-Morrow, E. A. (2007). The Senior Odyssey: Participant experiences of a program of social and intellectual engagement. *Activities, Adaptation & Aging*, 31(3), 31–49.

Pesce, C., Cereatti, L., Forte, R., Crova, C., & Casella, R. (2011). Acute and chronic exercise effects on attentional control in older road cyclists. *Gerontology*, 57(2), 121–128. http://dx.doi.org/10.1159/000314685.

Rane-Szostak, D., & Herth, K. A. (1995). Pleasure reading, other activities, and loneliness in later life. *Journal of Adolescent & Adult Literacy*, 39(2), 100–108.

Resnick, B. (2001). A prediction model of aerobic exercise in older adults living in a continuing-care retirement community. *Journal of Aging & Health*, 13(2), 287.

Rice, M. C., Katzel, L. I., & Waldstein, S. R. (2010). Sex-specific associations of depressive symptoms and cardiovascular risk factors in older adults. *Aging & Mental Health*, 14(4), 405–410. http://dx.doi.org/10.1080/13607860903586185.

Rudman, D. L., Friedland, J., Chipman, M., & Sciortino, P. (2006). Holding on and letting go: The perspectives of pre-seniors and seniors on driving self-regulation in later life. *Canadian Journal on Aging/La Revue Canadienne Du Vieillissement*, 25(01), 65–76.

Schaefer, S., & Schumacher, V. (2011). The interplay between cognitive and motor functioning in healthy older adults: Findings from dual-task studies and suggestions for intervention. *Gerontology*, 57(3), 239–246. http://dx.doi.org/10.1159/000322197.

Seligman, M. E., Steen, T. A., Park, N., & Peterson, C. (2005). Positive psychology progress: Empirical validation of interventions. *American Psychologist*, 60(5), 410.

Swartzberg, J. (2004). Mental aerobics. *University of California at Berkeley Wellness Letter*, 20(4), 3.

Swoap, R. A., Norvelt, N., Graves, J. E., & Pollock, M. L. (1994). High versus moderate intensity aerobic exercise in older adults: Psychological and physiological effects. *Journal of Aging & Physical Activity*, 2(4), 293–303.

Teixeira, C., Gobbi, L., Corazza, D., Stella, F., Costa, J., & Gobbi, S. (2012). Non-pharmacological interventions on cognitive functions in older people with mild cognitive impairment (MCI). *Archives of Gerontology & Geriatrics*, 54(1), 175–180. http://dx.doi.org/10.1016/j.archger.2011.02.014.

Tsantali, E., Tsolaki, M., Economides, D., & Paraskeuaidis, N. (2008). The retrogression of the Alzheimer's disease for 5 years through a cognitive rehabilitation intervention. A case report. *Annals of General Psychiatry*, 7(1), S354.http://dx.doi.org/10.1186/1744859X-7-S1-S354.

United Nations, Women Coordination Division. (2012). Between gender and ageing: The status of the world's older women and progress since the Madrid International Plan of Action on Ageing. Retrieved from: <http://www.un.org/womenwatch/osagi/ianwge2012/Between-Gender-Ageing-Report-Executive-Summary-2012.pdf>.

Vaillant, J., Vuillerme, N., Martigné, P., Caillat-Miousse, J., Parisot, J., Nougier, V., et al. (2006). Balance, aging, and osteoporosis: Effects of cognitive exercises combined with physiotherapy. *Joint Bone Spine*, 73(4), 414–418. http://dx.doi.org/10.1016/j.jbspin.2005.07.003.

Valenzuela, M., & Sachdev, P. S. (2009). Harnessing brain and cognitive reserve for the prevention of dementia. *Indian Journal of Psychiatry*, 51, 16–21.

Van Schaik, P., Blake, J., Pernet, F., Spears, I., & Fencott, C. (2008). Virtual augmented exercise gaming for older adults. *Cyberpsychology & Behavior*, 11(1), 103–106.

Verbrugge, L. M. (1990). The twain meet: Empirical explanations of sex differences in health and mortality. In M. G. Ory & H. R. Warner (Eds.), *Gender, health, and longevity: Multidisciplinary perspectives* (pp. 159–199). New York, NY: Springer.

Vidovich, M. R., Shaw, J., Flicker, L., & Almeida, O. P. (2011). Cognitive activity for the treatment of older adults with mild Alzheimer's Disease (AD)–PACE AD: Study protocol for a randomised controlled trial. *Trials*, 12(1), 47–53. http://dx.doi.org/10.1186/1745-6215-12-47.

Vohs, K. D., & Baumeister, R. F. (Eds.). (2011). *Handbook of self-regulation: Research, theory, and applications*. New York, NY: Guilford Press.

Weaver, R. L., II, & Kosan, J. (1992). Mental aerobics: Just for the fun of it. *Clearing House*, 65(3), 167–171.

Wurm, S., Warner, L. M., Ziegelmann, J. P., Wolff, J. K., & Schüz, B. (2013). How do negative self-perceptions of aging become a self-fulfilling prophecy? *Psychology and Aging*, 28(4), 1088–1097.

Yamamoto, M., Izumi, I., & Aso, Y. (2012). Relationship between cognition and activities of daily living in elderly women with mild cognitive impairment in Japan. *International Journal of Clinical Medicine*, 3, 251–253. http://dx.doi.org/10.4236/ijcm.2012.34050.

Zhou, J., & Oldham, G. R. (2001). Enhancing creative performance: Effects of expected developmental assessment strategies and creative personality. *The Journal of Creative Behavior*, 35(3), 151–167.

PHYSICAL HEALTH IN WOMEN'S AGING

Relevant chapters

5   *Physical Changes and Self-Perceptions in Women's Aging*   87

6   *Aging Women and Health Longevity*   101

7   *Importance of Daily Physical Activity for Older Women*   121

The second section of the book examines issues related to women's physical health changes as they age. Beyond the physical aspect of aging, this section examines ways to optimize this developmental process from both a functional and sociopsychological perspective. From a proactive aging perspective, it is important for aging women and those that care for them to understand these physical aging changes experienced by women within a social and cultural context. The purpose of this section of the book is to review research on women's physical aging issues across different locations of the world. It is important to make this examination of cross-cultural differences and similarities in women's aging trajectories in order to identify effective strategies to support positive aging outcomes for this aging subpopulation. Practical ways for women to adapt to physical aging in light of cultural, social, and familial contextual factors is examined. Across chapters in this section, factors determining physical aging outcomes from a positive aging perspective across a woman's life span will be examined.

Physical Changes and Self-Perceptions in Women's Aging

Global Fact: *The fact that women's life expectancy is greater than men's means that health problems that increase with age, such as disability, affect a greater number of women worldwide.*
—**United Nations, Women Coordination Division report (2012)**

Women's adaptive reactions to physical aging, and the associated social standards of attractiveness tied to these aging changes, are significant to the understanding of positive aging outcomes for a global aging population. One such issue is self-perception of personal aging among diverse groups of women.

AGING WOMEN AND THEIR BODY IMAGE

Aging women are concerned about their appearance (eg, Gosselink, Cox, McClure, & De Jong, 2008). Although aging women are often not the focus of body image research and interventions an argument can be made that body dissatisfaction might be expected to increase as women age given that most women are moving away from (not toward) the societal norm of beauty (Becker, Diedrichs, Jankowski, & Werchan, 2013).

Older adults often have more exposure to media (such as television viewing) than younger adults; however, they do not appear to be as susceptible to internalizing the social norms portrayed in the media (Bedford & Johnson, 2006; Hummert, Garstka, O'Brien, Greenwald, & Mellott, 2002). However, in a study that investigated the portrayal of 829 characters across 100 movies, it was found that older women were underrepresented on the big screen and when they were depicted in significant roles, the women were more negatively portrayed (on dimensions such as "attractiveness," "friendliness," and "character goodness") relative to their male counterparts (Bazzini, McIntosh, Smith, Cook, & Harris, 1997).

Although aging women are seldom the target of body image interventions several research studies have revealed that older women have levels of body dissatisfaction that parallel younger women (eg, Pruis & Janowsky, 2010). Bedford and Johnson (2006) found no difference in the prevalence of body image dissatisfaction between younger (ages 19–23) and older (ages 65–74) women. In a series of interviews conducted on women between the ages of 20 and 80, women across the life span acknowledged that they use different techniques (eg, exercise, food restriction, and cosmetic surgery) to maintain, or aspire toward, a certain body size (Reel, SooHoo, Summerhays, & Gill, 2008) and that as women age they still prefer a thinner body image when responding to line-drawing figures (Ferraro et al., 2008). Indeed, different research studies have demonstrated that body dissatisfaction remains stable throughout the life span; however, other important facets of an unhealthy body image decreased with age (eg, Tiggemann, 2004). For example, as women age they tend to experience less appearance-related anxiety and disordered eating behaviors (eg, Tiggemann & Lynch, 2001) and the relationship between body dissatisfaction and self-esteem weakens as women age (Webster & Tiggemann, 2003).

There appears to be a reprioritization as women age from an emphasis on physical attractiveness to an emphasis on being healthy (eg, Augustus-Horvath & Tylka, 2011; Leichty & Yarnal, 2010). Age may, therefore, offer some adaptive protection against a negative body image (Peat, Peyerl, & Muehlenkamp, 2008). Although Fooken (1994) found that body image was a more significant predictor of sexual interest in aging adults than was physical health. Interestingly, women in midlife who reported the highest levels of body dissatisfaction were also more likely to be from a higher social class (McLaren & Kuh, 2004).

"Gerontophobia," or the fear of growing old, appears to play a role in women's self-evaluation. And, it appears that culture perpetuates gerontophobia by selling products that help people look young or at least not to look so old (eg, Oberg & Tornstam, 1999). Lewis and Cachelin (2001) reported a positive relationship between fear of growing old and disordered eating behaviors, and Sabik (2013) found that perceptions of ageism and lower body self-image were related to lower psychological well-being for women in their sixties. Further, in focus groups where women were asked to respond to questions about "beauty culture" a clear theme emerged in that women, especially as they age, were negatively affected by the Western ideal of what it means to be beautiful (Gosselink et al., 2008). Gupta (1990) and Gupta and Schork (1993) showed that age-related concerns were related to a desire for thinness and late onset anorexia nervosa. Slevic and Tiggemann (2010) concluded that "aging anxiety" among middle-aged women predicted, in part, attitudes toward cosmetic surgery. Indeed, many middle-aged women indicated some level of anxiety about the aging process and a decline in levels of attractiveness (Barrett & Robbins, 2008).

PSYCHOLOGICAL MECHANISMS AND COGNITIVE BIASES THAT INFLUENCE SELF-PERCEPTIONS

One way that aging women may attempt to evaluate themselves is by relying on social comparison and/or temporal comparison (ie, whether the evaluation of self improves or deteriorates over time) (Zell & Alicke, 2009). Aging women may engage in selectively evaluating with whom they compare themselves (Wood, 1989), a process of strategic comparison known as "downward social comparison" (Festinger, 1954).

QUOTES FROM FAMOUS, POSITIVELY AGING WOMEN

I think it's nice to age gracefully.
OK, you lose the youth, a certain stamina and dewy glow,
but what you gain on the inside as a human being is wonderful:
the wisdom, the acceptance and the peace of mind. It's a fair exchange.
—*Cherie Lunghi, Actress*

Nature gives you the face you have at twenty;
it is up to you to merit the face you have at fifty.
—*Coco Chanel, Fashion Designer*

It is sad to grow old but nice to ripen.

—*Brigitte Bardot, Actress*

This evaluative process has been shown to be an adaptive strategy where people selectively choose to evaluate themselves against others who are in a worse position (eg, Taylor, Wood, & Lichtman, 1983). Researchers have demonstrated that downward social comparison can help protect the self-esteem of aging adults (eg, Kohn & Smith, 2003; Rickbaugh & Tomlinson-Keasey, 1997) and that social comparison (both upward and downward) has a considerable influence on the well-being of older women (Heidrich & Ryff, 1993) and helps to "maintain the illusion of youth" (Rodeheaver & Stohs, 1991). Frieswijk, Buunk, Steverink, and Slates (2004) reported that frail, older adults benefited the most from downward social comparison when they viewed the target as different from her/himself. In one study, Peck and Merighi (2007) found that social comparison accounted for a significant amount of variance associated with physical and mental health suggesting that social comparison plays a critical role in influencing longevity and decreasing depressive symptomatology.

Temporal comparison, may also play a role in how aging adults evaluate themselves and some researchers have argued that social comparison happens more frequently earlier in life while temporal comparisons take precedence in later life (eg, Suls & Mullen, 1984); however, research by Robinson-Whelen and Kiecolt-Glaser (1997) showed no difference in these strategies between "young-old" and "older-old" adults. Specifically, if comparing oneself to a younger version where things might be considered "better" or an older version where one might anticipate that things will be "worse" may cause older adults to make a negative assessment (eg, Suls, Marco, & Tobin, 1991).

TIPS FOR WOMEN'S AGING WELL

1. Have a regular health checkup (physical, dental, mental).
2. Do not put limitations on yourself—explore hobbies and options.
3. Take care of yourself and "listen" to your body.
4. Apply your accumulated wisdom in life decision-making.
5. See yourself as a "work in progress."

The role of "rosy retrospection," a form of memory bias, may also play a role in allowing aging adults to maintain a positive self-concept in that they may focus on positive rather than negative memories when recounting the past (eg, Storm & Jobe, 2012). For example, in one study participants who were asked to reminisce about past accomplishments showed higher coping self-efficacy and less anxiety than groups who were not asked to reminisce (Rybarczyk & Auerback, 1990). Reis-Bergan, Gibbons, Gerrard, and Ybema (2000) concluded that older women who reminisced about the past had an influence on how they responded to (upward and downward) social comparison and this is especially true for women who reported being currently dissatisfied with the status of their life.

A person's physical characteristics (gender, age, appearance) is the most obvious aspect of a person during an initial interaction and an abundant amount of research in Social Psychology offers many examples of people relying on physical appearance and concluding that "what is beautiful is good." For instance, attractive individuals are believed to possess other socially desired characteristics (eg, interesting, sincere, and modest; Dion, Berschied, & Walster, 1972), known as the "halo effect of attractiveness" (Thorndike, 1920). Interestingly, even babies as young as two months old show a preference for attractive over unattractive faces

(Langlois et al., 1987). Eagly and colleagues conducted a meta-analysis and demonstrated that physical attractiveness has the strongest influence on ratings of social competence (Eagly, Ashmore, Makhijani, & Longo, 1991). Larose and Standing (1998) hypothesized that older adults would be less susceptible to the halo effect because "age should bring wisdom," therefore reducing this judgmental bias; however, their study revealed that older adults were just as likely to make this judgmental error as younger adults. Zebrowitz and Franklin (2014) found results similar to Larose and Standing (1998) and extended their line of research to demonstrate that older adults also respond in a more stereotypical way to faces that are closer to their own age.

A influence of a person's appearance has applied implications as well, namely that research has shown that appearance has been cited as one of the strongest influences of employee selection and some argue might be the newest form of discrimination, referred to as "lookism" (eg, Warhurst, van den Broek, Hall, & Nickson, 2009). In fact, some researchers have argued that women have the dubious distinction of being in "triple jeopardy" because they may be discriminated against because of their age and/or gender ("gendered ageism") and/or physical appearance ("lookism") (Granleese & Sayer, 2006).

THINK ABOUT IT!

Do you think the recent trend for advertisers to show "real" women (eg, Dove advertisements) in their ads will help alleviate body image issues for women? Why or why not?

Some questions to consider:

1. Can we empirically study this?
2. How would you design a study to assess the differences between "real" (or "everyday") women and "supermodels"? What would be the independent variable? What would be the dependent (outcome) variable?
3. Is there a better way, other than an experimental design, to answer this question?

THE "CULTURE" OF YOUTH

Aging, rather than being viewed as a natural sequence in life, is often regarded instead as a "disease" or something that needs to be treated. Aging adults are spending a great deal of money on procedures in an attempt to reverse and/or thwart the outward signs of age on their appearance (eg, Honigman & Castle, 2006). In fact, billions of dollars are spent every year on beauty products that are intended to help a woman look younger longer (eg, Huang & Miller, 2007) while research by Eriksen (2012) indicated that women who had undergone cosmetic surgery did *not* feel better about themselves, did not report feeling "younger than their years," or experience less anxiety associated with aging when compared with women who had not had cosmetic surgery. Conversely, in a series of interviews, women who had undergone cosmetic surgery indicated that they were more secure with their image relative to women who had no surgery.

CHECK IT OUT!

It is important to understand our unconscious (implicit) attitudes about aging, because these internalized attitudes about aging can meaningfully impact how we age. Please take a moment to take an *Implicit Association Test* (IAT). The test is designed to uncover attitudes that may not be readily available or that people may be unwilling to report (ie, implicit attitudes). The IAT covers a wide range of topics, such as disability and age.

To take the Age IAT, go here: https://implicit.harvard.edu/implicit/selectatest.html and select "Age IAT." What did you learn about your personal attitudes toward aging? Were you surprised?

In an extensive review of the literature, Sarwer, Wadden, Pertschuk, and Whitaker (1998) found a discrepancy between the psychological outcomes expressed by cosmetic surgery patients as a function of methodology. Specifically, interviews of cosmetic surgery patients suggested psychopathology whereas on more standardized measures, cosmetic surgery patients yielded more "normal" response patterns. Women who had cosmetic surgery downplayed the role that the media had on their decision to have surgery (Goodman, 1994). Hurd (1999) conducted interviews with women who were 61–92 years old and found a contradiction between the endorsement of beauty norms yet acknowledging that health concerns take precedence over physical attractiveness. Similarly, another qualitative study interviewed a sample of women who were 60–69 years old, and the interviewees expressed being "content" with their appearance and body but still conveyed a desire to change their appearance (Leichty, 2012).

As women age, they seem to express the greatest dissatisfaction with their face whereas younger women seems to care more about the shape of their bodies (Goodman, 1994). Franzoi and Koehler (1998) showed that older adults had less positive attitudes toward their facial attractiveness (eg, lips, eyes) than younger adults. Not surprisingly, Botulinum toxin type A ("Botox") injections have become among the most common procedure of all, with a 703% increase from 2000 to 2013 (plastic surgeon statistics report). Anesthetic surgery, which is the "reshaping of normal structures" (Allen, 2003) is more common among aging adults than transformative surgery, which is done to restructure a physical feature such as a "nose job."

Buss (1989) has shown that males prefer mates who possess characteristics that signal "reproductive capacity,"; however, females were more likely to prefer males who possess "resource acquisition." In a sample of personal advertisement, researchers found that men explicitly sought women who were younger than them and this pattern of finding was more obvious among older men whereas women often sought men who were older than them (Buss, 1989; Wiederman, 1993). Stimson, Wase, and Stimson (1981) argued that the concept of "beauty" is more restrictive for aging women than for aging men. As women age, they tend to be devalued more so than men and this phenomenon is known as "gendered ageism" (Moore, 2009). Graying hair and aging skin seem to be viewed differently for men and women, and women are more likely to be described as "old" but men as "distinguished" (Porter, 2003). These gender differences have implications for the acceptance of age-related changes and normative societal beliefs about the role of aging for men and women (Allen, 2003).

SUMMARY

A number of different factors may work independently or interact to influence how an aging woman feels about her body. A large body of literature suggests that older women experience as much body dissatisfaction as younger women although they may not be the target of interventions and treatments as often as younger women. On the positive side, however, even though dissatisfaction levels seem to remain fairly stable throughout the life span, older women appear to be less susceptible to the negative effects (eg, decreased self-esteem) of body dissatisfaction; it appears that age offers some protection in this aspect.

Fear of aging also seems to play a significant role in how well older women adapt to the aging process. Specifically, those women who fear aging seem to be the most at risk for maladaptive behaviors (eg, a dysfunctional drive for thinness). Several psychological mechanisms (social comparison, temporal comparison, and reminiscence) may also help aging women maintain their positive view of self by allowing them to make favorable evaluations. Of course, these mechanisms are not always straight forward and this line of research continues to grow. Arguably, the best-researched area involves the notion that our society is obsessed with a culture of youth, and this is reflected in the growing rates of cosmetic surgery, and other antiaging products as well as the depiction of older women in the media (either absent or unfavorably portrayed).

DISCUSSION QUESTIONS

1. What is the difference between social comparison and temporal comparison? Describe an example of each and how it might help an older woman feel more confident in her appearance.
2. What is the relationship between the societal "messages" about aging and women's own aging self-perception?
3. What is "lookism" and how might it relate to women's attitudes about personal aging? Is lookism a cultural phenomenon that occurs within specific cultures or is it more of a "universal" issue?
4. What is one major difference between the physical attributes we ascribe to aging men versus women?
5. What might be some ways that family and peers can positively influence a woman's self-perception as she ages?
6. What role can community education offer in facilitating positive aging perceptions for women?
7. How early should education talk about positive development-related self-perceptions for women?
8. Are men and women different in their aging self-perceptions? If so, why?
9. Are there cultural differences in how women regard their aging trajectory? If yes, why?
10. If you were to develop a support program for women, how would you design it to best create positive aging?

TEST YOUR KNOWLEDGE!

Take the following body image test to assess your aging-related perceptions:

http://www.seemypersonality.com/personality.asp?p=Self-Perception-Test#q1

SUPPLEMENTAL BOOK READINGS

Over the past decades, there have been many books written on the topic of women's physical aging and associated reactions underlying positive aging attitudes. Here are some recommended *additional readings*:

Champ, J., & Moore, C. (2005). *Ripe: The truth about growing older and the beauty of getting on with your life.* New York, NY: Atria Books.
The authors do a great job in examining the many different reactions women have on aging from a humorous perspective. They encourage women to accept the aging process for sharing and understanding stories of other women going through the same journey. The myriad of information is offered that acknowledges the many different stages of life that women go through with a very strong message of personal acceptance and self-love. The authors of the book challenge women and the broader society to appreciate the beauty that can be found in women in the advanced stages of life.

Clarke, L.H. (2010). *Facing age: Women growing older in anti-aging culture.* Lanham, MD: Rowman & Littlefield Publishers.
From the findings of interviews with aging women conducted over a 10-year period, the author discusses feminist theories about aging, the aging body, attitudes toward feelings of femininity, and the aging "self." Importantly, the author does acknowledge the presence of medical interventions designed to be the quick fix toward women's anxiety toward physical aging and acknowledges that these options may not be for every woman. Culture and society unfairly characterize women in later life as potentially less feminine and less beautiful when, in actuality, women are simply transforming into a different type of beauty.

Carter, J. (1998). *The virtues of aging.* New York, NY: Ballantine Books.
This book raises an important social issue, in that society's attitude toward physical aging may be a dramatic form of ageism that is not as recognized or confronted as other "isms" in society. The author suggests that there are many virtues of aging which are not acknowledged and this translates into a lower social valuation of older women and men in society. This disempowerment of an aging segment of society creates many other devastating social ramifications (eg, age discrimination in the workplace) which undermine their ability to achieve positive aging. The message of this book is important for women who feel that they may be faced with double jeopardy issues of being discriminated against because of being both a woman and being older, for example.

SUPPLEMENTAL AGING VIDEOS

For learning purposes, the use of videos can be very beneficial for both instructors and readers. Here are some recommended *supplemental videos*:

Different video links on aging health: http://www.healthvideo.com/sitemap.php (Format: Website)
This is a great website that offers short videos on different aging-related health.

Younger Next Year: The New Science of Aging (Format: DVD)
This DVD examines the science of aging, both physically and mentally. Question posed through the content video is whether you can achieve as an aging woman a more physically fit status that will help you live a longer and healthier life. The signs of aging would suggest that you can be functionally younger than you are chronologically through proper regime of diet and exercise. This is an empowering message for normatively aging women whose life expectancy is typically longer than their male counterparts.

Dr Andrew Weil's Healthy Aging (Format: DVD)
Dr Weil suggests that older adults engage in many different types of physical activities (eg, yoga) in order to challenge their physical capabilities and engage their minds for a more "holistic" wellness result. The content of the video is very engaging and has a nice summary of points at the very end of the DVD to reiterate the main points communicate by Dr Weil. The basic message of the DVD is for older adults to be active participants in life and make proactive choices to engage physically, cognitively, and socially for basic health. This positive attitude translates into greater self-acceptance of the aging process.

ADDITIONAL INFORMATION LINKS

The following are some recommended *supplemental Internet links*:

Alzheimer's Foundation website: http://www.alzfdn.org/BrainHealth/successfulaging.html/

AARP website: http://www.aarp.org/health/

Centers for Disease Control and Prevention website: http://www.cdc.gov/aging/

Mature Resources website: http://www.matureresources.org/

NIA/NIH website: http://www.nia.nih.gov/health/

Tao Institute website: http://www.taosinstitute.net/positive-aging-newsletter/

References

Allen, D. B. (2003). Aesthetic and reconstructive surgery in the aging patient. *Archives of Surgery, 138*(10), 1099–1105. http://dx.doi.org/10.1001/archsurg.138.10.1099.

Augustus-Horvath, C. L., & Tylka, T. L. (2011). The acceptance model of intuitive eating: A comparison of women in emerging adulthood, early adulthood and middle adulthood. *Journal of Counseling Psychology, 58*, 110–125. http://dx.doi.org/10.1037/a0022129.

Barrett, A. E., & Robbins, C. (2008). The multiple sources of women's aging anxiety and their relationship with psychological distress. *Journal of Aging and Health, 20*, 32–65.

Bazzini, D., McIntosh, W., Smith, S., Cook, S., & Harris, C. (1997). The aging women in popular film: Underrepresented, unattractive, unfriendly, and unintelligent. *Sex Roles, 36*(7/8), 531–543. http://dx.doi.org/10.1007/BF02766689.

Becker, C. B., Diedrichs, P., Jankowski, G., & Werchan, C. (2013). I'm not just fat, I'm old: Has the study of body image overlooked "old talk"? *Journal of Eating Disorders, 1*(6), 1–12. http://dx.doi.org/10.1186/2050-2974-1-6.

Bedford, J., & Johnson, S. (2006). Societal influences on body image dissatisfaction in younger and older women. *Journal of Women & Aging, 18*(1), 41–55. http://dx.doi.org/10.1300/J074v18n01_04.

Buss, D. M. (1989). Sex differences in human mate preferences: Evolutionary hypotheses tested in 37 cultures. *Behavioral and Brain Sciences, 12*, 1–49.

Dion, K., Berschied, E., & Walster, E. (1972). What is beautiful is good. *Journal of Personality and Social Psychology, 24*(3), 285–290.

Eagly, A., Ashmore, R., Makhijani, M., & Longo, L. (1991). What is beautiful is good, but…: A meta-analytic review of research on the physical attractiveness stereotype. *Psychological Bulletin, 110*(1), 109–128.

Eriksen, S. (2012). To cut or not to cut: Cosmetic surgery usage and women's age-related experiences. *International Journal of Human Development, 74*(1), 1–24. http://dx.doi.org/10.2190/-AG.74.1.a.

Ferraro, F. R., Muehlenkamp, J., Paintner, A., Wasson, K., Hager, T., & Hoverson, F. (2008). Aging, body image, and body shape. *The Journal of General Psychology, 135*(4), 379–392. http://dx.doi.org/10.3200/GENP.135.4.379-392.

Festinger, L. (1954). A theory of social comparison processes. *Human Relations, 7*, 117–140. http://dx.doi.org/10.1177/001872675400700202.

Fooken, I. (1994). Sexuality in the later years - the impact of health and body-image in a sample of older women. *Patient Education and Counseling, 23*(3), 227–233. http://dx.doi.org/10.1016/0738-3991(94)90038-8.

Franzoi, S. L., & Koehler, V. (1998). Age and gender differences in body attitudes: A comparison of young and elderly adults. *International Journal of Aging and Human Development, 47*(1), 1–10.

Frieswijk, N., Buunk, B. P., Steverink, N., & Slates, J. P. (2004). The effects of social comparison information on the life satisfaction of frail older persons. *Psychology and Aging, 19*(1), 183–190. http://dx.doi.org/10.1037/0882-7974.19.1.183.

Goodman, M. (1994). Social, psychological, and developmental factors to women's receptivity to cosmetic surgery. *Journal of Aging Studies, 8*(4), 375–396. http://dx.doi.org/10.1016/08904065-(94)90010-8.

Gosselink, C., Cox, D., McClure, S. J., & De Jong, M. L. (2008). Ravishing or ravaged: Women's relationships with women in the context of aging and Western beauty culture. *Journal of Aging and Human Development, 66*(4), 307–327. http://dx.doi.org/10.2190/AG.66.4.c.

Granleese, J., & Sayer, G. (2006). Gendered ageism and lookism: Triple jeopardy for female academics. *Women in Management Review, 21*(6), 500–517. http://dx.doi.org/10.1177/-0950017011426313.

Gupta, M. A. (1990). Fear of aging: A precipitating factor in late onset anorexia nervosa. *International Journal of Eating Disorders, 9*, 221–224. http://dx.doi.org/10.1002/1098-108X.

Gupta, M. A., & Schork, N. J. (1993). Aging-related concerns and body image: Possible future implications for eating disorders. *International Journal of Eating Disorders, 14*, 481–486. http://dx.doi.org/10.1002/1098-108X.

Heidrich, S. M., & Ryff, C. D. (1993). The role of social comparisons processes in the psychological adaptation of elderly adults. *Journal of Gerontology, 48*(3), 127–136. http://dx.doi.org/10.1093/geronj/48.3.P127.

Honigman, R., & Castle, D. (2006). Aging and cosmetic enhancement. *Clinical Interventions and Aging, 1*(2), 115–119.

Huang, C. K., & Miller, T. A. (2007). The truth about over-the-counter topical anti-aging products: A comprehensive review. *Aesthetic Surgery Journal, 4*, 413–415. http://dx.doi.org/10.1016/j.asj.2007.05.005.

Hummert, M. L., Garstka, T. A., O'Brien, L. T., Greenwald, A. G., & Mellott, D. S. (2002). Using the implicit association test to measure age differences in implicit social cognitions. *Psychology and Aging, 17*(3), 482–495.

Hurd, L. C. (1999). Older women's body image and embodied experience: An exploration. *Journal of Women & Aging, 12*(3–4), 77–97.

Kohn, S., & Smith, G. (2003). The impact of downward social comparison processes on depressive symptoms in older men and women. *Ageing International, 28*(1), 37–65. http://dx.doi.org/10.1007/s12126-003-1015-7.

Langlois, J., Roggman, L., Casey, R., Ritter, J., Rieser-Danner, L., & Jenkins, V. (1987). Infant preferences for attractive faces: Rudiments of a stereotype? *Developmental Psychology, 23*(3), 363–369.

Larose, H., & Standing, L. (1998). Does the halo effect occur in the elderly? *Social Behavior and Personality: An International Journal, 26*(2), 147–150.

Leichty, T. (2012). "Yes, I worry about my weight… but for the most part I'm content with my body": Older women's body dissatisfaction alongside contentment. *Journal of Women Aging, 24*(1), 70–88. http://dx.doi.org/10.1080/08952841.2012.638873.

Leichty, T., & Yarnal, C. (2010). Older women's body image: A life course perspective. *Aging and Society, 30*(7), 1197–1218. http://dx.doi.org/10.1017/S0144686X10000346.

Lewis, D., & Cachelin, F. (2001). Body image, body dissatisfaction, and eating attitudes in midlife and elderly women. *Eating Disorders: The Journal of Treatment & Prevention, 9*(1), 29–39.

McLaren, L., & Kuh, D. (2004). Body dissatisfaction in midlife. *Journal of Women & Aging, 1*, 35–54. http://dx.doi.org/10.1300/J074v16n01_04.

Moore, S. (2009). No matter what I did I would still end up in the same position: Age as a factor defining older women's experience of labour market participation. *Work, Employment and Society, 23*, 655–662. http://dx.doi.org/10.1177/0950017009344871.

Oberg, P., & Tornstam, L. (1999). Body images of men and women of different ages. *Ageing and Society, 19*(5), 629–644. http://dx.doi.org/10.5878/002423.

Peat, C., Peyerl, N., & Muehlenkamp, J. (2008). Body image and eating disorders in older adults: A review. *The Journal of General Psychology, 135*(4), 343–358. http://dx.doi.org/0.3200/-GENP.135.4.343-358.

Peck, M., & Merighi, J. (2007). The relation of social comparison to subjective well-being and health status in older adults. *Journal of Human Behavior in the Social Environment, 16*(3), 121–142. http://dx.doi.org/10.1300/10911350802107827.

Porter, N. B. (2003). Sex plus age discrimination: Protecting older women workers. *Denver University Law Review, 81*, 79–111.

Pruis, T., & Janowsky, J. (2010). Assessment of body image in younger and older women. *The Journal of General Psychology, 137*(3), 225–238.

Reel, J. J., SooHoo, S., Summerhays, J. F., & Gill, D. L. (2008). Age before beauty: An exploration of body image in African-American and Caucasian adult women. *Journal of Gender Studies, 17*(4), 321–330. http://dx.doi.org/10.1080/09589230802419963.

Reis-Bergan, M., Gibbons, F., Gerrard, M., & Ybema, J. (2000). The impact of reminiscence on socially active elderly women's reactions to social comparisons. *Basic and Applied Social Psychology, 22*(3), 225–236.

Rickbaugh, C. A., & Tomlinson-Keasey, C. (1997). Social and temporal comparisons in adjustment to aging. *Basic and Applied Social Psychology, 19*, 307–328.

Robinson-Whelen, S., & Kiecolt-Glaser, J. (1997). The importance of social versus temporal comparison appraisals among older adults. *Journal of Applied Social Psychology, 27*(11), 959–966. http://dx.doi.org/10.1111/j.1559-1816.1997.tb00281.x.

Rodeheaver, D., & Stohs, J. (1991). The adaptive misperception of age in older women: Sociocultural images and psychological mechanisms of control. *Educational Gerontology, 17*(2), 141–156.

Rybarczyk, B., & Auerback, S. (1990). Reminiscence interviews as stress management interventions for older patients undergoing surgery. *The Gerontologist, 30*(4), 522–528.

Sabik, N. J. (2013). Ageism and body esteem: Associations with psychological well-being among late-middle aged African American and European American women. *The Journal of Gerontology, 70*(2), 189–199. http://dx.doi.org/10.1093/geronb/gbt080.

Sarwer, D. B., Wadden, T. A., Pertschuk, M. J., & Whitaker, L. A. (1998). The psychology of cosmetic surgery: A review and reconceptualization. *Clinical Psychology Review, 18*(1), 1–22. http://dx.doi.org/10.1016/S02727358(97)00047-0.

Slevic, J., & Tiggemann, M. (2010). Attitudes toward cosmetic surgery in middle-aged women: Body image, aging anxiety, and the media. *Psychology of Women Quarterly, 34*, 65–74. http://dx.doi.org/10.1111/j.1471-6402.2009.01542.x.

Stimson, A., Wase, J., & Stimson, J. (1981). Sexuality and self-esteem among the aged. *Research on Aging, 3*(2), 228–239.

Storm, B., & Jobe, T. (2012). Retrieval induced forgetting predicts failure to recall negative autobiographical memories. *Psychological Science, 23*(11), 1356–1363. http://dx.doi.org/10.1177/-095679-7612443837.

Suls, J., Marco, C., & Tobin, S. (1991). The role of temporal comparison, social comparison, and direct appraisal in the elderly's self-evaluation of health. *Journal of Applied Social Psychology, 21*(14), 1125–1144.

Suls, J., & Mullen, B. (1984). Social and temporal bases of self-evaluation in the elderly: Theory and evidence. *International Journal of Aging and Human Development, 18*(2), 111–120.

Taylor, S., Wood, J., & Lichtman, R. (1983). It could be worse: Selective evaluation as a response to victimization. *Journal of Social Issues, 39*(2), 19–40.

Thorndike, E. L. (1920). A constant error in psychological ratings. *Journal of Applied Psychology, 4*(1), 25–29. http://dx.doi.org/10.1037/h0071663.

Tiggemann, M. (2004). Body image across the adult life span: Stability and change. *Body Image, 1*, 29–41. http://dx.doi.org/10.1177/1359105306065013.

Tiggemann, M., & Lynch, J. (2001). Body image across the lifespan in adult women: The role of self-objectification. *Developmental Psychology, 37*(2), 243–253. http://dx.doi.org/10.1037/00121-649.37.2.243.

United Nations, Women Coordination Division. (2012). Between gender and ageing: The status of the world's older women and progress since the Madrid International Plan of Action on Ageing. Retrieved from: <http://www.un.org/womenwatch/osagi/ianwge2012/Between-Gender-Ageing-Report-Executive-Summary-2012.pdf>.

Warhurst, C., van den Broek, D., Hall, R., & Nickson, D. (2009). Lookism: The new frontier of employment discrimination? *Journal of Industrial Relations, 51*(1), 131–136. http://dx.doi.org/10.1177/0022185608096808.

Webster, J., & Tiggemann, M. (2003). The relationship between women's body satisfaction and self-image across the life span: The role of cognitive control. *The Journal of Genetic Psychology: Research and Theory on Human Development, 164*(2), 241–252. http://dx.doi.org/10.1080/00221320309597980.

Wiederman, M. (1993). Evolved gender differences in mate preferences: Evidence from personal advertisements. *Ethology and Sociobiology, 14*(5), 331–351. http://dx.doi.org/10.1016/0162-3095(93)90003-Z.

Wood, J. V. (1989). Theory and research concerning social comparison of personal attributes. *Psychological Bulletin, 106,* 231–248. http://dx.doi.org/apa.org/journals/bul/106/2/231.

Zebrowitz, L., & Franklin, R. (2014). The attractiveness halo effect and the babyface stereotype in older and younger adults: Similarities, old age accentuation, and OA positivity effects. *Experimental Aging Research, 40*(3), 375–393. http://dx.doi.org/10.1080/0361073X.2014.897151.

Zell, E., & Alicke, M. (2009). Self-evaluation effects of temporal and social comparison. *Journal of Experimental Social Psychology, 45*(1), 223–227. http://dx.doi.org/10.1016/j.jesp.2008.09.007.

6

Aging Women and Health Longevity

Global Fact: *The number of people aged 80 years or older will have almost quadrupled between 2000 and 2050 to 395 million... On average, women live six to eight years longer than men.*

— **World Health Organization (2014)**

Common beliefs about aging are beginning to evolve as more empirical work is being conducted in the area of aging. Poor health and loss of autonomy are not necessary inevitable outcomes of growing older. Many situational and genetic factors play a significant role in how well a woman ages, or if she will age successfully. As the global population is predominantly living longer than ever before, the goals of aging women (and men) may be shifting from living longer to increasing the quality of life. Several factors, mostly modifiable, have been identified, as important antecedents to better health and longevity, those factors as well as potential interventions will be discussed in this chapter.

The concept of "positive" aging has garnered a fair amount of research attention since Baker (1958) first introduced the concept about half a decade ago. The construct of positive aging has been refined and expanded upon over time (eg, Depp & Jeste, 2006), and Rowe and Kahn (1987) popularized the idea of "successful" aging by putting forth a convincing case arguing that what people perceived as inevitable effects of aging actually had more to do with disease processes than age, per se. Rowe and Kahn suggested that older adults who were "successful agers" would not demonstrate diseases associated with advanced age and that positive aging, as opposed to "usual aging," may be influenced by environmental factors (eg, exercise, social support). In an updated definition to their original idea of positive aging, Rowe and Kahn (1998) suggested that successfully aging adults should meet three criteria: absence of disease and risk factors for disease; physical and mental functioning; and active engagement.

Women and Positive Aging.
DOI: http://dx.doi.org/10.1016/B978-0-12-420136-1.00006-2

Using these criteria; however, has led to a discrepancy between self-reported (subjective) and objective (eg, Rowe & Kahn's model) reports of positive aging (Phelan, Anderson, Lacroix, & Larson, 2004), with self-reports indicating more instances of positive aging; about 50% using self-report and 19% using Rowe and Kahn's criteria (eg, Strawbridge, Wallhagen, & Cohen, 2002). Similarly, Montross and colleagues (2006) demonstrated that in a sample of community-dwelling adults aged 60 and over, 92% rated themselves as aging successfully versus 5% when using Rowe and Kahn's criteria.

Research has demonstrated, in part, that quality of life is not always dependent upon being disease free in older age (Wong, 1989). In short, a unified definition of positive aging has yet to be reached in the field of gerontology (eg, Montross et al., 2006) but both subjective and objective measures help to gain a fuller picture of what it means to age success-fully and remain healthy over time. Although, many of the factors associated with positive aging are considered modifiable (eg, remaining active), Austin (1991) has argued that not every individual has equal access to resources to help ensure that the transition into older adulthood will be a successful one. For instance, some social factors (eg, poverty, lack of access to education, residency in rural areas, social isolation, and developmental delays) provide limited opportunities for older women to age well (eg, Cattan, White, Bond, & Learmouth, 2005).

INCOME

Socioeconomic status has consistently been shown to be associated with facets of positive aging and longevity. Unfortunately, women of age 65 and older are almost twice as likely to have a low socioeconomic status compared to older men (Lee & Shaw, 2008). In a fairly extensive meta-analysis investigating the relationship between several variables and subjective well-being in later life, which tapped into three different dimensions of life satisfaction, happiness, and self-esteem, Pinquart and Sorensen (2000) found that socioeconomic status was positively related to all three aspects of subjective well-being. Furthermore, in a 10-year follow-up study of older adults, those identified as the most success-ful agers were from a higher socioeconomic status (Kaplan et al., 2008). Berkman et al. (1993) grouped older adults into "high," "medium," or "impaired" functioning and found that those adults with less money were three times more likely to be categorized as "impaired." Guralnik and Kaplan (1989) asked a cohort of individuals a number of health-related questions and grouped those who scored in the top 20% as "healthy aging," these individuals were compared to the remainder of the cohort;

higher family income, as well as other variables such as being of normal weight or being a nonsmoker, predicted high functioning 19 years later.

Individuals from lower socioeconomic groups have more health-related issues (eg, Huguet, Kaplan, & Feeny, 2008), such as frailty (Szanton, Seplaki, Thorpe, Allen, & Fried, 2010) and higher mortality rates (Bassuk, Berkman, & Amick, 2002). Furthermore, older adults from lower socioeconomic status appear to receive poorer medical treatment, such as being prescribed too many prescription drugs (Odubanjo, Bennett, & Feely, 2004). Thus, income levels serve as a strong predictor of health and longevity.

WORDS OF WISDOM

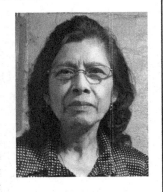

Herminia, a Guatemalan native, came to the United States over 15 years ago. At age 60, she considers herself to be pretty health conscious, although she has been battling gastritis for the last three years. She is dealing with this medical issue by eating healthy and by exercising.

Herminia maintains a healthy diet by consuming plenty of fruits and vegetables on a daily basis. In addition, she always meets her doctor to ensure that she is on the right track. Although, Herminia's parents did not struggle with gastritis, her daughter and granddaughter battle with gastritis as she does. Herminia wishes she would have handled her health concern better by being more cautious and aware of the situation. In the beginning, she took her health concern lightly and did not take enough measures to prevent further medical concerns. Herminia's lifestyle has drastically changed since she was a young adult. In her country, she struggled to make ends meet. She married young and worked long hours and admits that she did not eat three meals a day.

Coming to the United States was a complete blessing for her because now she always has food on the table, making her lifestyle more positive. Herminia advises other women to eat healthy and to be aware of their eating habits. For starters, she recommends that all women have at least three meals a day. Not only is physical health important, but mental health as well. She advises other women to not let others' bad habits influence your lifestyle.

QUOTES FROM FAMOUS, POSITIVELY AGING WOMEN

Whenever I go to New York or any European country,
they say: "Nawal, why don't you get a facelift?"
I tell them, "I am proud of my wrinkles.
Every wrinkle on my face tells the story of my life.
Why should I hide my age?"

—*Nawal El Saadawi, Egyptian Author*

When a noble life has prepared old age,
it is not decline that it reveals, but the first days of immortality.

—*Muriel Spark, English Novelist*

In the end, long life is the reward, strength, and beauty.

—*Grace Paley, American Author*

CHECK IT OUT!

The United States Office of Disease Prevention and Health Promotion launched an initiation for *Healthy People 2020*, one of the goals focuses specifically on older adults with the explicit goal to "improve the health, function and quality of life of older adults." Check out the website: www.healthypeople.gov/2020/topics-objectives/topic/older-adults

This website provides objectives (eg, "Reduce the proportion of older adults who have moderate to severe functional limitations"); interventions and resources ("Recommendations to increase physical activities in communities"); and provides a national profile of older adults. This website is a good resource for practitioners, older adults, and/or family/ friends who are interested in empirically based recommendations to help increase or maintain the heath and functional status of an aging person.

SOCIAL SUPPORT

Social support is generally and broadly defined as the offering of help performed by significant others for an individual (eg, Thoits, 2011). Social support can be categorized into three types: instrumental (eg, supplying tangible items,); informational (eg, offerings advice and helping to solve problems); and emotional (providing moral support, encouragement, etc.) (eg, House & Kahn, 1985). The relationship between social support and longevity and health is well established, such that greater perceived support is associated with more positive outcomes (eg, Berkman, Leo-Summers, & Horwitz, 1992; Ell, Nishimoto, Mediansky, Mantell, & Hamovitch, 1992).

A robust body of literature has shown that married individuals have lower mortality rates than unmarried people. For example, Kaplan and Kronick (2006) used the National Health and Interview Survey (NHIS) to determine if there was a relationship between marital status and longevity and found that the rates of death were highest for individuals who were (currently) unmarried than those individuals who were currently married and those individuals who were never married had the highest rates of premature mortality. This pattern of results was true for both male and female but the "never married effect" was weaker for females. Further, the change in status from married to unmarried is associated with an increase in poor health behaviors (Umberson, 1992). Stereotypical gender norms may also influence perceived and actual support given to a spouse as married men report more support from their spouse than do married women (Kristofferzon, Löfmark, & Carlsson, 2003) and women are more likely than are men to "control" the health behaviors of others (Umberson, 1992). Men report receiving emotional support primarily from their spouse; however, women receive more emotional support from their children, close relatives, and friends (Gurung, Taylor, & Seeman, 2003). In a large-scale study (sample size about 3500), older adults (age 65–84) were interviewed once at baseline and then again 12 years later in an effort to determine factors that contributed to positive aging, despite the number of predictors that were investigated only a few were able to predict positive aging, among these were having one's spouse still alive (Ross & Havens, 1991).

Friedman (1993) suggested that family versus nonfamily support, for older women may lead to differing outcomes. For example, nonfamily emotional and instrumental support was associated with lower positive affect and less life satisfaction. Likewise, Shor, Roelfs, and Yogev (2013) utilized meta-analysis to examine the relationship between social support and longevity and health and revealed that perceived social support from family members was associated with better outcomes than support from friends. Family relationships, in particular, may serve as a buffer for illness.

Interestingly, older adults living in rural areas may be at an increased risk for poor health, in part, because of their lack of access to a reliable social support network (eg, Johnson, 1996) and higher levels of education are related to a larger social support network (Ajrouch, Blandon, & Antonucci, 2005). Indeed, some research has shown that as individuals move into late adulthood the less educated become more deprived of social support relative to college-educated older adults (Fischer & Beresford, 2015) and these items in turn lead to poorer outcomes among aging women.

Promisingly, some work has shown that elderly patients perceive their social support to be available and reliable and are satisfied with the level of support provided by their network of friends and family (eg, Hildingh, Segesten, & Fridlund, 1997). One study demonstrated that around 90% of women who had recently undergone surgery indicated that they had a social network who provided them with support (Hildingh & Fridlund, 1997). As individuals age, the number of friends that they report do not usually decrease and evaluations of support from those friends become more positive (eg, Schnittker, 2007). Although the research is clear about the link between social support and health and longevity, older adults report being satisfied with their social network.

EDUCATION

The relationship between educational achievement and health and longevity is well established. Pinsky, Leaverton, and Stokes (1987) in a longitudinal design explored which factors lead people to survive longer and report good overall functioning compared to those individuals with premature mortality and poorer overall functioning. Of a number of potential factors (eg, alcohol consumption, cigarette smoking, education), the only significant predictor of good health-related functioning besides chronological age was education and, not surprisingly, education was positively associated with reports of good functioning. In Berkman and colleagues' study (Berkman et al., 1993), older adults who were categorized as "low functioning" were less likely than "high functioning" older adults to have completed high school. In one study of 70- to 75-year-olds, theoretical models were tested to examine which factors could predict cognitive change over a 2 to 2½-year period, of the 22 variables tested, four variables were predictors of cognitive change in that 2-year period: self-efficacy, pulmonary flow rate, physical activity, and, importantly educational achievement (Albert et al., 1995). Relatedly, blue-collar work and low education levels have been associated with dementia-related diseases (eg, Fratiglioni, Winblad, & von Strauss, 2007).

Although, cognitive decline was once presumed to be an expected outcome of aging, Gould, Reeves, Graziano, and Gross (1999) have found that adults (primates) are capable of growing new neurons (ie, neurogenesis) throughout the entire duration of their life. This line of research is the first to demonstrate that neurons that have died or are damaged are capable of producing more. Additionally, aging adults can practice certain cognitive strategies to increase the ability to age successfully as it relates to cognitive functioning (Vance et al., 2008).

Interestingly, Ross and Wu (1996) have shown that the gap in health-related areas increases among those individuals with high and low educational achievement as age increases. In other words, the differences in health outcomes are more discriminating in older age between higher and lower educated adults. Although, intelligence is a slightly different construct than educational attainment, some researchers (eg, Gottfredson & Deary, 2004) have shown that childhood IQ can predict mortality and disease in adulthood. Finally, negative affect may mediate the relationship between education and positive aging, such that higher educational achievement is associated with decreased levels of negative affect (Meeks & Murrell, 2001).

HEALTHY CHOICES: SMOKING AND PHYSICAL ACTIVITY

In short, adults who make healthy choices in terms of smoking (or more specifically, lack thereof), and physical exercise report more enjoyment and satisfaction with life and tend to have fewer incidences of disease, disability, and premature mortality. In fact, McGinnis and Foege (1993) showed that the two leading (nongenetic) factors that contribute to death are tobacco use and physical inactivity. Ferrucci and colleagues (1999) argued that no other intervention has a greater likelihood of improving health status in aging adults than the cessation of smoking and the promotion of physical exercise and these measures may be the most cost-effective way to reduce healthcare expenses.

In more specific examples, older adults who fell into a "high functioning" group exercised more and smoked less than an "impaired functioning" group (Berkman et al., 1993) and women who were "nonsmokers" survived about 1.5 to 3.5 years longer than women who were "smokers" but the length of survival was dependent on the degree of physical activity (Ferrucci et al., 1999).

Physical Activity

Many empirical studies reveal that physical activity may be the single best thing that one can do to increase the chances of positive aging and that almost all diseases that lead to disability in aging adults can be explained, in large part, by the absence of physical activity (Williamson & Pahor, 2010). In short, the role of physical activity on health, well-being, and longevity cannot be understated. Physically inactive adults were significantly more likely to have some sort of disability in the year(s) prior to death than adults who regularly engaged in physical activity (Ferrucci et al., 1999; Leveille, Guralnik, Ferrucci, & Langlois, 1999).

Physical activity does not have to be extensive in order to make great gains, exercise programs that include walking have been shown to lead to increased cognitive functioning for older adults (eg, Weuve, Kang, Manson, Breteler, Ware, & Grodstein, 2004), and this pattern of results holds true even when controlling for potential confounding factors such as educational achievement, tobacco use, and other comorbid conditions (Yaffe, Barnes, Nevitt, Lui, & Covinsky, 2001). The relationship between physical activity and health status is linear, such that the more physically active a person is, the more positive the health gains (eg, Lee & Skerrett, 2001; Warburton, Nicol, & Bredin, 2006). Indeed moderate and high levels of exercise were associated with a 1.5 to 3.5 year increase in life expectancy and 1.3 to 3.3 increase of living without cardiovascular disease in women. (Franco et al., 2005) and moderate levels of physical activity showed an increase in disability-free years and this effect was greater with higher levels of physical activity (both groups were compared to low physical activity older adults) (Nusselder et al., 2008).

One group of researchers investigated healthy women at baseline (ie, those women who were free of major chronic diseases) and then again when (if) they turned 70 years old. Women who had higher physical activity levels at midlife were significantly more likely to enjoy a "successful survival" (ie, free of chronic disease, no physical or cognitive impairment, and no mental health issues) than those with a more sedentary lifestyle (Sun et al., 2010), active older adults also report greater happiness levels (Menec, 2003). Women who change their physical activity levels between a baseline and follow-up measures had lower mortality rates than women who remained sedentary over time; however, the influence of exercise was less evident for women aged 75 and older (Gregg et al., 2003). And, women who increased their levels of activity showed a reduction (by about 25%, or more) of risk of death (Oguma, Sesso, Paffenbarger, & Lee, 2002).

Smoking Behavior

The benefits of never smoking, or quitting smoking, even at an advanced age have been consistently and reliably established. Not surprisingly, smoking reduces life expectancy and those who quit smoking live longer, on average, than those who continue to smoke (eg, Ozasa et al., 2008).

Quitting tobacco use prior to the age of 40 reduced the chances of dying from a smoking-related illness by almost 90% (Centers for Disease Control and Prevention, 2014). About 25 years ago, lung cancer became the leading cause of cancer among women, a record previously held by breast cancer (Centers for Disease Control and Prevention, 2008). The health implication of tobacco use may be greater for females as a large percentage of women in their 50s and 60s report being "current" rather than "former" smokers but the opposite pattern holds true for aging men (King, Taylor, & Haskell, 1990) and the pattern of cessation in older adults was consistently higher for men than for women (Husten et al., 1997).

Smoking cigarettes has an expansive range of health implications such as premature mortality (eg, Jha et al., 2013; Rogers & Powell-Griner, 1991), an increase in cognitive-related impairments (Anstey, von Sanden, Salim, & O'Kearney, 2007), stroke, heart attack (Centers for Disease Control and Prevention, 2008), and depression (McClave et al., 2009). Thus, smoking cigarettes has an enormous influence on whether women will enjoy health and longevity.

TRY IT OUT!

How long will you live? Take the following longevity quiz to get an estimate of your life span as a function of your (current) daily lifestyle choices. The quiz takes into account certain factors that are known to be associated with longevity such as physical activity, eating and drinking habits, and family medical history: http://www.northwesternmutual. com/games/longevity

Some things to consider:

1. Were you surprised by your results? Why or why not?
2. What is the one factor that you can easily change to help lead a more healthy life?
3. Each longevity question provides information based on current research. What information was most interesting or surprising to you?

INTERVENTIONS

Research suggests that positive aging may be predicted by factors that occur before midlife suggesting that people have some influence over their health and longevity (Vaillant & Mukamal, 2001) and that adults may benefit from interventions well before old age. Likewise, given that many older women may be low income the interventions should be cost-effective and community based in an effort to capitalize on social support (Shapiro & Taylor, 2002). Interventions that have been tailored to meet the needs of the individual also appear to be the most effective in term of changing behavior (Greaney et al., 2008; Rimer et al., 1994).

Given the relationship between social support and quality of life for aging adults, it is important to identify the most positive ways to utilize support. Interventions that attempt to focus on social support should take into account the differing association between perceived support and gender (Pérez-Garcia, Ruiz, Sanjuan, & Reuda, 2011) as evidence shows that men and women respond to social support in differing ways (eg, Caetano, Silva, & Vettore, 2013) and men and women rely on different people for support (eg, spouse versus friends and children).

A number of social support interventions have shown promise but the differing effects of one-on-one, professional and peer lead support still need to be examined in order to determine the types of interventions that are most effective under certain life circumstances (eg, Dickens, Richards, Greaves, & Campbell, 2011; Findlay, 2003). As noted earlier, however, many older adults are satisfied with the level of support that they receive from their friends and family (eg, Hildingh et al., 1997).

Older adults may be unable and/or unwilling to increase their educational achievement in older age; however, attempts can be made to increase their cognitive functioning. Clearly, cognitive functioning is an important component of positive aging, health, and longevity. One line of work that has shown encouraging results without associated negative side effects (as may be the case with pharmaceutical interventions) is cognitive behavioral interventions, such as memory training (Shumaker, Legault, & Coker, 2006). ACTIVE (Advanced Cognitive Training for Independent and Vital Elderly) focuses on such cognitive behavior interventions by using cognitive training. For example, in one case, older adults may be asked to identify objects on a computer screen at speeds that increase over time. ACTIVE demonstrated some positive outcomes for aging adults over a 5-year span of time (Willis et al., 2006). Finally, Vance et al. (2008) argued that healthcare professionals are in critical positions for relaying information about measures to increase cognitive function. Specifically, cognitive activities should be challenging and novel such that the activity should make the participants "brain sweat" in order to make the greatest strides.

As previously discussed the promotion of exercise and cessation of cigarette smoking may be the most effective prescription for positive aging. The cessation of smoking behavior in older adults raises a unique set of challenges versus cessation in younger cohorts, as it appears that older adults subscribe to inaccurate beliefs about smoking, such as believing that there is "no benefit to quitting at an advanced age" (Donze, Ruffieux, & Cornuz, 2007). Thus, attempts should be made to make sure older adults are properly informed regarding the benefits (even in older age) of quitting smoking. A number of interventions to promote physical activity have shown remarkable results with a number of these demonstrating that social support is a key factor to increasing physical activity levels, especially for older woman (eg, Booth, Owen, Bauman, Clavisi, & Leslie, 2000; Seefeldt, Malina, & Clark, 2002).

SUMMARY

No single variable is responsible for quality of life and longevity; however, most of the variables that are related to positive aging are modifiable (eg, exercise, smoking cessation). The relationships between factors such as income, social support, education, physical activity, and cigarette smoking are well established and robust. Care should be taken to properly advise aging adults, especially the "young-old" as steps can be taken to ensure more positive aging. The tailoring of programs should provide a more powerful intervention for aging adult women.

DISCUSSION QUESTIONS

1. What role does physical activity play in increasing the changes of health and longevity?
2. What is the role of education programs to assist older women to age successfully?
3. What are some ways that an aging woman can increase her cognitive capacity as she ages?
4. What are some of the differences between men and women, in terms of social support, as they age?
5. Are there gender-specific activities that best support women's positive aging?
6. Some factors associated with health and longevity can be changed (eg, increasing physical activity); however, others are not as malleable (eg, education level, socioeconomic status). Can anything be done to help women who have not achieved higher levels of education and/or socioeconomic status to age successfully?
7. How does early education help to increase health longevity for women?
8. How might tailoring intervention programs be more beneficial than using a "one-size-fits-all" approach?
9. How does social support influence (other) positive aging factors (eg, smoking cessation, physical exercise)? Can social support be used to design a more successful intervention? How?
10. If you were to design a positive aging intervention, which factors would be the most important? Why?

TEST YOUR KNOWLEDGE!

Research the Japanese island of Okinawa. The elderly Okinawans have both the longest and healthiest life expectancy in the world. Specifically, Okinawans do NOT seem to have diseases often associated with aging (eg, stroke, heart disease). Consequently, many researchers are interested in learning more about genetic and lifestyle choices among Okinawans.

Check out this website about the Okinawa Centenarian study: http://www.okicent.org/

Consider some of the following questions:

1. What are some of the factors that this population has in common?
2. Is it possible to apply these changes to the Western way of living?
3. How is this consistent (or inconsistent) with the factors discussed in this chapter?

SUPPLEMENTAL BOOK READINGS

Over the past decades, there have been many books written on the topic of women and health longevity. Here are some recommended *additional readings*:

Willcox, B. J., Willcox, D. C., & Suzuki, M. (2002). *The Okinawa program: How the world's longest-lived people achieve everlasting health—and how you can too.* New York, NY: Harmony.

   The authors present information about aging health and longevity based upon finding from the Okinawa Centenarian Study which was sponsored by the Japanese Ministry. The authors, experts in the field, suggest specific exercise, diet, and lifestyle factors to be followed beginning with a 4-week "Turnaround Plan" with an easy-to-follow exercise and diet plan (100 recipes).

Angel, J. L., Fernando Torres-Gil (Editor), & Kyriakos Markides (Editor) (2012). *Aging, health, and longevity in the Mexican-origin population.* New York, NY: Springer.

   Aging, Health, and Longevity in the Mexican-Origin Population raises an important issue of examining the bi-national perspective of aging adults of Mexican origin who are faced with increasing disabilities and long-term care needs. This segment of the US population is growing but their needs have not been adequately addressed in community program and public policies. This book is relevant to older women in this cultural context, as well as other cultural groups of need, who are in need of support resources for their positive aging outcomes.

Landry, R. (2014). *Live long, die short: A guide to authentic health and successful aging*. Austin, TX: Greenleaf Book Group Press.
The author encourages readers to do a "lifestyle inventory" to assess a woman's health status. After completing the checklist, Dr Landry offers 10 tips to change personal health for positive aging. This is a great resource for both laypeople, caregivers, and practitioners who desire to achieve positive aging and shift perspectives on what it means to get "older" in society.

Pfeiffer, E. (2013). *Winning strategies for successful aging*. New Haven, CT: Yale University Press.
The book presents advice on how to live life to the fullest in an easy-to-follow manner. The book outlines practical ways to achieve and optimize positive independence, mental well-being, financial stability, social engagement, and physical health status. The author also emphasizes older adults having an active sexual life and incorporating spirituality into one's daily activities. Finally, the author discusses the need to have a "good death." This is a wonderful resource and a practical guide for aging women who are looking for ways to change their lifestyle in a balanced, holistic manner. The book is filled with anecdotes and poems supporting the theoretical ideas presented.

Wykle, M. L., Whitehouse, P. J., & Morris, D. L. (Editors) (2004). *Successful aging through the life span: Intergenerational issues in health*. New York, NY: Springer Publishing Company.
This book explores concepts and practices for productive aging. The book's authors suggest ways to improve the aging process and, across topics, empower older adults to be more proactive in improving this process on a personal and societal level. Chapters presented examine multigenerational issues in positive aging. Importantly, the content of the book also examines how the physical and social environment of an older adult can be optimized to support positive aging outcomes for all involved.

Robbins, J. (2006). *Healthy at 100: The scientifically proven secrets of the world's healthiest and longest-lived peoples*. New York, NY: Random House.
This book is a great, "user-friendly" informational resource for adults and caregivers interested in advice for better diet and exercise regimes. Some of the advice may be more light-hearted in nature than based on empirical evidence but it is an entertaining book with a positive message about what it means to positively

age. Older women may be interested in the general optimistic message communicated through the content of the topics presented.

Giampapa, V. C. (2003). *Breaking the aging code: Maximizing your DNA function for optimal health and longevity*. Addison, IL: Basic Health Publications.

The author explains aging on a cellular level, and examines the impact of environmental toxins and other "assaults" to progressive aging changes in the human body. The author suggests a pro-active approach to aging, using exercise, diet, and "mind-body" techniques to reduce potential cellular damage and to optimize healthy aging from the cellular level outward.

SUPPLEMENTAL AGING VIDEOS

For learning purposes, the use of videos can be very beneficial for both instructors and readers. Here are some recommended *supplemental videos*:

Different video links on aging health: http://www.healthvideo.com/sitemap.php (Format: Website)

This is a great website that offers short videos on different aging-related health.

Different videos on human development: http://www.learner.org (Format: Website)

Supported by the Annenberg Foundation, this website offers several video series on human development and aging. Videos are approximately 60 min in length.

Health & Wellness among Older Adults: Challenges and Strategies (Format: DVD)

This DVD offers practical advice regarding how to prevent serious health conditions through preventative strategies. The program empowers aging adults to "know thyself" in terms of functional strengths and weaknesses. This message is great for older women who may need to optimize their positive aging outcomes through increased activities and behaviors related to personal strengths.

How to Live Forever (Format: DVD)

Description: An interesting documentary exploring the issue of different perspectives and lifestyle factors underlying the issue of living "forever." The social, practical, and ethical concerns underlying this intriguing topic are discussed from researchers and other people in society. The meaning of aging is debated, as well as an important distinction between quality of life and quantity of life.

ADDITIONAL INFORMATION LINKS

The following are some recommended *supplemental Internet links*:

Administration on Aging website: http://www.aoa.gov/AoARoot/ AoA_Programs/Tools_Resources/diversity.aspx/

American Society on Aging website: http://www.asaging.org/ diversity/

Centers for Disease Control and Prevention website: http://www.cdc. gov/physicalactivity/downloads/growing_stronger.pdf

NIA/NIH website: http://www.nia.nih.gov/about/minority-aging-and-health-disparities

References

Ajrouch, K. K., Blandon, A. Y., & Antonucci, T. C. (2005). Social networks among men and women: The effects of age and socioeconomic status. *Journal of Gerontology, 60*(6), 311–317.

Albert, M. S., Jones, K., Savage, C. R., Berkman, L., Seeman, T., Blazer, D., et al. (1995). Predictors of cognitive change in older persons: MacArthur studies of successful aging. *Psychology and Aging, 10*(4), 578.

Anstey, K. J., von Sanden, C., Salim, A., & O'Kearney, R. (2007). Smoking as a risk factor for dementia and cognitive decline: A meta-analysis of prospective studies. *American Journal of Epidemiology, 166*, 367–378.

Austin, C. D. (1991). Aging well: What are the odds? *Generations, 15*(1), 73–75.

Baker, J. L. (1958). The unsuccessful aged. *Journal of the American Geriatrics Society, 7*, 570–572.

Bassuk, S. S., Berkman, L. S., & Amick, B. C. (2002). Socioeconomic status and mortality among the elderly: Findings from four U.S. communities. *American Journal of Epidemiology, 155*(6), 520–533.

Berkman, L., Leo-Summers, L., & Horwitz, R. I. (1992). Emotional support and survival after myocardial infarction – A prospective, population-based study of the elderly. *Annals of Internal Medicine, 117*(12), 1003–1009.

Berkman, L., Seeman, T. E., Albert, M., Blazer, D. G., Kahn, R. L., & Mohs, R. (1993). High, usual and impaired functioning in community-dwelling older men and women: Findings from the MacArthur Foundation Research Network on successful aging. *Journal of Clinical Epidemiology, 46*(10), 1129–1140.

Booth, M., Owen, N., Bauman, A., Clavisi, O., & Leslie, E. (2000). Social–cognitive and perceived environment influences associated with physical activity in older Australians. *Preventive Medicine, 31*, 15–22.

Caetano, S. C., Silva, C., & Vettore, M. (2013). Gender difference in the association of perceived social support and social network with self-rated health status among older adults: A population based study in Brazil. *BMC Geriatrics, 13*, 122.

Cattan, M., White, M., Bond, J., & Learmouth, A. (2005). Preventing social isolation and loneliness among older people: A systematic review of health promotion interventions. *Ageing & Society, 25*(1), 41–67.

Centers for Disease Control and Prevention. (2008). Smoking-attributable mortality, years of potential life lost, and productivity losses – United States, 2000–2004 <http://www.cdc.-gov/mmwr/-preview/mmwrhtml/mm5745a3.htm>.

Centers for Disease Control and Prevention. (2014). Tobacco-related mortality <http://www.cdc.-gov/tobacco/-data_statistics/fact_sheets/health_effects/tobacco_related_mortality/>.

Depp, C. A., & Jeste, D. V. (2006). Definitions and predictors of successful aging: A comprehensive review of larger quantitative studies. *American Journal of Geriatric Psychiatry*, 14, 6–20.

Dickens, A., Richards, S., Greaves, C., & Campbell, J. (2011). Interventions targeting social isolation in older people: A systematic review. *BMC Public Health*, 11, 647–669.

Donze, J., Ruffieux, C., & Cornuz, J. (2007). Determinants of smoking and cessation in older women. *Age and Ageing*, 36(1), 53–57.

Ell, K., Nishimoto, R., Mediansky, L., Mantell, J., & Hamovitch, M. (1992). Social relations, social support and survival among patients with cancer. *Journal of Psychosomatic Research*, 36(6), 531–541.

Ferrucci, L., Izmirlian, G., Leveille, S., Phillips, C. L., Corti, M., Brock, D. B., et al. (1999). Smoking, physical activity, and active life expectancy. *American Journal of Epidemiology*, 149(7), 645–653.

Findlay, R. (2003). Interventions to reduce social isolation amongst older people: Where is the evidence? *Ageing and Society*, 23(5), 647–658.

Fischer, C. S., & Beresford, L. (2015). Changes in support networks in late middle age: The extension of gender and educational difference. *The Journal of Gerontology*, 70(1), 123–131.

Franco, O. H., deLaet, C., Peeters, A., Jonker, J., Mackenbach, J., & Nusselder, W. (2005). Effects of physical activity on life expectancy with cardiovascular disease. *Archives of Internal Medicine*, 165(20), 2355–2360.

Fratiglioni, L., Winblad, B., & von Strauss, E. (2007). Prevention of Alzheimer's disease and Dementia: Major findings from the Kungsholmen project. *Physiological Behavior*, 92(1–2), 98–104.

Friedman, M. (1993). Social support sources and psychological well-being in older women with Heart disease. *Research in Nursing & Health*, 16(6), 405–413.

Gottfredson, L. S., & Deary, I. J. (2004). Intelligence predicts health and longevity, but why? *Current Directions in Psychological Science*, 13(1), 1–4.

Gould, E., Reeves, A. J., Graziano, M. S. A., & Gross, P. C. G. (1999). Neurogenesis in the neocortex of adult primates. *Science*, 286(l), 548–552.

Greaney, M. L., Riebe, D., Garber, C. E., Rossi, J. S., Lees, F. D., Burbank, P. A., et al. (2008). Long-term effects of a stage-based intervention for changing exercise intentions and behavior in older adults. *The Gerontologist*, 4(4), 358–367.

Gregg, E. W., Cauley, J. A., Stone, K., Thompson, T. J., Bauer, D. C., Cummings, S. R., et al. (2003). Relationship of changes in physical activity and mortality among older women. *JAMA*, 289(18), 2379–2386.

Guralnik, J. M., & Kaplan, G. A. (1989). Predictors of healthy aging: Prospective evidence from the Alameda County study. *American Journal of Public Health*, 79, 703–708.

Gurung, R., Taylor, S., & Seeman, T. (2003). Accounting for changes in social support among married older adults: Insights from the MacArthur Studies of successful aging. *Psychology and Aging*, 18(3), 487–496.

Hildingh, C., & Fridlund, B. (1997). Social network and experiences of social support among women 12 months after their first myocardial infarction. *International Journal of Rehabilitation and Health*, 3(2), 131–142.

Hildingh, C., Segesten, K., & Fridlund, B. (1997). Elderly persons' social network and need for social support after their first myocardial infarction. *Scandinavian Journal of Caring Sciences*, 11(1), 3–4.

House, J. S., & Kahn, R. L. (1985). Measures and concepts of social support. In S. Cohen & L. Syme (Eds.), *Social support and health* (pp. 83–108). San Diego, CA: Academic Press.

Huguet, N., Kaplan, M. S., & Feeny, D. (2008). Socioeconomic status and health-related quality of life among elderly people: Results from the joint Canada/United States survey of health. *Social Science & Medicine, 66*, 803–810.

Husten, C. G., Shelton, D. M., Chrismon, J. H., Lin, Y. W., Mowery, P., & Powell, F. A. (1997). Cigarette smoking and smoking cessation among older adults. United States 1965–1994. *Tobacco Control, 6*, 175–180.

Jha, P., Ramasundarahettige, C., Landsman, V., Rostrom, B., Thun, M., Anderson, R., et al. (2013). 21st century hazards of smoking and benefits of cessation in the United States. *The New England Journal of Medicine, 368*(4), 341–350.

Johnson, J. (1996). Social support and physical health in the rural elderly. *Applied Nursing Research, 9*(2), 61–66.

Kaplan, M. S., Huguet, N., Orpana, H., Feeny, D., McFarland, B. H., & Ross, N. (2008). Prevalence and factors associated with thriving in older adulthood: A 10-year population based study. *The Journals of Gerontology, 63*(10), 1097–2004.

Kaplan, R. M., & Kronick, R. G. (2006). Marital status and longevity in the United States population. *Journal of Epidemiology and Community Health, 60*, 76–765.

King, A. C., Taylor, C. B., & Haskell, W. L. (1990). Smoking in older women: Is being female a "risk factor" for continued cigarette use? *JAMA, 150*(9), 1841–1846.

Kristofferzon, M., Löfmark, R., & Carlsson, M. (2003). Myocardial infarction: Gender differences in coping and social support. *Journal of Advanced Nursing, 44*(4), 360–374.

Lee, I. M., & Skerrett, P. J. (2001). Physical activity and all-cause mortality: What is the dose-response relation? *Medicine and Science in Sports and Exercise, 33*(6), 459–471.

Lee, S., & Shaw, L. (2008). *From work to retirement: Tracking changes in women's poverty.* Washington, DC: AARP. Retrieved from <http://www.aarp.org/research/assistance/-lowincome/2008_03_poverty.html>.

Leveille, S. G., Guralnik, J. M., Ferrucci, L., & Langlois, J. A. (1999). Aging successfully until death in old age: Opportunities for increasing active life expectancy. *American Journal of Epidemiology, 149*(7), 654–664.

McClave, A. K., Dube, S. R., Strine, T. W., Kroenke, K., Caraballo, R. S., & Mokdad, A. H. (2009). Associations between smoking cessation and anxiety and depression among U.S. adults. *Addictive Behaviors, 34*(6–7), 491–497.

McGinnis, J. M., & Foege, W. H. (1993). Actual causes of death in the United States. *JAMA, 12*, 2207–2212.

Meeks, S., & Murrell, S. A. (2001). Contribution of education to the health and life satisfaction in older adults mediated by negative affect. *Journal of Aging and Health, 13*, 92–119.

Menec, V. (2003). The relation between everyday activities and successful aging: A 6-year longitudinal study. *The Journal of Gerontology, 58*(2), 74–82.

Montross, L. P., Depp, C., Daly, J., Reichstadt, J., Golshan, S., Moore, D., et al. (2006). Correlates of self-rated successful aging among community-dwelling older adults. *American Journal of Geriatric Psychiatry, 14*, 43–51.

Nusselder, W. J., Looman, C. W., Franco, O. H., Peeters, A., Slingerland, A. S., & Mackenbach, J. P. (2008). The relation between no-occupational physical activity and years lived with and without disability. *Journal of Epidemiology and Community Health, 62*(9), 823–828.

Odubanjo, E., Bennett, K., & Feely, J. (2004). Influence of socioeconomic status on the quality of prescribing in the elderly – A population based study. *British Journal of Clinical Pharmacology, 58*(5), 496–502.

Oguma, Y., Sesso, H. D., Paffenbarger, R. S., & Lee, I. M. (2002). Physical activity and all cause mortality in women: A review of the evidence. *British Journal of Sports Medicine, 36*, 162–172.

Ozasa, K., Katanoda, K., Tamakoshi, A., Sato, H., Tajima, K., Suzuki, T., et al. (2008). Reduced life expectancy due to smoking in large-scale cohort studies in Japan. *Journal of Epidemiology, 18*(3), 111–118.

Pérez-Garcia, A., Ruiz, M., Sanjuan, P., & Reuda, B. (2011). The association of social support and gender with life satisfaction, emotional symptoms and mental adjustment in patients following a first cardiac coronary event. *Stress and Health, 27*(3), e252–e260.

Phelan, E. A., Anderson, L. A., Lacroix, A. Z., & Larson, E. B. (2004). Older adults' views of successful aging-how so they compare with researchers' definitions? *Journal of the American Geriatrics Society, 52*(2), 211–216.

Pinquart, M., & Sorensen, S. (2000). Influences of socioeconomic status, social network, and competence on subjective well-being in later life: A meta-analysis. *Psychology & Aging, 15*(2), 187–224.

Pinsky, J. L., Leaverton, P. E., & Stokes, J. (1987). Predictors of good function: The Framingham study. *Journal of Chronic Diseases, 40,* 1595–1675.

Rimer, B. K., Orleans, C. T., Fleisher, L., Cristinzio, S., Resch, N., Telepchak, J., et al. (1994). Does tailoring matter? The impact of a tailored guide on ratings and short-term smoking-related outcomes for older smokers. *Health Education Research, 9*(1), 69–84.

Rogers, R. G., & Powell-Griner, E. (1991). Life expectancies of cigarette smokers and non-smokers in the United States. *Social Science & Medicine, 32*(10), 1151–1159.

Ross, C. E., & Wu, C. (1996). Education, age, and the cumulative advantage in health. *Journal of Health and Social Behavior, 37,* 104–120.

Ross, N. P., & Havens, B. (1991). Predictors of successful aging: A twelve-year study of Manitoba elderly. *American Journal of Public Health, 81,* 63–69.

Rowe, J. W., & Kahn, R. L. (1987). Human aging: Usual and successful. *Science, 237,* 143–149.

Rowe, J. W., & Kahn, R. L. (1998). *Successful aging.* New York, NY: Pantheon.

Schnittker, J. (2007). Look (closely) at all the lonely people: Age and the social psychology of social support. *Journal of Aging and Health, 19*(4), 659–682.

Seefeldt, V., Malina, R., & Clark, M. (2002). Factors affecting levels of physical activity in adults. *Sports Medicine, 32*(3), 143–168.

Shapiro, A., & Taylor, M. (2002). Effects of a community-based early intervention program on the subjective well-being, institutionalization, and mortality of low-income elders. *The Gerontologist, 42*(3), 334–341.

Shor, E., Roelfs, D. J., & Yogev, T. (2013). The strength of family ties: A meta-analysis and meta-regression of self-reported social support and mortality. *Social Networks, 35*(4), 626–638.

Shumaker, S. A., Legault, C., & Coker, L. H. (2006). Behavior-based interventions to enhance cognitive functioning and independence in older adults. *JAMA, 296*(23), 2852–2854.

Strawbridge, W. J., Wallhagen, M. I., & Cohen, R. D. (2002). Successful aging and wellbeing: Self-rated compared with Rowe and Kahn. *Gerontologist, 42,* 727–733.

Sun, Q., Townsend, M. K., Okereke, O. I., Franco, O. H., Hu, F. B., & Grodstein, F. (2010). Physical activity at midlife in relation to successful survival in women at age 70 years or older. *JAMA, 170*(2), 194–201.

Szanton, S. L., Seplaki, C. L., Thorpe, R. J., Allen, J. K., & Fried, L. P. (2010). Socioeconomic status is associated with frailty: The women's health and aging studies. *Journal of Epidemiological Community Health, 64,* 63–67.

Thoits, P. (2011). Mechanisms linking social ties and support to physical and mental health. *Journal of Health and Social Behavior, 52*(2), 145–161.

Umberson, D. (1992). Gender, marital status and the social control of health. *Social Science & Medicine, 34*(8), 907–917.

Vaillant, G. E., & Mukamal, K. (2001). Successful aging. *The American Journal of Psychiatry, 158*(6), 839–847.

Vance, D. E., Webb, M. N., Marceaux, J. C., Viamonte, S. M., Foote, A. W., & Ball, K. K. (2008). Mental stimulation, neural plasticity, and aging: Directions for nursing research and practice. *The Journal of Neuroscience Nursing, 40*(4), 241–249.

Warburton, D. E. R., Nicol, C. W., & Bredin, S. S. D. (2006). Health benefits of physical activity: The evidence. *CMAJ, 174*(6), 801–809.

Weuve, J., Kang, J., Manson, J. E., Breteler, M. M. B., Ware, J., & Grodstein, F. (2004). Physical activity, including walking, and cognitive function in older women. *JAMA, 292*(12), 1454–1461.

Williamson, J., & Pahor, M. (2010). Evidence regarding the benefits of physical exercise. *JAMA Internal Medicine, 170*(2), 124–125.

Willis, S. L., Tennstedt, S. L., Marsiske, M., Ball, K., Elias, J., Koepke, K. M., et al. (2006). Long term effects of cognitive training on everyday functional outcomes in older adults. *JAMA, 296*(23), 2805–2814.

Wong, P. T. P. (1989). Personal meaning and successful aging. *Canadian Psychology, 30,* 516–525.

World Health Organization. (2014). Facts about ageing. Retrieved from: <http://www.who. int/ageing/about/facts/en/>.

Yaffe, K., Barnes, D., Nevitt, M., Lui, L., & Covinsky, K. (2001). A prospective study of physical activity and cognitive decline in elderly women: Women who walk. *JAMA, 161*(14), 1703–1708.

7

Importance of Daily Physical Activity for Older Women

Global Fact: *The majority of the world's older persons (51 percent) live in urban areas. By 2025, this is expected to climb to 62 percent of older persons, although large differences exist between more and less developed regions.*
—*Global Aging* **(2001)**

As with mental aerobics, the "use it or lose it" principle will be applied to the important factor of being physically active in later life for women's positive aging. In addition to identifying factors that support aging women's physical activity, "holistic" activity outcomes of being mentally, socially, and psychologically engaged within one's social environment for women will be discussed.

BEING ACTIVE IS A QUALITY-OF-LIFE ISSUE

Older adults are the least physically active age group relative to all other age groups (Centers for Disease Control and Prevention, 2003). A sedentary lifestyle has been shown to be an independent risk factor for health issues (eg, King, 2001). The aging population, and women specifically, face unique physical challenges as they age (eg, falling). Vertinsky (1995) argued that many aging women hold stereotypes and assumptions about physical activity, such as an inaccurate assessment of risk that prevents them from engaging in regular physical exercise. Likewise, O'Brien (2000) interviewed about 150 older women (aged 70 and over) and found that many of these women held misconceptions about physical activity and did not necessarily believe that the benefits outweigh the cost of engaging in exercise.

TEST YOURSELF!

Older Women's Activity Questionnaire

Source: Rantanen, T., Guralnik, J. M., Sakari-Rantala, R., Leveille, S., Simonsick, E. M., Ling, S., & Fried, L. P. (1999). Disability physical activity and muscle strength in older women: The women's health and aging study. *Archives of Physical Medicine and Rehabilitation, 80*, 130–135.

1. Number of blocks walked in past week (circle one choice):
   0 weeks   1 to 5 blocks   >=6 blocks
2. Number of flights of stairs climbed in past week (circle one choice):
   0 weeks   2 to 21 flights   >=6 flights
3. Heavy household chores in past 2 weeks (circle one choice):
   no   yes
4. Heavy outdoor work chores in past 2 weeks (circle one choice):
   no   yes
5. Regular exercise in past 2 weeks (circle one choice):
   no   yes
6. Dancing in past 2 weeks (circle one choice):
   no   yes
7. Bowling in past 2 weeks (circle one choice):
   no   yes

Scoring:	Finding	Points
1. number of blocks walked in past week	0	0
	1 to 5	1
	>=6	2
2. number of flights of stairs climbed in past week	0	0
	2 to 21	1
	>=22	2
3. heavy household chores in past 2 weeks	No	0
	Yes	1
4. heavy outdoor work chores in past 2 weeks	No	0
	Yes	1
5. regular exercise in past 2 weeks	No	0
	Yes	1
6. dancing in past 2 weeks	No	0
	Yes	1
7. bowling in past 2 weeks	No	0
	Yes	1

Total Points: 0 = very inactive, 1–3 points = very inactive, 4 >= moderately active

In sum, these women perceived themselves to be "physically vulnerable." The data generally support that younger adults are more physically active than older adults and men are more physically active than women (Lubben, Weiler, & Chi, 1989). Therefore, it is not surprising to learn that significantly more female than male older adults report being physically inactive (Booth, Owen, Bauman, Clavisi, & Leslie, 2000).

Physical inactivity among aging women is problematic, as studies have reliably shown numerous benefits associated with physical fitness in the aging population. These benefits include increased endurance (eg, Keysor & Jette, 2001; Purath, Buchholz, & Kark, 2009), increased cognitive functioning (eg, Anstey & Smith, 1999; Colcombe & Kramer, 2003), enhanced brain volume (eg, Colcombe et al., 2006), improved quality of life (Koltyn, 2001), improved mood (Arent, Landers, & Etnier, 2000) and decreased depression (Christmas & Andersen, 2000; Singh, Clements, & Singh, 2001).

QUOTES FROM FAMOUS, POSITIVELY AGING WOMEN

Even though I'm not a competitive athlete,
I have to still maintain things and try to keep myself fit
because I am at that age where I need to make sure
to get those regular checkups and make sure everything is intact.
—*Jackie Joyner-Kersee, Olympic Athlete*

Beautiful young people are accidents of nature,
but beautiful old people are works of art.
—*Eleanor Roosevelt, Presidential First Lady and Activist*

The most important thing to do as you age is to stay physically active.
Lots of people just throw in the towel if they can't do
what they used to do, and that's terrible.
—*Jane Fonda, Actress, Activist, and Exercise Video Icon*

THE INFLUENCE OF PHYSICAL ACTIVITY ON THE BRAIN

The physical benefits of a routine and appropriate exercise program are numerous and it has been demonstrated that there is linear association between exercise and health status (Warburton, Nicol, & Bredin, 2006). In some cases, "virtual" age may be reduced by 20 years as a function of physical activity (Shephard, 1998). In a compelling longitudinal study, which lasted approximately 8 years, women who reported the most physical activity (in this case, the number of blocks walked/stairs climbed) were also the least likely to have cognitive impairment (Yaffe, Barnes, Nevitt, Lui, & Covinsky, 2001). Erickson and colleagues (2010) demonstrated, through experimental design, that aerobic (ie, cardio-vascular) exercise increased hippocampal volume thus reversing age-related loss by over a year. Finally, aerobic exercise is thought to be effective in thwarting brain aging and dementia, in that, aging adults who were physically fit had improved cognitive scores, larger hippo-campal volume, and reduced risk of dementia (Ahlskog, Geda, Graff-Radford, & Petersen, 2011).

Several researchers have demonstrated the profound effect of exercise on older women's well-being (eg, Williams & Lord, 1997). Strawbridge, Deleger, Roberts, and Kaplan (2002) conducted a persuasive longitudinal study that lasted 5 years and included around 2000 (50–94-year-olds, at baseline) participants. The researchers found that even when controlling for factors such as age, financial stress, and social relationships, greater physical activity was associated with less depression. Similarly in a sam-ple of older adults with low or high depression, both groups benefited (in terms of alleviated symptomatology) from aerobic (but not resistance) exercise (Penninx et al., 2002) and it may be the case that aging women benefit more than men, in terms of the lessening of depression symp-tomatology, from exercise (Lindwall, Rennemark, Halling, Berglund, & Hassmen, 2007).

THE INFLUENCE OF PHYSICAL ACTIVITY ON THE BODY

Milton et al. (2008) conducted a study where they randomly assigned older adults of ages 58–78 years to either an experimental/functional exercise or a traditional exercise condition. The experimental/functional exercise condition was intended to approximate work done around the home, such as carrying a laundry basket. Adults who were placed in the functional exercise condition scored significantly better in upper and lower body strength, respiratory endurance, and balance. An additional benefit of this research is that functional exercise programs are inexpen-sive to implement and designed to be done at home. Brach et al. (2003) also found that women who were consistently active had the best func-tional status and women who were consistently inactive had the worst functional status.

FACTORS THAT SUPPORT PHYSICAL ACTIVITY

There are several factors which can support the daily physical activity of women over the life span. These factors can be implemented through social programs and community-based education initiatives for women on a global basis.

Sense of Community

The social component of exercising with friends and/or family significantly increases motivation to engage in physical fitness, indeed, social support is a strong predictor of physical activity among aging adults (Booth et al., 2000). Gill and Overdorf (1994) concluded that both younger and older adult women who regularly exercise both acknowledged that health and physical activity were important to them; however, aging women were more likely to value the social aspects of exercise whereas younger women were more likely to value exercise as a means to control one's weight. Cousins (1996) purported that social reinforcement did the best job of predicting exercise among aging women. Similarly, research has found that different predictors are important for different stages of exercise (ie, "beginning" versus "maintaining" an exercise regime); however, long-term exercise behavior (measured at 12 months after beginning the exercise routine) was best predicted by social support for physical activity (Litt, Kleppinger, & Judge, 2002).

Research suggests that aging adults appear to benefit the most when they have a small circle of close friends (eg, Carstensen, Gross, & Fung, 1998), naturally then programs can take advantage of this by offering incentives for signing up for a class with close friends or family members (Godbey, Burnett-Wolle, & Chow, 2007). Dorgo, Robinson, and Bader (2009) conducted a study where older adults who were taking part in a fitness program were either paired with their peers or a professional (ie, a kinesiology student). Those adults who were paired with a peer demonstrated significantly better outcomes of physical and social health than individuals who were paired with a nonpeer mentor. Likewise, Ginis, Nigg, and Smith (2013) found no difference between peer- and professional-pairings for increasing physical activity suggesting that the implementation of exercise programs may be made more cost-effective and easier to implement by relying on resources already available (ie, peers). Social support for exercise appears to be most promising for older women who are transitioning from a sedentary to an active lifestyle; however, "regular exercisers" rely less on social support to help maintain their activity level (Eyler et al., 1999).

WORDS OF WISDOM

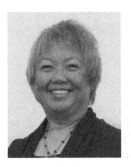

Lily retired one year ago at the age of 61 to take care of her husband who is fighting a disease called Peripheral Neuropathy. This debilitating disease causes loss of feeling in nerve endings. Since the symptoms have worsened, Lily's husband has been working from home where Lily takes care of him. Lily and her husband have been married for over 30 years. "He is my best friend," Lily stated. Before Lily's husband was diagnosed with Peripheral Neuropathy, Lily battled health issues of her own. At age 52, Lily suffered from a minor stroke. She recovered fully and, thankfully, has not experienced any devastating side effects. Shortly after her stroke, Lily slipped on ice and broke her ankle. This caused her to be immobile for some time. Then, at age 55, Lily was diagnosed with Type-2 diabetes. Lily was told she would have to go on medication to maintain her blood sugar level but Lily refused. Lily's doctor said she would need to exercise every day for an hour.

Since 2011, Lily has been working with a personal trainer. She has lost 50 pounds, has maintained a healthy and stable blood sugar level, and is no longer considered diabetic. Lily does not take medication, but instead "pumps iron."

Now, at the age of 62, Lily can dead lift 135 pounds, leg press 200 pounds, and free squat 115 pounds. Lily sword fights once a week with her grandson, and works out at least five to six times per week. She loves to stay active and is always seeking ways to stay physically involved in her daily activities. Lily advises women who are not regular exercisers to at least try to stay active—get up and walk around for 30 min a day. Take the extra trip up and down the stairs. Exercise has changed Lily's life. She wants other women to change their life, too. In Lily's words, "No excuses. Don't give up, and stay active!"

TRY IT OUT!

The *Age of Champions* documentary is "an award-winning PBS documentary following five competitors who sprint, leap, and swim for gold at the National Senior Olympics." The seniors interviewed have some interesting insights about competition, and the documentary highlights athletes who would arguably be considered successfully aging adults. Go online and check out the trailer: http://ageofchampions.org/

After you view the video clip, consider the following questions:

1. Are there any gender differences between the portrayals of the senior Olympians? If so, what are they?
2. What are the similarities and difference of the portrayal of the senior Olympians compared to traditional older athletes? Why is that important to understand?
3. What lessons from this video clip can be applied to all women across the world in terms of their daily activities?
4. What is the message about positive aging from this video clip?
5. After you viewed the video clip, what did you learn that surprised you? Why?
6. How can you apply the information you learned in order to better interact with older adults in your community?

Motivation

Interestingly, the motivation to work out differs depending on a number of factors. One study identified mobility as a factor that determines the underlying motivation to work out. For example, those with limited/impaired mobility stated that they were more likely to work out to manage any type of disease symptoms, while those who were more mobile cited "health promotion" and "positive experiences related to exercise" as motivating their exercise routine (Rasinaho, Hirvensalo, Leinonen, Lintunen, & Rantanen, 2006).

Aging adults who remain physically active and healthy as they age (dubbed "successfully aging adults") may use activity and competition as a coping mechanism in that it gives them a sense of meaning and purpose to one's life (O'Brien & Conger, 1991). One important way to support these initiatives is to understand potential barriers so they can be addressed and prevented.

BARRIERS TO WORKING OUT

Several research studies have sought to identify the unique barriers that exist to working out among aging adults. One study found that "caregiving duties" and "lack of energy" were consistently among the topmost reported obstacles (King et al., 2000). An expert panel was asked to make a determination of what personal factors might predict the initiation and adherence to an exercise plan among aging adults. The panel concluded that the top two personal characteristics were current health status and a history of exercise (Boyette et al., 2002). Several research studies (eg, Shepard, 1994; Williams & Lord, 1995) have shown that poor health and compromised mobility, especially among aging adults, are barriers to engaging in exercise.

Several constructs, such as self-efficacy and attitude toward exercise, are associated with regular exercise behavior (Rhodes et al., 1999). Different factors (eg, self-efficacy, social support, and age) influence adherence to an exercise regime throughout the duration of the exercise program (Brassington, Stienza, Perczek, DiLorenzo, & King, 2002). Jancey et al. (2007) demonstrated that individuals who dropped out of an exercise program tended to be from a lower socioeconomic background, were more likely to be overweight, and had lower self-efficacy scores (ie, related to walking) and higher loneliness scores. In one cross-sectional study of women who were between the ages of 20 and 85, age was inversely related to exercise self-efficacy scores (Sidney, Niinimaa, & Shepard, 1983). Finally, one study that explored barriers to achieving 10,000 steps per day among aging women found that women who did not meet the goal of 10,000 steps had lower self-efficacy scores than those women who did meet their goal (Hall & McAuley, 2010).

Neid and Franklin (2002) identified major barriers to working out for aging adults as well as approaches to counteract those barriers. The barriers include: low self-efficacy, poor attitude, discomfort, disability, poor balance, fear of injury, lack of social support, fixed income, environmental factors, cognitive decline, and poor health. Some recommendations to address these barriers include the utilization of assistive devices when working out, the use of a physical therapist or the employment of another person who can supervise the physical activity (at least initially), the recruitment of friends and/or others who can encourage/work out with the person, varying the intensity and range of exercise, and having the person begin small and then increase the intensity of the workout, as able. Phillips, Schneider, and Mercer (2004) offered similar recommendations, such as promotion of a gradual progression of exercise, socialization, and adapting exercises. These recommendations are especially important for aging adults who have some sort of physical impairment.

Finally, some past research (eg, Lee, 1993) suggested that aging women may be hesitant to attend classes and/or the gym and expressed concern over changing in a public locker room. One analysis revealed that aging adults were hesitant to go to the gym because they were embarrassed by their appearance, nervous about the competitive environment at the gym, or slowing down a group exercise class (Costello, Kafchinski, Vrazel, & Sullivan, 2011).

HOW MUCH PHYSICAL ACTIVITY SHOULD I DO?

Source: Womanshealth.gov

http://womenshealth.gov/publications/our-publications/fact-sheet/physical-activity.html

Health benefits are gained by doing the following each week:

- 2 h and 30 min of moderate-intensity aerobic physical activity *or*
- 1 h and 15 min of vigorous-intensity aerobic physical activity *or*
- A combination of moderate and vigorous-intensity aerobic physical activity *and*
- Muscle-strengthening activities on 2 or more days

This physical activity should be in addition to your routine activities of daily living, such as cleaning or spending a few minutes walking from the parking lot to your office.

Moderate Activity

During moderate-intensity activities you should notice an increase in your heart rate, but you should still be able to talk comfortably. An example of a moderate-intensity activity is walking on a level surface at a brisk pace (about 3 to 4 miles per hour). Other examples include ballroom dancing, leisurely bicycling, moderate housework, and waiting tables.

Vigorous Activity

If your heart rate increases a lot and you are breathing so hard that it is difficult to carry on a conversation, you are probably doing vigorous-intensity activity. Examples of vigorous-intensity activities include jogging, bicycling fast or uphill, singles tennis, and pushing a hand mower.

TIPS FOR WOMEN'S PHYSICAL ACTIVITIES

1. Choose activities that you enjoy.
2. Create a sensible list of activities to accomplish.
3. Be realistic about your physical limits.
4. Challenge yourself to keep improving within your capabilities.
5. Find someone to share the physical activities with.

Although, it should be noted that more than half of the aging adults who exercised regularly reported working out at the gym while only about a quarter reported working out at home (Bethancourt, Rosenberg, Beatty, & Arterburn, 2014). Several research projects have demonstrated that older adults are more likely to use the gym if they can exercise at her/his own pace, believe the staff to be competent, and they can work out with/feel supported by their peers (eg, Lübcke, Martin, & Hellström, 2012).

RECOMMENDATIONS/INTERVENTIONS

There is some evidence to suggest (eg, Gregg et al., 2003) that current physical activity levels are a better predictor of mortality rates and disease reduction than previous (ie, earlier in life) activity levels. Specifically, aging women who began an exercise program (ie, are currently physically active), even if they had been sedentary in their earlier life, had longevity rates comparable to aging women who had a history of being active. The reverse of this relationship also appears to hold true in that women who were physically active but became sedentary had mortality rates similar to women who had been sedentary most of their lives. There also is a clear link between an older adult's cognitive functioning and daily physical exercise (eg, Erickson et al., 2011; Weuve et al., 2008). Nelson et al. (2007) argued that given the myriad benefits of a regular physical activity, interventions to promote exercise should be widely implemented. In addition, improved mood and mental health have been found to result from such physical activities with older adults (Arent et al., 2000; Penninx et al., 2002; Shephard, 1998).

In general, the promotion of regular exercise should focus on both community-based and individual-level interventions, and the interaction between the two (Satariano & McAuley, 2003). Schutzer and Graves (2004) suggested that because older adults generally place a great deal of trust in their physician's opinion, doctors can play an important role in promoting and maintaining a physical exercise routine for their patients. Indeed, advice from a physician to increase exercise habits was a major predictor for aging adults to change their exercise behavior (Thomas et al., 2002). Interestingly, participants who were given a "prescription" to work out on a notepad were more likely to work out than individuals who were given the same advice verbally (Swinburn, Walter, Arroll, Tilyard, & Russell, 1998).

Active Start, a community-based fitness program, is one particular intervention that has received support for their programming. Specifically, those individuals who were a part of *Active Start* performed significantly better on all measures of performance (ie, strength, flexibility, and balance) than they did prior to the start of the program (Yan, Wilbur, & Aguirre, 2009). A similar intervention, *CHAMPS* (Community Health Activities Model Programming for Seniors) found that the promotion of exercise in already existing community-based programs leads to better results for those adults in the intervention group. Not surprisingly the intervention group was more active than the nonintervention group but the intervention group also scored higher on a measure of self-esteem and those participants who remained in the program for six months also reported better psychological well-being and less anxiety and depression than older adults who did not remain in the program for that period of time (Stewart et al., 1997).

Workplace interventions are also successful at promoting an active lifestyle (eg, Striik, Proper, van der Beek, & van Mechelen, 2012) and aging workers indicate that they feel positive about the intervention (Strijk, Proper, van der Beek, & van Mechelen, 2011). The most successful interventions capitalize on social support from friends and family, take into account initial levels of fitness, and allow for control over the exercise activity (Seefeldt, Malina, & Clark, 2002). Finally, the theory of planned behavior, which investigates the single and combined effects of behavioral beliefs, perceived behavioral control, and normative beliefs on the likelihood that a person will engage in a specific behavior (eg, exercise) may be a good starting point to designing exercise interventions for aging women (eg, Conn, Tripp-Reimer, & Maas, 2003). In short, behavioral intentions (eg, intent to exercise) can be positively predicted from a person's attitude toward performing the behavior, subjective norms (ie, what do others think about the behavior?), and perceived behavioral control (ie, how easy or difficult is it to perform the behavior?); thus behavior intentions are the single strongest predictors of engaging in a behavior (eg, Ajzen, 1991).

Wilcox, Castro, King, Housemann, and Brownson (2000) argued that interventions designed to increase physical activity in older women must take into account different contextual factors that may act as perceived barriers to working out. Specifically, rural and urban women perceive different obstacles to working out (eg, lack of sidewalks versus crime, respectively). In the same way, characteristics of particular neighbors predict the probability that older adults will walk for exercise. Predictably, the more walkable the neighborhood, the greater the increase in the number of older adults who reported walking as a daily activity (Berke, Koepsell, Moudon, Hoskins, & Larson, 2007).

Several studies have converged and arrived at the conclusion that empowerment is a potent mechanism for promoting exercise (eg, O'Brien & Vertinski, 1991). Specifically, Hardcastle and Taylor (2005) purported that older women whose self-concept included the label of "exerciser" felt empowered and had a fulfilled sense of well-being. Further, nursing home patients who were encouraged to increase control over their own health had greater activity levels than those who were not encouraged (Rodin, 1986).

SUMMARY

Although the benefits of physical exercise for aging women are well-documented many older women still lead a comparatively sedentary lifestyle. In order to implement appropriate interventions for aging women, social (eg, the presence/absence of peers), individual (eg, self-efficacy), and environmental (eg, access to safe walking paths) factors need to be considered, as well as, the interaction among these factors. Several interventions have been shown to be successful in increasing physical activity levels among aging women. The most successful among these interventions tend to focus on social capital. The major barriers to working out should be kept in mind when recommending exercise for older women and an effort should be made to attenuate concerns about physical activity and giving aging women an accurate assessment of risk (and benefits) associated with routine physical activity. Even women who begin a fitness routine much later in life still reap the benefits of a physically active lifestyle.

DISCUSSION QUESTIONS

1. Compare and contrast a "traditional" gym and a "medical fitness" gym (eg, Galter Life Center in Chicago). Consider the following questions:
   a. How might a medical fitness center be more appealing to an older adult?
   b. Are there different types of group classes offered at the two facilities?

c. What kinds of professionals are employed at the two different gyms? Do gyms employ professionals who have a background in providing services to aging adults?

2. What role does education play in encouraging women to be more physically active into later life?

3. How can communities outreach to older women in their area to encourage greater physical activity on a daily basis?

4. Do television commercials and media advertisements about physical health "target" or ignore the needs of aging women?

5. Should our knowledge about the aging body influence the design of exercise equipment and/or exercise programs for older women? If yes, how so?

6. From a cultural perspective, are there diversity issues related to the appropriateness of aging and physical activity for women? Give examples to explain your answer.

7. Are there gender differences to consider in designing a physical activity program? Why is this important to consider in supporting women's positive aging experiences through physical activities?

8. How can technology assist in helping aging women to remain fit?

9. Can a woman increase her level of physical activity as she ages? What role does family and/or peer support play in this activity transition process?

10. If you are designing a physical activity program for diverse women as they age, what factors would you take into consideration?

TEST YOUR KNOWLEDGE!

As mentioned in the chapter, virtual age can be decreased by as many as 20 years as a result of physical activity. How well are you doing in your own life? Find out by calculating your virtual age. Your virtual age is calculated based on lifestyle (eg, exercise, food) choices.

Go to: http://www.sonnyradio.com/realage.htm

1. Is there a difference between your "real" and "virtual" age? If yes, how so?

2. Can you identify one or two areas in your life where you can do better?

3. Why is this important to understand? How can this be applied in different ways?

SUPPLEMENTAL BOOK READINGS

Over the past decades, there have been many books written on the importance of older women engaging in physical activities on a daily basis. Here are some recommended *additional readings*:

Amini, S. B. (2012). *Accelerometer determined physical activity in older women: A descriptive study.* Saarbrücken, Germany: Lambert Academic Publishing.

> This is a research study which examines the best exercise activities for aging women. This research thesis explains the results of a descriptive study designed which examined the optimal level of physical activity (amount and intensity) to best support positive aging health for women.

Gambert, S. R. (2010). *Be fit for life: A guide to successful aging.* Hackensack, NJ: World Scientific Publishing Company.

> The book is a great self-help resource for aging women wishing to improve their physical quality of life. The author offers practical advice on how to avoid physical illnesses, slow the aging process, and generally assume a "preventative" tactic in reacting to aging process. Positive advice regarding exercise, diet, and lifestyle changes to promote more positive aging outcomes is offered.

Knopf, K. (2005). *Stretching for 50+: A customized program for increasing flexibility, avoiding injury, and enjoying an active lifestyle.* Berkeley, CA: Ulysses Press.

> Stretching exercise to help older adults who are 50 years of age or older with agility, balance, and overall physical strength is presented in an easily understandable manner through step-by-step text and photos. Proper stretching can help reduce older women's daily bodily aches and pain as well as help increase their level of daily physical (and associated mental) functioning. The implications toward ways to enhance women's positive aging outcomes are apparent through the great activities presented in the book's content.

SUPPLEMENTAL AGING VIDEOS

For learning purposes, the use of videos can be very beneficial for both instructors and readers. Here are some recommended *supplemental videos*:

Aging with Attitude: The Impact of Exercise on Quality of Life (Format: DVD)
> The DVD explores the benefits of regular physical activity on improving adults' physical functioning in their daily activities, and

their associated general functional capacity (eg, accomplishment of ADLs). Increasing knowledge and practice in regarding older adults and exercise will help both the aging population and the broader society (eg, healthcare program demands).

Exercise: A Video from the National Institute on Aging (Format: DVD) This video is interesting because it was developed by the US Government's National Institute on Aging for older adults. This is a very well-done video which presents in easily understandable terms muscle-toning exercises for total body health. The exercises are designed to help older adults with improving overall physical strength, muscle tone, balance, and flexibility. All the exercises are also designed with limited mobility seniors, only based on activities that can be done in a seat or by standing in place.

ADDITIONAL INFORMATION LINKS

The following are some recommended *supplemental Internet links*:

Alzheimer's Foundation website: http://www.alzfdn.org/BrainHealth/successfulaging.html/

AARP website: http://www.aarp.org/health/

Centers for Disease Control and Prevention website: http://www.cdc.gov/aging/

Mature Resources website: http://www.matureresources.org/

NIA/NIH website: http://www.nia.nih.gov/health/

Tao Institute website: http://www.taosinstitute.net/positive-aging-newsletter/

References

Ahlskog, J., Geda, Y., Graff-Radford, N., & Petersen, R. (2011). Physical exercise as a preventive or disease-modifying treatment of dementia and brain aging. *Mayo Clinic Proceedings, 86*(9), 876–884.

Ajzen, I. (1991). The theory of planned behavior. *Organizational Behavior and Human Decision Processes, 50*, 179–211.

Anstey, K., & Smith, G. (1999). Interrelationships among biological markers of aging, health, activity acculturation, and cognitive performance in late adulthood. *Psychology and Aging, 14*(4), 605–618.

Arent, S., Landers, D., & Etnier, J. (2000). The effects of exercise on mood in older adults: A meta-analytic review. *Journal of Ageing and Physical Activity, 8*, 407–430.

Berke, E., Koepsell, T., Moudon, A., Hoskins, R., & Larson, E. (2007). Associations of the built environment with physical activity and obesity in older persons. *American Journal of Public Health, 978*(3), 486–492.

Bethancourt, H. J., Rosenberg, D. E., Beatty, T., & Arterburn, D. E. (2014). Barriers to and facilitators of physical activity program use among older adults. *Clinical Medicine and Research, 12*(1–2), 10–20.

Booth, M., Owen, N., Bauman, A., Clavisi, O., & Leslie, E. (2000). Social-cognitive and perceived environment influences associated with physical activity in older Australians. *Preventive Medicine, 31*, 15–22.

Boyette, L., Lloyd, A., Boyette, J., Watkins, E., Furbush, L., Dunbar, S., et al. (2002). Personal characteristics that influence exercise behavior of older adults. *Journal of Rehabilitation Research and Development, 39*(1), 95–103.

Brach, J. S., Fitzgerald, S., Newman, A. B., Kelsey, S., Kuller, L., Van Swearingen, J. M., et al. (2003). Physical activity and functional status in community-dwelling older women: A 14-year prospective study. *Archives of Internal Medicine, 163*(21), 2565–2571.

Brassington, G., Stienza, A., Perczek, R., DiLorenzo, T., & King, A. (2002). Intervention-related cognitive versus social mediators of exercise adherence in the elderly. *American Journal of Preventive Medicine, 23*(2), 80–86.

Carstensen, L., Gross, J., & Fung, H. (1998). The social context of emotional experience. In K. W. Schaie & M. P. Lawton (Eds.), *Annual review of gerontology and geriatrics: Focus on emotion and adult development* (pp. 325–352). New York, NY: Springer.

Centers for Disease Control and Prevention, (2003). Prevalence of physical activity, including lifestyle activities among adults in the United States, 2000–2001. *MMWR, 52*, 764–769.

Christmas, C., & Andersen, R. A. (2000). Exercise and older patients: Guidelines for the clinician. *Journal of the American Geriatric Society, 48*(3), 318–324.

Colcombe, S., Erickson, K., Scalf, P., Kim, J., Prakash, R., McAuley, E., et al. (2006). Aerobic exercise training increases brain volume in aging humans. *Journal of Gerontology, 11*, 1166–1170.

Colcombe, S., & Kramer, A. F. (2003). Fitness effects on the cognitive function of older adults: A meta-analytic study. *Psychological Science, 14*(2), 125–130.

Conn, V., Tripp-Reimer, T., & Maas, M. (2003). Older women and exercise: Theory of planned behavior beliefs. *Public Health Nursing, 20*(2), 153–163.

Costello, E., Kafchinski, M., Vrazel, J., & Sullivan, P. (2011). Motivators, barriers, and beliefs regarding physical activity in an older adult population. *Journal of Geriatric Physical Therapy, 34*(3), 138–147.

Cousins, O. S. (1996). Exercise cognition among elderly women. *Journal of Applied Sport Psychology, 8*(2), 131–145.

Dorgo, S., Robinson, K. M., & Bader, J. (2009). The effectiveness of a peer-mentored older adult fitness program on perceived physical, mental, and social function. *Journal of the American Academy of Nurse Practitioners, 21*(2), 116–122.

Erickson, K. I., Voss, M. W., Prakash, R. S., Basak, C., Szabo, A., Chaddock, L., et al. (2011). Exercise training increases size of hippocampus and improves memory. *Proceedings of the National Academy of Sciences of the United States of America, 108*(7), 3017–3022. http://dx.doi.org/10.1073/pnas.1015950108.

Eyler, A., Brownson, R., Donatelle, R., King, A., Brown, D., & Sallis, J. (1999). Physical activity social support and middle-and older-aged minority women: Results from a U.S. survey. *Social Science & Medicine, 49*, 781–789.

Gill, K., & Overdorf, V. (1994). Incentives for exercise in younger and older women. *Journal of Sports Behavior, 17*(2), 87–97.

Ginis, K. A., Nigg, C., & Smith, A. L. (2013). Peer-delivered physical activity interventions: An overlooked opportunity for physical activity promotion. *Translational Behavioral Medicine, 3*(4), 434–443.

Global Aging. (2001). The ageing of the world's population. Retrieved from: <http://www.globalaging.org/waa2/documents/theagingoftheworld.htm>.

Godbey, G., Burnett-Wolle, S., & Chow, H. (2007). New ideas for promoting physical activity among middle age and older adults. *Journal of Physical Education, Recreation & Dance, 78*(7), 22–26.

Gregg, E., Cauley, J., Stone, K., Thompson, T., Bauer, D., Cummings, S., et al. (2003). Relationship of changes in physical activity and mortality among older women. *JAMA, 289*(18), 2379–2386.

Hall, K., & McAuley, E. (2010). Individual, social environmental and physical environmental barriers to achieving 10,000 steps per day among older women. *Health Education Research, 25*(3), 478–488.

Hardcastle, S., & Taylor, A. (2005). Finding an exercise identity in an older body: "It's redefining yourself and working out who you are." *Psychology of Sport and Exercise, 6*(2), 173–188.

Jancey, J., Lee, A., Howat, P., Clarke, A., Wang, K., & Shilton, T. (2007). Reducing attrition in physical activity programs for older adults. *Journal of Aging and Physical Activity, 15*(2), 152–165.

Keysor, J. J., & Jette, A. M. (2001). Have we oversold the benefit of late-life exercise? *Journal of Gerontology, 56*(7), M412–M423.

King, A. (2001). Interventions to promote physical activity by older adults. *Journal of Gerontology, 56*(2), 36–46.

King, A., Castro, C., Wilcox, S., Eyler, A., Sallis, J., & Brownson, R. (2000). Personal and environmental factors associated with physical inactivity among different racial–ethnic groups of U.S. middle-aged and older-aged women. *Health Psychology, 19*(4), 354–364.

Koltyn, K. (2001). The association between physical activity and quality of life in older women. *Women's Health Issues, 11*(6), 471–480.

Lee, C. (1993). Attitudes, knowledge, and stages of change: A survey of exercise patterns in older Australian women. *Health Psychology, 12*, 476–480.

Lindwall, M., Rennemark, M., Halling, A., Berglund, J., & Hassmen, P. (2007). Depression and exercise in elderly men and women: Findings from the Swedish national study on aging and care. *Journal of Aging and Physical Activity, 15*(1), 41–55.

Litt, M., Kleppinger, A., & Judge, J. (2002). Initiation and maintenance of exercise behavior in older women: Predictors form the social learning model. *Journal of Behavioral Medicine, 25*(1), 83–97.

Lubben, J., Weiler, P., & Chi, I. (1989). Gender and health difference in the health practices of the elderly poor. *Journal of Clinical Epidemiology, 42*(8), 725–733.

Lübcke, A., Martin, C., & Hellström, K. (2012). Older adults' perceptions of exercising in a senior gym. *Activities, Adaptation & Aging, 36*(21), 131–146.

Milton, D., Porcari, J., Foster, C., Gibson, M., Udermann, B., Greany, J., et al. (2008). The effect of functional exercise training on functional fitness levels of older adults. *Gundersen Lutheran Medical Journal, 5*(1), 4–8.

Neid, R., & Franklin, B. (2002). Promoting and prescribing exercise for the elderly. *American Family Physician, 65*(3), 419–426.

Nelson, M., Rejeski, J., Blair, S., Duncan, P., Judge, J., King, A., et al. (2007). Physical activity and public health in older adults: Recommendation from the American College of Sports Medicine and the American Heart Association. *Medicine and Science in Sports and Exercise, 39*, 1435–1445.

O'Brien, S. (2000). "My heart couldn't take it": Older women's beliefs about exercise benefits and risks. *Journal of Gerontology: Psychological Science, 55*(5), 283–294.

O'Brien, S., & Conger, P. (1991). No time to look back: Approaching the finish line of life's course. *The International Journal of Aging and Human Development, 33*, 75–87.

O'Brien, S., & Vertinski, P. (1991). Unfit survivors: Exercise as a resource for aging women. *Gerontologist, 3*, 347–357.

Penninx, B. W., Rejeski, W. J., Pandya, J., Miller, M. E., DiBari, M., Applegate, W. B., et al. (2002). Exercise and depressive symptoms: A comparison of aerobic and resistance exercise effects on emotional and physical function in older persons with high and low depressive symptomatology. *Journal of Gerontology, 57*(2), 124–132.

Phillips, E., Schneider, J., & Mercer, G. (2004). Motivating elders to initiate and maintain exercise. *Archives of Physical Medicine and Rehabilitation, 85*(3), S52–S57.

Purath, J., Buchholz, S. W., & Kark, D. L. (2009). Physical fitness assessment of older adults in the primary care setting. *Journal of the American Academy of Nurse Practitioners, 21*(2), 101–107.

Rantanen, T., Guralnik, J. M., Sakari-Rantala, R., Leveille, S., Simonsick, E. M., Ling, S., et al. (1999). Disability physical activity and muscle strength in older women: The women's health and aging study. *Archives of Physical Medicine and Rehabilitation, 80*, 130–135.

Rasinaho, M., Hirvensalo, M., Leinonen, R., Lintunen, T., & Rantanen, T. (2006). Motives for and barriers to physical activity among older adults with mobility limitations. *Journal of Aging and Physical Activity, 15*, 90–102.

Rhodes, R., Martin, A., Taunton, M., Rhodes, E., Donnelly, M., & Elliot, J. (1999). Factors associated with exercise adherence among older adults. *Sports Medicine, 28*(6), 397–411.

Rodin, J. (1986). Aging and health: Effects of the sense of control. *Science, 233*, 1271–1276.

Satariano, W., & McAuley, E. (2003). Promoting physical activity among older adults: From ecology to the individual. *American Journal of Preventive Medicine, 25*(3), 184–192.

Schutzer, K., & Graves, S. (2004). Barrier and motivations to exercise in older adults. *Preventive Medicine, 39*(5), 1056–1061.

Seefeldt, V., Malina, R., & Clark, M. (2002). Factors affecting levels of physical activity in adults. *Sports Medicine, 32*(3), 143–168.

Shepard, R. J. (1994). Determinants of exercise in people aged 65 years and older. In R. K. Dishman (Ed.), *Advances in exercise adherence* (pp. 343–360). Champaign, IL: Human Kinetics.

Shephard, R. J. (1998). Aging and exercise. In T. D. Fahey (Ed.), *Encyclopedia of sports medicine and science*. Internet Society for Sport Science. <http://sportsci.org>.

Sidney, K. H., Niinimaa, V., & Shepard, R. J. (1983). Attitudes toward exercise and sports: Sex and age differences, and changes with endurance training. *Journal of Sports Sciences, 1*, 195–210.

Singh, N. A., Clements, K. M., & Singh, M. A. (2001). The efficacy of exercise as a long-term antidepressant in elderly subjects: A randomized, controlled trial. *Journal of Gerontology, 56*(8), 497–504.

Stewart, A., Mills, K., Sepsis, P., King, A., McLellan, B., Roitz, K., et al. (1997). Evaluation of CHAMPS, a physical activity promotion program for older adults. *Annals of Behavioral Medicine, 19*(4), 353–361.

Strawbridge, W., Deleger, S., Roberts, R., & Kaplan, G. (2002). Physical activity reduces the risk of subsequent depression for older adults. *American Journal of Epidemiology, 156*(4), 328–334.

Strijk, J., Proper, K., van der Beek, A., & van Mechelen, W. (2011). A process evaluation of worksite vitality intervention among aging hospital workers. *International Journal of Behavioral Nutrition and Physical Activity, 10*(8), 1–9.

Striik, J., Proper, K., van der Beek, A., & van Mechelen, W. (2012). A worksite vitality intervention to improve older workers' lifestyle and vitality-related outcome: Results of a randomized controlled trial. *Journal of Epidemiological Community Health, 66*(11), 1071–1078.

Swinburn, B. A., Walter, L. G., Arroll, B., Tilyard, M. W., & Russell, D. G. (1998). The green prescription study: A randomized controlled trial of written exercise advice provided by general practitioners. *American Journal of Public Health, 88*, 288–291.

Thomas, R., Kottke, T. E., Brekke, M., Brekke, L., Brandel, C., Aase, L. A., et al. (2002). Attempts at changing dietary and exercise habits to reduce risk of cardiovascular disease: Who's doing what in the community? *Preventive Cardiology, 5*(3), 102–108.

Vertinsky, P. (1995). Stereotypes of aging women and exercise: A historical perspective. *Journal of Aging and Physical Activity, 3*(3), 223–237.

Warburton, D., Nicol, C. W., & Bredin, S. (2006). Health benefits of physical activity: The evidence. *Canadian Medical Association Journal, 174*(6), 801–809.

Weuve, J., Kang, J., Manson, J., Breteler, M., Ware, J., & Grodstein, F. (2008). Physical activity, including walking, and cognitive function in older women. *Journal of the American Medical Association, 22,* 1454–1461.

Wilcox, S., Castro, C., King, A., Housemann, R., & Brownson, R. (2000). Determinants of leisure time physical activity in rural compared with urban older and ethnically diverse women in the United States. *Journal of Epidemiological Community Health, 54,* 667–672.

Williams, P., & Lord, S. R. (1995). Predictors of adherence to a structured exercise program for older women. *Psychology of Aging, 10,* 617–624.

Williams, P., & Lord, S. R. (1997). Effects of group exercise on cognitive functioning and mood in older women. *Australian and New Zealand Journal of Public Health, 21*(1), 45–52.

Yaffe, K., Barnes, D., Nevitt, M., Lui, L., & Covinsky, K. (2001). A prospective study of physical activity and cognitive decline in elderly women: Women who walk. *Archives of Internal Medicine, 161*(14), 1703–1708.

Yan, T., Wilbur, K., & Aguirre, R. (2009). Do sedentary older adults benefit from community-based exercise? Results from the active start program. *The Gerontologist, 49*(6), 847–855.

WOMEN'S DIVERSE AGING EXPERIENCES

Relevant chapters

8   *Diversity among Older Women*   143

9   *Expansion of Women's Roles in Later Life*   169

10   *The Role of Social Relationships for Aging Women*   185

11   *Women's Sexuality in Later Life*   201

The third section of the book examines issues related to women's socialization and associated roles as they age. As the global population of aging women in many different countries continues to rise in number and associated longevity trends, it is important to better understand their social roles and personal identities (eg, sexual identity) as they develop into later life. Only through this enhanced understanding can effective interventions be developed and administered to serve women in communities. From a positive aging perspective, it is important for aging women to acknowledge the impact of their diverse social roles within and across cultures as they influence opportunities to age well. The purpose of this section of the book is to review research on women's diverse lifespan experiences as a function of gender, sexual identity, culture, and other factors that may affect their positive aging processes and/or outcomes. If better understood, community-support program and related services (eg, healthcare services) can be designed to meet the unique needs of diverse groups of older women. Practical ways for women to adapt to changes in women's roles in light of cultural, social, and familial contextual factors are examined. Across chapters in this section, diversity factors determining positive aging outcomes in a woman's later life will be examined.

8

Diversity among Older Women

Global Fact: *Ageing occupies connecting chambers within the development landscape, interacting with global patterns in labour and capital markets, governmental pensions, services, and traditional support systems, all which are further shaped by technological change and cultural transformations.*

—*Global Aging (2001)*

From a positive aging perspective, better understanding factors underlying women's aging perceptions and experiences over time can be used to then create more effective support programs and policies within communities (eg, Reichstadt, Sengupta, Depp, Palinkas, & Jeste, 2010). It is important to understand what positive aging means in today's world, and how one defines positive aging depends upon many different diversity-related factors (Aldwin & Gilmer, 2013; Butler, Fuji, & Sasaki, 2011).

There are potentially as many definitions of "positive aging" as there are diverse aging women in the world (Bogunovic, 2011; Butt & Beiser, 1987). The concept of "diversity" itself can be defined in many ways, such as within and across racial/ethnic groups, living environments, cultures, and levels of performance functioning (eg, Ayotte, Allaire, & Whitfield, 2012). If different societies, and associated cultures, are going to make communities more "age friendly" for women, the understanding of their diversity issues is important to examine from many different perspectives (Bradshaw, 1999; Hrostowski, 2010; Iwamasa & Iwasaki, 2011; Troutman, Nies, & Bentley, 2011). Only through this thoughtful examination can there be "better aged" societies across the world (Arai, Ouchi, Yokode, Ito, & Uematsu, et al., 2012). Litwin (2005) emphasizes the importance of understanding factors that are universal in nature that can be generalizable to many different communities and cultures for there to be successful interventions in supporting an aging population. Effective positive aging

143

interventions should encompass social, physical, and environmental elements within a woman's living circumstance (Lee, Lan, & Yen, 2011; Pruchno, Hahn, & Wilson-Genderson, 2012).

Nimrod and colleagues (Nimrod, 2011; Nimrod & Kleiber, 2007; Nimrod & Rotom, 2012) purported that it is more important to examine patterns of change and continuity within an aging adult's developmental trajectory to best understand positive aging outcomes (ie, Innovation Theory of Successful Aging). Similarly, Hank (2011) studied the differential factors underlying quality-of-life perceptions among European older adults, and concluded that changing functional capability was a critical factor in determining these feelings.

As lifespan factors predicting an individual's positive aging change, it is vital to realize that some predictors related to positive aging can shift in importance from cohort to cohort. For example, Piccinin et al. (2013) examined the relationship between an aging adult's educational attainment and the maintenance of cognitive functioning. Interestingly, there was no direct relationship found, and this has important implications toward assumptions about predictive factors which could be much more complex and individualistic in effect than previously assumed.

Potentially, there could be multiple and diverse meanings of positive aging as a function of equally diverse perspectives and cultural contexts. For example, Liang and Luo (2012) proposed the concept of "harmonious" aging as a way to define positive aging from a cross-cultural perspective. Alternately, Baltes and Baltes (1990) examined positive aging in terms of how an aging woman (or man) adopts strategies to maintain functioning in daily activities through a conscious process of identifying activities that the older adult is best at ("selective optimization") with associated adaptive adjustments ("compensation").

Phelan, Anderson, LaCroix, and Larson (2004) made the important point that older adults and researchers may have different perspectives regarding the meaning of positive aging. This insight is important to acknowledge, and emphasizes the need to have older women be a part of the consultation process in developing programs, services, or other public policies intended to help support their positive aging needs. Dionigi, Horton, and Bellamy (2011) investigated the meaning of aging among a sample of older women with different physical activity capabilities. Their research suggests that there is a strong need to examine what is important in terms of quality-of-life needs of aging women to then create effective and supportive interventions to optimize their aging outcomes. Both Glover (1998) and Hazzard (2013) emphasized that many "personal" meanings exist regarding what it means to have a good quality of life for aging adults. Matching one's aging-related areas of expertise, needs, and preferences to potential environmental resources determines the best options to be chosen to support positive aging (eg, disability-related capabilities; Minkler & Fadem, 2002).

Communities' programs and services should be sensitive to this concept and allow flexibility of options for older women in order to optimize their feelings of personal control and mastery within a cultural context (Hopman-Rock & Westhoff, 2002). The process of understanding "fit" is both an internal and an external process of information gathering. From a Continuity theory perspective (Atchley, 1989), it is vital that an aging woman participates in a process of self-examination to determine personal goals, motivations, and age-related perceptions in order to best decide on approaches to achieving positive aging outcomes. This examination of "self" is influenced by our immediate social networks of family members, friends, and other "relevant" social contacts (eg, coworkers). Nimrod (2011) researched older adults' social activities within online communities and other social networks to examine their impact on older adults' feelings of positive aging and social engagement. This is an interesting idea because it certainly expands the definition of culture as it impacts one's aging.

Beyond our immediate social network is the influence of the culture in which we live; this may include more than one culture that we identify with and are influenced by. It is important to examine in many different ways how culture influences our perceptions of aging identity, social resources, and other factors which impact the degree to which a woman can successfully age (eg, Cohen et al., 2006).

Public policies and programs offered to support women's aging are important to scrutinize to avoid potential bias or discrimination that limit opportunities for women across their life spans. For example, the research of both Freedman and Iwata-Weickgennant (2011) focused on cultural influences on older women's feelings of optimism and happiness. How society defines "appropriate" aging reactions and coping mechanisms for aging women have a significant impact upon their own self-concept and aging-adjustment reactions (Hyde, Nee, Howlett, Butler, & Drennan, 2011; Osorio-Parraguez, 2013; Strauss, 2011).

In response to the complexity of this positive aging focus, there is the need for a comprehensive cross-cultural model that encompasses many different factors related to aging (Eaton et al., 2012), incorporating both "micro" (self) to "macro" (culture, society) perspectives. The following is a proposed model reflecting a more "holistic" perspective on different levels of factors impacting women's positive aging:

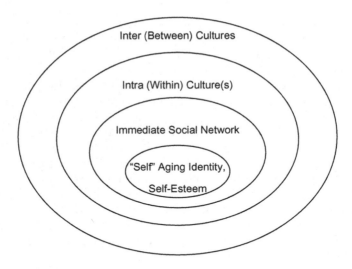

There has been a growing movement to better understand important individual differences in the aging experience for women across their life span (eg, McCann Mortimer, Ward, & Winefield, 2008). This understanding can help communities empower middle-aged and older women to optimize their aging over time (eg, social support networks; Saucier, 2004). The role of culture on the aging experience cannot be understated; it impacts the very meaning of aging from an older adult's perspective (Litwin, 2006; Torres, 2003, 2009).

While aging seems to be a series of losses beyond one's control, better understanding of how older women attempt to maintain personal identity through behavioral strategies (eg, self-care regimes; Leach & Schoenberg, 2008; coping with partner violence; Stöckl, Watts, & Penhale, 2012) can assist in developing effective training programs for/interventions within communities to assist with positive aging outcomes. Baltes and colleagues (eg, Smith & Baltes, 1993) purported the influence of three aging events that can significantly influence aging trajectories: "Normative biological events" relate to the genetic inherited characteristics of one's family lineage that impacts a woman's aging as it unfolds, "normative historical events" relate to the Cold War–related generational experiences that shape a woman's aging path as she gets older, and "nonnormative events" relate to the very unique characteristics that shape the diversity of aging.

DIVERSITY AND QUALITY-OF-LIFE PERCEPTIONS

Within a broad cultural definition, there are many unique quality-of-life factors derived from one's beliefs and values (Molzahn, Kalfoss,

Schick Makaroff, & Skevington, 2011). Over a period of 12 years, Roos and Havens (1991) investigated social factors predicting positive aging outcomes for adults living in the Manitoba region. Women and men living in this region of the world have interesting perspectives toward women and diversity issues across different regions of the world. How cultural relevancy, diversity issues, and positive aging for women are assessed is an important factor to consider when investigating different adjustment issues with culturally diverse older women (eg, Iranian immigrants to Sweden; Torres, 2009). Cultural relevance toward aging successfully has direct implications toward the design and implementation of public policies and laws regarding older citizens (Torres-Gil & Rudinica, 2012).

Kleyman (2006) argued that it is important to understand the potentially different aging trajectories of adults living in diverse urban settings for tailored community outreach efforts. Further, effective support services and other community resources (eg, educational programs) must be developed with the understanding of what it means to "age" and associated resiliency responses within a specific culture (eg, Middle Eastern culture; Litwin, 2009) (rural Midwest; Stark-Wroblewski, Edelbaum, & Bello, 2008). This logic extends to specific community-based programs developed for diverse groups of aging women. The planning and administration of support services and community-based programs must be grounded in research on diverse aging female populations within different geographical locations of the world (eg, aging in the United States; Myers, 2013) and different life circumstances (eg, elder abuse programs in Israel; Rabi, 2006).

The assessment of positive aging outcomes, such as feelings of positive life satisfaction in later-life, needs to take into account both objective (eg, functional capability) and subjective (eg, self-rated health) assessments of different groups of aging women (Cernin, Lysack, & Lichtenberg, 2011). The importance of this concept of examining both objective and subjective factors cannot be understated in better understanding positive outcomes for aging women. Understanding the complexity of aging experiences for diverse women across the world will only help create more effective assessments of diverse aging groups for intervention purposes (Kampfe, 2000).

It is equally important to understand how aging adjustment experiences subsequently affect one's sense of "self" and ego identity (eg, transition to retirement; Teuscher, 2010). Similarly, the role of productive activities on a frequent basis can play a significant part in shaping women's positive aging outcomes and should be encouraged. For example, Willcox, Willcox, Sokolowsky, and Sakihara (2007) observed women weavers in North Okinawa and how their role of productivity assisted in their positive aging attitudes and aging adjustment.

QUOTES FROM FAMOUS, POSITIVELY AGING WOMEN

No matter what age you are, or what your circumstances might be,
you are special, and you still have something unique to offer.
Your life, because of who you are, has meaning.

—*Barbara de Angelis, Writer*

Age is not measured by years. Nature does not equally distribute energy.
Some people are born old and tired while others are going strong at seventy.

—*Dorothy Thompson, Journalist*

It is time for parents to teach young people early on
that in diversity there is beauty and there is strength.
We all should know that diversity makes for a rich tapestry, and
we must understand that all the threads of that tapestry are
equal in value no matter their color.

—*Maya Angelou, National Poet Laureate*

WOMEN'S RACE, CULTURE, AND ETHNICITY FACTORS IN GETTING OLDER

As women age, their developmental experiences are shaped by their respective race, cultural, and ethnic identities (Twigg & Martin, 2015). How older women are valued and regarded is influenced by society's reactions to their social status within the community (eg, Thomas, Hardy, Cutcher, & Ainsworth, 2014). Societal promotion of positive aging outcomes is determined by others' reactions to the older woman's identity as being "older" in addition to being a "woman" and of a certain race, ethnicity, and culture (Krainitzki, 2014; Laceulle & Baars, 2014). Communities can become positive and supportive entities for aging women through the eradication of biased attitudes and practices.

Interestingly, a "similar to me" bias may have a positive influence on how communities share in the support and caregiving of aging women within the community (eg, African-American culture and prevalence of nonbiological family caregivers) (Powers & Whitlatch, 2014) but, increasingly, there is also a need to acknowledge the reality of a growing multiethnic, multiracial aging population (eg, Aleman, Fitzpatrick, Tran, & Gonzalez, 2014). Internalized self-identity (eg, cultural identity of aging) can influence how aging women engage in social interactions and/or exhibit societal "self" presentations (eg, Twigg & Majima, 2014). Understanding older women's internalized and dynamically changing "aging paradigm" from a diversity (eg, cultural and/or cohort) perspective is an ethical imperative for community outreach programs, educational initiatives, and other services (eg, new attitude of "senior coolness;" Zimmermann & Grebe, 2014). For example, "cohort" or generational difference between women's aging experiences across the world is important to analyze.

GENERATIONAL EXPERIENCES SHAPING WOMEN'S AGING

Baltes and colleagues (eg, Baltes, Cornelius, & Nesselroade, 1979) emphasized the role of cohort as a factor shaping one's aging outcomes. Historical events guiding and shaping a woman's development across a life span can have a profound effect on the probability of achieving positive aging. Generational opportunities for educational and career growth also influence how well a woman may age and more recent works of women have certainly improved their projected aging trajectories (eg, degree attainment; Isopahkala-Bouret, 2015). Again, communities and broader world societies must acknowledge this influential factor when considering current and future aging trends of women on a national and international level.

What are the examples of generational experiences that have shaped women's aging in many different cultures? Certainly, changes in public policies for many industrialized countries have helped improve women's quality of life but there is still room for improvement (eg, women's health; Borrell et al., 2014). Unfortunately in many different countries across the world, women have not equally experienced the same improvements that have been seen in more industrialized nations (Keck & Sikkink, 2014; Stromquist, 2014). The differential experiences of social status, resources, and protection through community-based public policies have influenced the nature of aging for many women across the world.

SOCIETAL STATUS FOR OLDER WOMEN

Over history, the role of women and their associated social status has shifted and become potentially more complex as a function of living circumstances and culture (eg, Katz & Monk, 2014). One might argue, in many different cultures, that the responsibilities of women have multiplied, but there has not been an equivocal gain in terms of social power with the acquisition of multiple roles (Kulik, 2015). The valuation of women in society needs to become more of a priority, especially as these women transition to roles of dependency in later life. There is always the concern of "double jeopardy" bias in how women are regarded and treated, regarded as less valued (unfairly) because of being both a woman and an older adult. This bias cannot be tolerated. Instead, women across the world need to be valued for exactly those reasons of being an active, contributory member of society as a woman who has lived a long life. For women to value their personal aging journey, it is important for society to communicate that they are valued as they age and that aging is a positive transition in their lives. This does require a cultural "shift" for many different countries that directly or indirectly communicate a message of youth valuation and aging discouragement.

In order to successfully age, societies across the world need to acknowledge the contributions and wisdom of older women. The woman's typical experience of aging is transitioning from a child being cared for to becoming a primary caregiver of one's parents. Across many cultures in the world, women are the "default" long-term caregivers within a family system and this role of caregiver can affect a woman's aging over time (eg, perceived burden among Chinese spousal caregivers; Chan & Chui, 2011). If we think about the many different physical, mental, and social challenges for a woman to be a caregiver over her life span, it certainly becomes apparent that there are many different stresses and strains, as well as growth experiences that occur within a woman's development over time. The contribution of this caregiver role within the micro family system, as well as the broader macro society cannot be understated and needs to be acknowledged. Further exacerbating the importance of this diversity role within women's life spans, their caregiving role responsibilities are usually multifaceted, multifocused, and several decades in duration. Through this acknowledgment of older women's benefit to communities, women can better accept and embrace their personal development into later life.

CHANGING LIVING SITUATIONS WITH AGING

Environmental demands ("environmental press"), accessibility and mobility needs are factors to consider when attempting to optimize an older woman's transition from one situation to another (eg, transitioning from independent living to assisted living) and their associated physical performance and/or mental health needs (eg, Lindemann et al., 2014). Environmental factors underlying and influencing older women's emotional, social, psychological, and physical resiliency reactions are significant influences, and associated interventions should be tailored in response to these dynamic factors impacting their positive aging (eg, tailored exercise program design; Hooker et al., 2005). In addition to more "internal" factors, support programs and other resources should incorporate aspects of religion, marital status, educational background, social economics, and motivational issues related to older women's interests and hobbies; community outreach programs need to take all these factors into account to optimize women's later-life adjustment to eldercare, retirement, health changes, and other later-life transitions (Padilla & Villalobos, 2007).

SEXUALITY AND GENDER IDENTITY IN LATER LIFE

When we think about individual difference factors, one factor rarely addressed or erroneously categorized is the sexuality of aging women (eg, stereotype of an oversexed "cougar;" Montemurro & Seifken, 2014). An important part of the aging self-concept, one's sexuality and associated identity shapes feelings about personal aging, feelings of belongingness, and relationship needs (Buttaro, Koeniger-Donohue, & Hawkins, 2014). Often, sexuality in later life is considered to be a moot issue, but, in fact, that belief is erroneous and potentially damaging to the self-esteem of aging women. How society reacts to aging women and their associated relationship needs and gender identity issues is important to explore because caregivers and other support resources must acknowledge this individual difference factor to better understand the holistic process of women aging over time.

Women's gender identity framed from a positive aging perspective is important to explore with practitioners offering education and/or support services for older women. For example, better understanding of the social support needs of aging lesbians and transgender women (Kimmel, 2014; Witten, 2015) is an ethical imperative for a caring society faced with aging populations from diverse backgrounds and lifespan experiences (Averett & Jenkins, 2012).

EDUCATION ACCESS

Education is the gateway to accessing job opportunities and associated socioeconomic benefits. Education for women should not simply be relegated to the time periods of early childhood to early adulthood, but rather regarded as a lifespan experience to help women positively adjust to later-life transitions (Merriam & Kee, 2014; Stromquist, 2014). From most societies, career training in middle age and later is a necessity as retirement becomes a less realistic option. As women age, their continued involvement in the workforce is a reality that necessitates continued career training (Arizpe & Aranda, 2014). Employers, educators, and community outreach programs must ethically offer this opportunity to a growing number of women facing the need for skill updating to remain competitive in the workforce environment.

QUALITY-OF-LIFE FACTORS

Physical and mental health and aging women. Research over the last decade has begun to more closely examine the relationship between physical and mental health and their influence on aging (eg, in Latin America; Palloni & McEniry, 2007) as well as the need to understand gender issues in research on health and aging (Perrig-Chiello & Hutchinson, 2010). There are two main factors predicting positive aging for both men and women: health and wealth. Women and men can exhibit differential patterns of nonnormative health patterns and associated "end-of-life" transitions that are influenced by cultural norms and attitudes (eg, Japan; Chan, Zimmer, & Saito, 2011). Disability trend in an aging population is one aspect of this "nonnormative" aging process that increasingly becomes normative in nature as women reach later stages of life and live healthier than ever before (Mendes de Leon, Eschbach, & Markides, 2011). As with aging men, diversity issues within the societal and genetic context can significantly influence older women's health-related status and associated physical and mental health outcomes in a meaningful manner (Ajrouch & Marshall, 2004; Duda et al., 2011).

Lee and Lee (2011) reported that there are significant gender-related differences among older South Koreans regarding mental health factors that determine quality-of-life outcomes in later-life adjustment. Gender differences in mental health across the life span are vital to understand for social support programs and community education interventions. The cultural context of a woman's mental health environment is important to acknowledge both within the United States (eg, Arab-American older adults; Ajrouch, 2007) and in other countries (eg, in Malaysia; Momtaz, Ibrahim, Hamid, & Yahaya, 2011; in Japan; Tiedt, 2013; in China; Zhang, Xu, Nie, Zhang, & Wu, 2012). Within cultures, differences in race, ethnicity, and other demographic factors create an even more complex picture related to lifespan issues of depression and other mental health outcomes. Across cultures, attention should be given to identify adjustment issues and the associated intervention provided by societies (eg, later-life marital relationship adjustment issues; Laganá, Spellman, Wakefield, & Oliver, 2011). If not addressed, negative mental health conditions can have an adverse impact on an older adult's daily functioning capability, such as memory functioning, that can impact the ability to live independently and engage in positive, active-life activities (Steffens, Fisher, Langa, Potter, & Plassman, 2009).

From a positive aging perspective, health education and community programs offering health screenings for aging women are vital to the health and well-being of the growing aging female population in many different countries across the world. The allocation of economic resources for the health of older women is certainly an issue to be scrutinized in countries across the world (eg, Al Hazzouri, Sibai, Chaaya, Mahfoud, & Yount, 2011; Szwarcwald, da Mota, Damarcena, & Pereira, 2011). Whether older women have access to diverse healthy foods, for example, due to economic status and geographical location should be addressed within communities (Hans and Tibetan older adults; Kimura et al., 2009).

An important diversity issue to examine among aging women is lifespan longevity. The social factors unique to women that determine their quality-of-life outcomes and extended physical health over time are important to identify (eg, Ailshire, Beltrán-Sánchez, & Crimmins, 2011). Mobility status is an important factor related to the social "power" of older women in different cultures and should be better understood within the social context of society as a quality-of-life outcome (Nilsson, Avlund, & Lund, 2010). Encouraging aging women's physical activity is an important "proactive" intervention to consider when thinking about ways to improve their positive aging processes and outcomes (Guedas, Hatmann, Martini, Borges, & Bernardelli, 2012). In creating appropriate physical "aerobics" activities for older women, it is an imperative that up-to-date research takes into account current issues of women's diet, physical role demands, and other health-related concerns (Kaur, Bains, & Kaur, 2012).

Aging women's financial resources/opportunities. As was discussed in the previous chapter, one of the two main factors predicting life satisfaction, and positive aging for many older adults is the factor of financial security and stability. One might argue that older women of past generations, and even today, are at a disadvantage in preparing for the expenses of healthcare retirement in later life because of unstable or deficient employment work histories and associated accumulated earnings over a lifetime (Teuscher, 2010). The wage gap between men's and women's earnings still exists today in many countries across the world and this disparity has serious implications toward older women's financial security and opportunities for personal growth.

Social support for older women. Across a woman's life span, it is important for her to depend upon many different sources of social support for both physical and psychosocial adjustment to the many developmental changes she will experience as she ages. Sources of support may range from a media to extended family systems, peers, friends, and the broader community in which she lives (Smith, Tobin, Robertson-Tchabo, & Power, 1995; Thanakwang, Ingersoll-Dayton, & Soonthorndhada, 2012). Emotional, social, psychological, and physical benefits from having such support cannot be understated as significant factors influencing a woman's aging trajectory (Kreager & Schröder-Butterfill, 2007; Litwin, 2009; McCandless, 1998).

Diversity-sensitive education and community outreach for women living in urban and rural communities are needed to maintain and optimize utilization of these resources for positive aging outcomes (Flood, 2005; Johnell & Fastbom, 2012; Kimura & Browne, 2009; McMullin, 2000; Minkler & Stone, 1985; Mokuau & Tomioka, 2010). The availability of positive, supportive social networks and social living environments to achieve optimal aging outcomes for older women, and men, within a specific cultural context needs more investigation regarding linkages to mental health outcomes (eg, older women in Singapore; Chan, Malhotra, Malhotra, & Østbye, 2011).

Societal attitudes toward aging women. The role of culture has a profound impact on what it means to be an aging woman in a specific culture, and broader society (Molzahn et al., 2011; Myers, 2013). How members of a society feel about their own aging process contributes to more pervasive treatment issues for aging women in the world (Saucier, 2004). It is important for societies across the world to examine their policies and programs intended to support and promote the positive growth of aging women into later life (eg, financial support programs; Ryser & Halseth, 2011; Shah, 2007). The examination may yield revelations related to a "double jeopardy" nature of biased attitudes and or discrimination toward older women (eg, understanding aging women's later-life sexuality; Thompson et al., 2011). Only through education about positive aging and the needs of aging citizenry can communities hope, to best support and promote the positive aging of women.

CHECK IT OUT!

Search the Internet to find resources and content related to a discussion of women's diversity issues into later life. In reviewing these websites, identify cultural and other environmental/lifestyle factors impacting aging women's life experiences and aging outcomes. As you are examining these factors, think about the following questions:

1. What are some interesting cultural differences among older women across the world?
2. What role does geographical location have on women's aging outcomes?

3. How do differences in social support resources impact aging women's positive growth?
4. Are there different family system dynamics regarding aging women's roles across cultures?
5. Were you surprised about what you learned? Why?

WORDS OF WISDOM

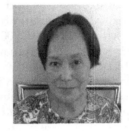

Francisca is a 65-year-old woman who was born in Guatemala. Her native language is Spanish and she came to the United States over 30 years ago. Throughout this time she has developed a diverse circle of friends. She has friends from different parts of the world such as El Salvador, China, and Ireland. Other than a language barrier, Francisca has not encountered many obstacles with other aging women, she is confident that the little English she knows allows her to communicate well with others who do not speak her native language.

Francisca states it is enjoyable to be able to have conversations with others about their culture and share the similarities across them. She finds it amazing that she is able to learn from others as she ages; she especially loves to get advice from diverse older women. Throughout her life she has received advice that she has found helpful, such as learning how to save money, raising her children, and knowing what is right and what is wrong.

Francisca is very thankful to be living in this country because it has given her things that she could not have in her home country. She benefits from living in a diverse environment because she learns something new from everyone she encounters. She advises younger women to appreciate diversity. She also advises younger women to try to get along with others and learn just like she has!

One might argue that women's positive aging trajectories may have very specific gender issues to be aware of for policy and program development purposes. From a biological perspective, women's experiences in aging are embedded within cultural contextual factors (Duay & Bryan,

2006). How a culture responds to a woman's aging (eg, educational programs) influences how she may perceive and interpret menopausal changes, physical changes (eg, physical appearance), and similar aging-related transitions. The cessation of fertility could be interpreted as a positive transition for aging women if that reflects the positive aging message transmitted through many sources of social feedback within the woman's culture and society at large. Jenkins and Marti (2012) argued that it is important to examine the postfeminist culture within many different societies that can have a significant impact upon how women feel about their fiscal aging and associated loss of youth. With biological changes, there are important social roles that are maintained, transformed, and/ or ended for older women within cultures (Dykstra, 2006). The diversity of experiences and needs for aging women is vital to understand from both a community-based (local) and a global perspective (Fiori, Consedine, & Magai, 2009; Guse & Masesar, 1999; Hutchinson & Nimrod, 2012; Kalavar & Jamuna, 2011; Kauffman, 2002).

To assume that all women experience similar aging events would be doing a disservice to an international aging female population and those who care for them. Individual difference factors of culture, genetics, available social resources and opportunities, among other factors significantly impact an older woman's quality of life and associated adjustment to personal aging (eg, Aranda et al., 2012). Only through this recognition of "fit" can support programs, legislation, and resources be best tailored to meet the needs of older adults and support their positive aging (Charpentier, Quéniart, & Jacques, 2008; Clark & Glicksman, 2012; Cutler, 1998; Davis-Berman, 2011; Kleyman, 2006).

SUMMARY

Many different factors related to the diversity of aging experiences for women were examined. It is important to acknowledge that the aging trajectories of women are very complex and are based upon personal, cultural, and geographical location issues. Combinations of factors dynamically interact to impact both the quantity and quality of years of women as they develop into later life. Potential growth experiences and learning opportunities need to be explored for aging women in order to create effective community-based educational and intervention programs to achieve these aims. Churches, institutions of higher education, and senior centers are among the many opportunities for such programs to be offered to women across communities in the world.

DISCUSSION QUESTIONS

1. What are the important individual difference factors which meaningfully shape how a woman ages?
2. What role does cultural identity play in the positive aging outcomes of women?
3. How might social support programs address the potentially diverse needs of an aging female population in many different countries across the world?
4. In today's society, how have women's roles changed and does this have implications toward their aging outcomes from a diversity perspective?
5. In the future, will there be the same or different diversity issues within the aging female population in the world?
6. How much do generational (cohort) experiences impact diverse women's aging experiences?
7. Taking diversity issues into consideration, how does this topic apply to the design of community outreach support program designed for aging women across the world? Give examples of factors to be considered.
8. Are there family issues to be understood that further explain how diverse women positively age? If so, what are they?
9. If women are varied in their backgrounds and interests, is it possible to create educational programs and support interventions for positive aging outcomes that are "universal" in focus?
10. Think about your own aging female family members and how there are similar and different aging trajectories. What individual-difference factors influenced their aging adaptation?

TEST YOUR KNOWLEDGE!

When thinking about the many different diversity issues of women's aging, it is very important to understand how aging is shown across the world. Take the following quiz about your knowledge regarding population aging: http://www.niapublications.org/quiz/index.php

---

SUPPLEMENTAL BOOK READINGS

Over the past decades, there have been many books written on the topic of diversity issues underlying women's aging experiences. Here are some recommended *additional readings*:

Mehrotra, C. M., Wagner, L. S., Fried, S., & Mehrotra, C. (2008). *Aging and diversity: An active learning experience*. New York, NY: Routledge.
> This text does a thorough job of reviewing the many different diversity factors which may meaningfully influence the aging trajectory of an aging adult. Gender and other unique environment, cultural, and cohort factors are discussed by the authors as they have implications toward quality-of-aging experiences. Pluralistic societies as a complex cultural context for aging are examined. Aging women from many different cultural and socio-environmental contexts would gain meaningful information from this resource book.

Cruikshank, M. (2013). *Learning to be old: Gender, culture, and aging*. Lanham, MD: Rowman & Littlefield Publishers.
> Learning how to be "old" in society is the primary message of this textbook. The adjustment process within cultural and societal attitudes toward aging is discussed. "Schema" development and shift related to how aging is perceived and treated is reflected in the topics discussed. This adaptation process of learning to become "old" in society relates to positive aging but is not a direct message through the book's content.

McCulloch, B. J. (1998). *Old, female, and rural*. New York, NY: Routledge.
> This book examines the meaning of existence and what it is like to age as a woman living in a rural environment. Issues of having access to dependable healthcare, living independently, having adequate contact with others for social support, and other quality-of-life factors are examined in the lives of these older women.

Gelfand, D. E. (2003). *Aging and ethnicity: Knowledge and services (second edition)*. New York, NY: Springer Publishing Co.
> Based on information from the US 2000 Census, this book examines a myriad of diversity issues impacting the quality-of-aging outcomes for diverse individuals. Many different aspects of sex, race, culture, economic status, education level, and lifestyle, among other individual-difference characteristics, are reviewed as significant factors requiring attention in the design and implementation of programs and services to support optimal aging. Aging women from diverse backgrounds would benefit from reading the book.

Cheng, S., Chi, I., Li, L. W., Woo, J., & Fung, H. H. (Editors) (2015). *Successful aging: Asian perspectives.* New York, NY: Springer Publishing Co.

This book does an interesting comparison of Eastern versus Western cultures and their differential impact on the aging of their populations. The chapters in the book examine cultural differences in family system dynamics, social and physical environments, beliefs and values, and lifestyle factors impacting the aging trajectories of women and men. The authors conclude by discussing the quality of aging within these two cultures. Aging women from different cultural backgrounds would benefit from the insights of the book.

Fishman, T. C. (2010). *Shock of gray: The aging of the world's population and how it pits young against old, child against parent, worker against boss, company against rival, and nation against nation.* New York, NY: Scribner.

The author brings an important point to the reader—the world is changing because the world is aging. This is a powerful statement that truly needs to be discussed in terms of eradicating ageism to bringing cohorts together under the shared experience of inevitable aging processes. From an international perspective, the author argues that a growing aging population necessitates a paradigm shift in how "old age" is understood as a life stage and its implications toward communities and public policies. Social change is needed on many different levels within many different countries. Intergenerational relationships and the sharing of resources are certainly social priorities which need to be made into a reality. Older women would be empowered by the message conveyed through the book's chapters.

Magnus, G. M. (2008). *The age of aging: How demographics are changing the global economy and our world.* Hoboken, NJ: Wiley.

The author makes the assertion that it is vital to acknowledge that most countries across the world will be significantly impacted by an aging population for the coming decades. With this demographic "aging" population shift across many countries will create a significant impact on the world economy. If societies are not in the process of addressing economic and associated social policies (eg, retirement pension systems) in response to this changing support ratio of younger to older generations, there will be a negative effect on their economic viability. This is an important issue for older women in many different countries of the world who will directly experience this effect on their economy.

SUPPLEMENTAL AGING VIDEOS

For learning purposes, the use of videos can be very beneficial for both instructors and readers. Here are some recommended *supplemental videos*:

Global aging: http://on.aol.com/video/global-aging-demographics-297733172 (Format: Website)
This is a great website that offers a short video on global aging.

How to Live Forever (2008) (Format: DVD)
The video examines the factors which may predict the lives of people who live to 100 and beyond.

ADDITIONAL INFORMATION LINKS

The following are some recommended *supplemental Internet links*:

American Federation for Aging Research website: http://www.afar.org/infoaging/

NIA Demography Centers website: http://agingcenters.org/

Administration on Aging website: http://www.aoa.gov/AoARoot/Aging_Statistics/index.aspx

World Health Organization website: http://www.who.int/ageing/about/facts/en/index.html

Centers for Disease Control and Prevention website: http://www.cdc.gov/mmwr/preview/mmwrhtml/mm5206a2.htm

United Nations website: http://www.un.org/esa/population/publications/Worldageing19502050/

U.S. Census Bureau website: http://www.census.gov/newsroom/releases/archives/aging_population/cb10-72.html

References

Ailshire, J. A., Beltrán-Sánchez, H., & Crimmins, E. M. (2011). Social characteristics and health status of exceptionally long-lived Americans in the health and retirement study. *Journal of the American Geriatrics Society, 59*(12), 2241–2248. http://dx.doi.org/10.1111/j.1532-5415.

Ajrouch, K. (2007). Resources and well-being among Arab-American elders. *Journal of Cross-Cultural Gerontology, 22*(2), 167–182. http://dx.doi.org/10.1007/s10823-006-9033-z.

Ajrouch, K., & Marshall, V. (2004). Aging and global diversity: Implications for health and practice. *The Gerontologist, 44*(1), 245–246.

Al Hazzouri, A., Sibai, A., Chaaya, M., Mahfoud, Z., & Yount, K. M. (2011). Gender differences in physical disability among older adults in underprivileged communities in Lebanon. *Journal of Aging & Health, 23*(2), 367–382. http://dx.doi.org/10.1177/0898264310385454.

Aldwin, C. M., & Gilmer, D. F. (2013). *Health, illness, and optimal aging: Biological and psychosocial perspectives*. Berlin, Germany: Springer Publishing Company.

Aleman, S., Fitzpatrick, T., Tran, T. V., & Gonzalez, E. (2014). *Therapeutic interventions with ethnic elders: Health and social issues*. New York, NY: Routledge.

Arai, H., Ouchi, Y., Yokode, M., Ito, H., Uematsu, H., Eto, F., et al. (2012). Toward the realization of a better aged society: Messages from gerontology and geriatrics. *Geriatrics and Gerontology International, 12,* 16–22. http://dx.doi.org/10.1111/j.447-0594.2011.00776.x.

Aranda, M. P., Chae, D. H., Lincoln, K. D., Taylor, R., Woodward, A., & Chatters, L. M. (2012). Demographic correlates of DSM-IV major depressive disorder among older African Americans, Black Caribbeans, and non-Hispanic Whites: Results from the national survey of American life. *International Journal of Geriatric Psychiatry, 27*(9), 940–947. http://dx.doi.org/10.1002/gps.2805.

Arizpe, L., & Aranda, J. (2014). Women workers in the strawberry agribusiness in Mexico: *Migration, women and social development*. Berlin, Germany: Springer International Publishing.7495

Atchley,, R. C. (1989). A continuity theory of normal aging. *The Gerontologist, 29*(2), 183–190. http://dx.doi.org/10.1093/geront/29.2.183.

Averett, P., & Jenkins, C. (2012). Review of the literature on older lesbians: Implications for education, practice, and research. *Journal of Applied Gerontology, 31*(4), 537–561. http://dx.doi.org/10.1177/0733464810392555.

Ayotte, B. J., Allaire, J. C., & Whitfield, K. E. (2012). Understanding within-group variability of everyday cognition in aging Black/African American adults: A mimic (multiple indicators, multiple causes) model approach. *Experimental Aging Research, 38*(5), 488–510. http://dx.doi.org/10.1080/0361073X.2012.726022.

Baltes, P. B., & Baltes, M. M. (1990). Psychological perspectives on successful aging: The model of selective optimization with compensation. In P. B. Baltes & M. M. Baltes (Eds.), *Successful aging: Perspectives from the behavioral sciences* (pp. 1–34). New York: Cambridge University Press.

Baltes, P. B., Cornelius, S. W., & Nesselroade, J. R. (1979). Cohort effects in developmental psychology. In J. R. Nesselroade & P. B. Baltes (Eds.), *Longitudinal research in the study of behavior and development*. New York, NY: Academic Press.

Bogunovic, O. (2011). Women and aging. *Harvard Review of Psychiatry, 19*(6), 321–324. http://dx.doi.org/10.3109/10673229.2011.630821.

Borrell, C., Palència, L., Muntaner, C., Urquía, M., Malmusi, D., & O'Campo, P. (2014). Influence of macrosocial policies on women's health and gender inequalities in health. *Epidemiologic Reviews, 36*(1), 31–48.

Bradshaw, R. (1999). The aging experience: Diversity and commonality across cultures. *Journal of Cross-Cultural Psychology, 30*(1), 131–132.

Butler, J. P., Fujii, M., & Sasaki, H. (2011). Balanced aging, or successful aging? *Geriatrics & Gerontology International, 11*(1), 1–2. http://dx.doi.org/10.1111/j.14470594.2010.00661.x.

Butt, D. S., & Beiser, M. (1987). Successful aging: A theme for international psychology. *Psychology and Aging, 2,* 87–94.

Buttaro, T. M., Koeniger-Donohue, R., & Hawkins, J. (2014). Sexuality and quality of life in aging: Implications for practice. *The Journal for Nurse Practitioners, 10*(7), 480–485.

Cernin, P. A., Lysack, C., & Lichtenberg, P. A. (2011). A comparison of self-rated and objectively measured successful aging constructs in an urban sample of African American older adults. *Clinical Gerontologist, 34*(2), 89–102. http://dx.doi.org/10.1080/07317115.2011.539525.

Chan, A., Malhotra, C., Malhotra, R., & Østbye, T. (2011). Living arrangements, social networks and depressive symptoms among older men and women in Singapore. *International Journal of Geriatric Psychiatry, 26*(6), 630–639. http://dx.doi.org/10.1002/gps.2574.

Chan, A., Zimmer, Z., & Saito, Y. (2011). Gender differentials in disability and mortality transitions: The case of older adults in Japan. *Journal of Aging & Health, 23*(8), 1285–1308. http://dx.doi.org/10.1177/0898264311408417.

Chan, C. F., & Chui, E. T. (2011). Association between cultural factors and the caregiving burden for Chinese spousal caregivers of frail elderly in Hong Kong. *Aging & Mental Health, 15*(4), 500–509. http://dx.doi.org/10.1080/13607863.2010.536139.

Charpentier, M., Quéniart, A., & Jacques, J. (2008). Activism among older women in Quebec, Canada: Changing the world after age 65. *Journal of Women & Aging, 20*(3/4), 343–360.

Clark, K., & Glicksman, A. (2012). Age-friendly Philadelphia: Bringing diverse networks together around aging issues. *Journal of Housing for the Elderly, 26*(1–3), 121–136. http://dx.doi.org/10.1080/02763893.2012.655662.

Cohen, G. D., Perlstein, S., Chapline, J., Kelly, J., Firth, K. M., & Simmens, S. (2006). The impact of professionally conducted cultural programs on the physical health, mental health, and social functioning of older adults. *The Gerontologist, 46*(6), 726–734.

Cutler, N. E. (1998). Preparing for their older years: The financial diversity of aging boomers. *Generations, 22*(1), 81–86.

Davis-Berman, J. (2011). Older women in the homeless shelter: Personal perspectives and practice ideas. *Journal of Women & Aging, 23*(4), 360–374. http://dx.doi.org/10.1080/08952841-.2011.611391.

Dionigi, R. A., Horton, S., & Bellamy, J. (2011). Meanings of aging among older Canadian women of varying physical activity levels. *Leisure Sciences, 33*(5), 402–419. http://dx.doi.org/10.1080/01490400.2011.606779.

Duay, D., & Bryan, V. (2006). Senior adults' perceptions of successful aging. *Educational Gerontology, 32*(6), 423–445. http://dx.doi.org/10.1080/03601270600685636.

Duda, R. B., Anarfi, J. K., Adanu, R. M. K., Seffah, J., Darko, R., & Hill, A. G. (2011). The health of the "older women" in Accra, Ghana: Results of the women's health study of Accra. *Journal of Cross-Cultural Gerontology, 26*, 299–314. http://dx.doi.org/10.1007/s10823-011-9148-8.

Dykstra, P. A. (2006). Off the beaten track: Childlessness and social integration in late life. *Research on Aging, 28*(6), 749–767.

Eaton, N. R., Krueger, R. F., South, S. C., Gruenewald, T. L., Seeman, T. E., & Roberts, B. W. (2012). Genes, environments, personality, and successful aging: Toward a comprehensive developmental model in later life. *Journals of Gerontology Series A: Biological Sciences & Medical Sciences, 67A*(5), 480–488.

Fiori, K., Consedine, N., & Magai, C. (2009). Late life attachment in context: Patterns of relating among men and women from seven ethnic groups. *Journal of Cross-Cultural Gerontology, 24*(2), 121–141. http://dx.doi.org/10.1007/s10823-008-9078-2.

Flood, M. (2005). A mid-range nursing theory of successful aging. *Journal of Theory Construction & Testing, 9*(2), 35–39.

Freedman, A., & Iwata-Weickgenannt, K. (2011). Count what you have now. Don't count what you don't have: The Japanese television drama around 40 and the politics of women's happiness. *Asian Studies Review, 35*(3), 295–313. http://dx.doi.org/10.1080/10357823.2011.602042.

Global Aging. (2001). The ageing of the world's population. Retrieved from: <http://www.globalaging.org/waa2/documents/theagingoftheworld.htm>.

Glover, R. J. (1998). Perspectives on aging: Issues affecting the latter part of the life cycle. *Educational Gerontology, 24*(4), 325–331.

Guedes, D. P., Hatmann, A. C., Martini, F. N., Borges, M. B., & Bernardelli, R. (2012). Quality of life and physical activity in a sample of Brazilian older adults. *Journal of Aging & Health, 24*(2), 212–226. http://dx.doi.org/10.1177/0898264311410693.

Guse, L. W., & Masesar, M. A. (1999). Quality of life and successful aging in long-term care: Perceptions of residents. *Issues in Mental Health Nursing, 20*, 527–539.

Hank, K. (2011). How "successful" do older Europeans age? Findings from share. *Journal of Gerontology: Social Sciences, 66B*(2), 230–236. http://dx.doi.org/10.1093/geronb/gbq089.

Hazzard, W. R. (2013). As a gerontologist enters old age. *Journal of the American Geriatrics Society, 61*(4), 639–640. http://dx.doi.org/10.1111/jgs.12176.

Hooker, S. P., Seavey, W., Weidmer, C. E., Harvey, D. J., Stewart, A. L., Gillis, D. E., et al. (2005). The California active aging community grant program: Translating science into practice to promote physical activity in older adults. *Annals of Behavioral Medicine, 29*(3), 155–165.

Hopman-Rock, M., & Westhoff, M. H. (2002). Development and evaluation of "aging well and healthily:" A health-education and exercise program for community-living older adults. *Journal of Aging and Physical Activity, 10*(4), 364–381.

Hrostowski, S. (2010). Diversity in aging America: Making our communities aging friendly. *Race, Gender & Class, 17*(3), 307–313.

Hutchinson, S. L., & Nimrod, G. (2012). Leisure as a resource for successful aging by older adults with chronic health conditions. *International Journal of Aging and Human Development, 74*(1), 41–65.

Hyde, A., Nee, J., Howlett, E., Butler, M., & Drennan, J. (2011). The ending of menstruation: Perspectives and experiences of lesbian and heterosexual women. *Journal of Women & Aging, 23*(2), 160–176. http://dx.doi.org/10.1080/08952841.2011.561145.

Isopahkala-Bouret, U. (2015). Graduation at age 50+: Contested efforts to construct "third age" identities and negotiate cultural age stereotypes. *Journal of Aging Studies, 35*, 1–9.

Iwamasa, G. Y., & Iwasaki, M. (2011). A new multidimensional model of successful aging: Perceptions of Japanese American older adults. *Journal of Cross-Cultural Gerontology, 26*, 261–278. http://dx.doi.org/10.1007/s10823-011-9147-9.

Jenkins, K. E., & Marti, G. (2012). Warrior chicks: Youthful aging in a postfeminist prosperity discourse. *Journal for the Scientific Study of Religion, 51*(2), 241–256. http://dx.doi.org/10.1111/-j.1468-5906.2012.01651.x.

Johnell, K., & Fastbom, J. (2012). Comparison of prescription drug use between community-dwelling and institutionalized elderly in Sweden. *Drugs & Aging, 29*(9), 751–758. http://dx.doi.org/10.1007/s40266-012-0002-7.

Kalavar, J., & Jamuna, D. (2011). Aging of Indian women in India: The experience of older women in formal care homes. *Journal of Women & Aging, 23*(3), 203–215. http://dx.doi.org/10.1080/08952841.2011.587730.

Kampfe, C. M. (2000). Characteristics of diversity and aging: Implications for assessment. *Journal of Applied Rehabilitation Counseling, 31*(1), 33–39.

Katz, C., & Monk, J. (2014). *Full circles: Geographies of women over the life course*. New York, NY: Routledge.

Kauffman, J. (2002). Looking at the past and the future of diversity and aging: An interview with E. Percil Stanford and Fernando Torres-Gil. *Generations, 26*(3), 74–78.

Kaur, G., Bains, K., & Kaur, H. (2012). Body composition, dietary intake and physical activity level of sedentary adult Indian women. *Food and Nutrition Sciences, 3*, 1577–1585. http://dx.doi.org/10.4236/fns.2012.311206.

Keck, M. E., & Sikkink, K. (2014). *Activists beyond borders: Advocacy networks in international politics*. Ithaca, NY: Cornell University Press.

Kimmel, D. (2014). Lesbian, gay, bisexual, and transgender aging concerns. *Clinical Gerontologist, 37*(1), 49–63.

Kimura, J., & Browne, C. V. (2009). Eldercare in a Filipino community: Older women's attitudes toward caregiving and service use. *Journal of Women & Aging, 21*(3), 229–243. http://dx.doi.org/10.1080/08952840903054815.

Kimura, Y., Okumiya, K., Sakamoto, R., Ishine, M., Wada, T., Kosaka, Y., et al. (2009). Comprehensive geriatric assessment of older adults highlanders in Qinghai, China IV: Comparison of food diversity and its relation to health of Han and Tibetan elderly. *Geriatrics & Gerontology International, 9*(4), 359–365. http://dx.doi.org/10.1111/j.1447-0594.2009.00543.x.

Kleyman, P. (2006). Looking ahead: Philadelphia study focuses on diversity in urban aging. *Aging Today, 27*(6), 7–8.

Krainitzki, E. (2014). Judi Dench's age-inappropriateness and the role of M: Challenging normative temporality. *Journal of Aging Studies, 29*, 32–40.

Kreager, P., & Schröder-Butterfill, E. (2007). Gaps in the family networks of older people in three Indonesian communities. *Journal of Cross-Cultural Gerontology, 22*, 1–25. http://dx.doi.org/10.1007/s10823-006-9013-3.

Kulik, L. (2015). The impact of multiple roles on the well-being of older women: Strain or enrichment?: *Women and aging*. Berlin, Germany: Springer International Publishing.5169

Laceulle, H., & Baars, J. (2014). Self-realization and cultural narratives about later life. *Journal of Aging Studies, 31*, 34–44.

Laganá, L., Spellman, T., Wakefield, J., & Oliver, T. (2011). Ethnic minority status, depression, and cognitive failures in relation to marital adjustment in ethnically diverse older women. *Clinical Gerontologist, 34*(3), 173–189. http://dx.doi.org/10.1080/07317115.201 1.554627.

Leach, C. R., & Schoenberg, N. E. (2008). Striving for control: Cognitive, self-care, and faith strategies employed by vulnerable Black and White older adults with multiple chronic conditions. *Journal of Cross-Cultural Gerontology, 23*, 377–399. http://dx.doi.org/10.1007/s10823-008-9086-2.

Lee, E., & Lee, J. (2011). Gender differences in predictors of mental health among older adults in South Korea. *International Journal of Aging & Human Development, 72*(3), 207–223. http://dx.doi.org/10.2190/AG.72.3.c.

Lee, P., Lan, W., & Yen, T. (2011). Aging successfully: A four-factor model. *Educational Gerontology, 37*(3), 210–227. http://dx.doi.org/10.1080/03601277.2010.487759.

Liang, J., & Luo, B. (2012). Toward a discourse shift in social gerontology: From successful aging to harmonious aging. *Journal of Aging Studies, 26*(3), 327–334.

Lindemann, U., Oksa, J., Skelton, D. A., Beyer, N., Klenk, J., Zscheile, J., et al. (2014). Effect of cold indoor environment on physical performance of older women living in the community. *Age and Ageing, 43*(4), 571–575.

Litwin, H. (2005). Correlates of successful aging: Are they universal? *International Journal of Aging & Human Development, 61*(4), 313–333.

Litwin, H. (2006). The path to well-being among elderly Arab Israelis. *Journal of Cross-Cultural Gerontology, 21*(1/2), 25–40. http://dx.doi.org/10.1007/s10823-006-9019-x.

Litwin, H. (2009). Understanding aging in a Middle Eastern context: The SHARE-Israel survey of persons aged 50 and older. *Journal of Cross-Cultural Gerontology, 24*(1), 49–62. http://dx.doi.org/10.1007/s10823-008-9073-7.

McCandless, N. J. (1998). Strengthening aging families: Diversity in practice and policy. *Journal of Comparative Family Studies, 29*(3), 607–608.

McCann Mortimer, P., Ward, L., & Winefield, H. (2008). Successful ageing by whose definition? Views of older, spiritually affiliated women. *Australian Journal on Ageing, 27*(4), 200–204.

McMullin, J. A. (2000). Diversity and the state of sociological aging theory. *The Gerontologist, 40*(5), 517–530.

Mendes de Leon, C. F., Eschbach, K., & Markides, K. S. (2011). Population trends and late-life disability in Hispanics from the Midwest. *Journal of Aging & Health, 23*(7), 1166–1188. http://dx.doi.org/10.1177/0898264311422100.

Merriam, S. B., & Kee, Y. (2014). Promoting community wellbeing: The case for lifelong learning for older adults. *Adult Education Quarterly, 64*(2), 128–144.

Minkler, M., & Fadem, P. (2002). "Successful aging:" A disability perspective. *Journal of Disability Policy Studies, 12*(4), 229–235.

Minkler, M., & Stone, R. (1985). The feminization of poverty and older women. *The Gerontologist, 25*(4), 351–357. http://dx.doi.org/10.1093/geront/25.4.351.

Mokuau, N., & Tomioka, M. (2010). Caregiving and older Japanese adults: Lessons learned from the periodical literature. *Journal of Gerontological Social Work, 53*(2), 117–136. http://dx.doi.org/10.1080/01634370903202868.

Molzahn, A. E., Kalfoss, M., Schick Makaroff, K., & Skevington, S. M. (2011). Comparing the importance of different aspects of quality of life to older adults across diverse cultures. *Age & Ageing, 40*(2), 192–199. http://dx.doi.org/10.1093/ageing/afq156.

Momtaz, Y. A., Ibrahim, R., Hamid, T. A., & Yahaya, N. (2011). Sociodemographic predictors of elderly's psychological well-being in Malaysia. *Aging & Mental Health, 15*(4), 437–445.

Montemurro, B., & Siefken, J. M. (2014). Cougars on the prowl? New perceptions of older women's sexuality. *Journal of Aging Studies, 28*, 35–43.

Myers, D. (2013). Diversity and aging in America. *Planning, 79*(3), 11–15.

Nilsson, C., Avlund, K., & Lund, R. (2010). Social inequality in onset of mobility disability among older Danes: The mediation effect of social relations. *Journal of Aging & Health, 22*(4), 522–541. http://dx.doi.org/10.1177/0898264309359684.

Nimrod, G. (2011). The fun culture in seniors' online communities. *Gerontologist, 51*(2), 226–237.

Nimrod, G., & Kleiber, D. A. (2007). Reconsidering change and continuity in later life: Toward an innovation theory of successful aging. *International Journal of Aging & Human Development, 65*(1), 1–22.

Nimrod, G., & Rotem, A. (2012). An exploration of the innovation theory of successful aging among older tourists. *Ageing & Society, 32*(3), 379–404. http://dx.doi.org/10.1017/S0144686X.1100033X.

Osorio-Parraguez, P. (2013). Health and widowhood: Meanings and experience of elderly women in Chile. *Health, 5*(8), 1272–1276. http://dx.doi.org/10.4236/health.2013.58173.

Padilla, Y. C., & Villalobos, G. (2007). Cultural responses to health among Mexican American women and their families. *Family & Community Health, 30*, S24–S33.

Palloni, A., & McEniry, M. (2007). Aging and health status of elderly in Latin America and the Caribbean: Preliminary findings. *Journal of Cross-Cultural Gerontology, 22*, 263–285. http://dx.doi.org/10.1007/s10823-006-9001-7.

Perrig-Chiello, P., & Hutchison, S. (2010). Health and well-being in old age: The pertinence of a gender mainstreaming approach in research. *Gerontology, 56*(2), 208–213. http://dx.doi.org/10.1159/-000235813.

Phelan, E. A., Anderson, L. A., LaCroix, A. Z., & Larson, E. B. (2004). Older adults' views of "successful aging"- How do they compare with researchers' definitions? *Journal of the American Geriatrics Society, 52*(2), 211–216. http://dx.doi.org/10.1111/j.15325415.2004.52056.x.

Piccinin, A. M., Muniz-Terrera, G., Clouston, S., Reynolds, C. A., Thorvaldsson, V., Deary, I. J., et al. (2013). Coordinated analysis of age, sex, and education effects on change in MMSE scores. *Journals of Gerontology Series B: Psychological Sciences & Social Sciences, 68*(3), 374–390.

Powers, S. M., & Whitlatch, C. J. (2014). Measuring cultural justifications for caregiving in African American and White caregivers. *Dementia* Online publication. http://dx.doi.org/10.1177/-1471301214532112.

Pruchno, R., Hahn, S., & Wilson-Genderson, M. (2012). Cigarette smokers, never-smokers, and transitions: Implications for successful aging. *International Journal of Aging and Human Development, 74*(3), 193–209.

Rabi, K. (2006). Israeli perspectives on elder abuse. *Educational Gerontology, 32*(1), 49–62. http://dx.doi.org/10.1080/03601270500338617.

Reichstadt, J., Sengupta, G., Depp, C. A., Palinkas, L. A., & Jeste, D. V. (2010). Older adults' perspectives on successful aging: Qualitative interviews. *The American Journal of Geriatric Psychiatry, 18*(7), 567–575.

Roos, N. P., & Havens, B. (1991). Predictors of successful aging: A twelve-year study of Manitoba elderly. *American Journal of Public Health, 81*(1), 63–68.

Ryser, L., & Halseth, G. (2011). Informal support networks of low-income senior women living alone: Evidence from Fort St. John, BC. *Journal of Women & Aging, 23*(3), 185–202. http://dx.doi.org/10.1080/08952841.2011.587734.

Saucier, M. G. (2004). Midlife and beyond: Issues for aging women. *Journal of Counseling & Development, 82*(4), 420–425.

Shah, A. (2007). Does long-term economic adversity affect older adults' suicide rates? A cross-national comparison. *International Psychogeriatrics, 19*(4), 788–789. http://dx.doi.org/10.1017/S1041610207005704.

Smith, G. C., Tobin, S. S., Robertson-Tchabo, E. A., & Power, P. W. (1995). *Strengthening aging families: Diversity in practice and policy.* Thousand Oaks, CA: Sage.

Smith, J., & Baltes, P. B. (1993). Differential psychological ageing: Profiles of the old and very old. *Ageing and Society, 13*(4), 551–587.

Stark-Wroblewski, K., Edelbaum, J. K., & Bello, T. O. (2008). Perceptions of aging among rural, Midwestern senior citizens: Signs of women's resiliency. *Journal of Women & Aging, 20*(3–4), 361–373. http://dx.doi.org/10.1080/08952840801985185.

Steffens, D. C., Fisher, G. G., Langa, K. M., Potter, G. G., & Plassman, B. L. (2009). Prevalence of depression among older Americans: The aging, demographics and memory study. *International Psychogeriatrics, 21*(5), 879–888. http://dx.doi.org/10.1017/S1041610209990044.

Stöckl, H., Watts, C., & Penhale, B. (2012). Intimate partner violence against older women in Germany: Prevalence and associated factors. *Journal of Interpersonal Violence, 27*(13), 2545–2564. http://dx.doi.org/10.1177/0886260512436390.

Strauss, J. R. (2011). Contextual influences on women's health concerns and attitudes toward menopause. *Health & Social Work, 36*(2), 121–127.

Stromquist, N. P. (2014). *Women in the third world: An encyclopedia of contemporary issues.* New York, NY: Routledge.

Szwarcwald, C., da Mota, J., Damacena, G., & Pereira, T. (2011). Health inequalities in Rio de Janeiro, Brazil: Lower healthy life expectancy in socioeconomically disadvantaged areas. *American Journal of Public Health, 101*(3), 517–523. http://dx.doi.org/10.2105/AJPH.2010.195453.

Teuscher, U. (2010). Change and persistence of personal identities after the transition to retirement. *International Journal of Aging & Human Development, 70*(1), 89–106. http://dx.doi.org/10.2190/AG.70.1.d.

Thanakwang, K., Ingersoll-Dayton, B., & Soonthorndhada, K. (2012). The relationships among family, friends, and psychological well-being for Thai elderly. *Aging & Mental Health, 16*(8), 993–1003. http://dx.doi.org/10.1080/13607863.2012.692762.

Thomas, R., Hardy, C., Cutcher, L., & Ainsworth, S. (2014). What's age got to do with it? On the critical analysis of age and organizations. *Organization Studies, 35*(11), 1569–1584.

Thompson, W. K., Charoa, L., Vahia, I. V., Depp, C., Allison, M., & Jeste, D. V. (2011). Association between higher levels of sexual function, activity, and satisfaction and self-rated successful aging in older postmenopausal women. *Journal of Applied Gerontology, 59*, 1503–1508.

Tiedt, A. D. (2013). Cross-national comparisons of gender differences in late-life depressive symptoms in Japan and the United States. *Journals of Gerontology Series B: Psychological Sciences & Social Sciences, 68*(3), 443–454.

Torres, S. (2003). A preliminary empirical test of a culturally-relevant theoretical framework for the study of successful aging. *Journal of Cross-Cultural Gerontology, 18*(1), 79–100.

Torres, S. (2009). Vignette methodology and culture-relevance: Lessons learned through a project on successful aging with Iranian immigrants to Sweden. *Journal of Cross-Cultural Gerontology, 24*, 93–114. http://dx.doi.org/10.1007/s10823-0099095-9.

Torres-Gil, F., & Rudinica, B. (2012). The 21st century realities of American politics, aging and diversity. *Aging Today, 33*(1), 9–14.

Troutman, M., Nies, M. A., & Bentley, M. (2011). Measuring successful aging in Southern Black older adults. *Educational Gerontology, 37*, 38–50. http://dx.doi.org/10.1080/0360 1277.2010.500587.

Twigg, J., & Majima, S. (2014). Consumption and the constitution of age: Expenditure patterns on clothing, hair and cosmetics among post-war 'baby boomers'. *Journal of Aging Studies, 30*, 23–32.

Twigg, J., & Martin, W. (Eds.). (2015). *Routledge handbook of cultural gerontology*. New York, NY: Routledge.

Willcox, D. C., Willcox, B. J., Sokolovsky, J., & Sakihara, S. (2007). The cultural context of "successful aging" among older women weavers in a northern Okinawan village: The role of productive activity. *Journal of Cross-Cultural Gerontology, 22*, 137–165. http://dx.doi.org/10.1007/s10823-006-9032-0.

Witten, T. M. (2015). Elder transgender lesbians: Exploring the intersection of age, lesbian sexual identity, and transgender identity. *Journal of Lesbian Studies, 19*(1), 73–89.

Zhang, L., Xu, Y., Nie, H., Zhang, Y., & Wu, Y. (2012). The prevalence of depressive symptoms among the older in China: A meta-analysis. *International Journal of Geriatric Psychiatry, 27*(9), 900–906. http://dx.doi.org/10.1002/gps.2821.

Zimmermann, H. P., & Grebe, H. (2014). "Senior coolness:" Living well as an attitude in later life. *Journal of Aging Studies, 28*, 22–34.

9

Expansion of Women's Roles in Later Life

Global Fact: *In many parts of the world it is not uncommon today to be part of a four-generation family, where the chronological rules for assuming the roles of grandparents or grandchildren are increasingly blurred. At the same time, more individuals are growing older outside of traditional family networks and are simulating family life through communities or primary groups.*

—Global Aging (2001)

Women have a midlife and later-life "journey" of self-exploration that involves many role transitions and changes (Wiggs, 2010). In discussing the many different evolving social roles of women as they age, it is invariably important to understand their expectations toward a healthy life span within and across these life roles (Cicirelli, 2011; Ferrucci, Schrack, Knuth, & Simonsick, 2012; Pakarinen, Raitanen, Kaaja, & Luoto, 2010). Evers, Klusmann, Schwarzer, and Heuser (2011) suggested that older adults' role-related activities involving engagement in active physical or mental functioning can meaningfully contribute to their positive aging outcomes. It is equally important to acknowledge how women's physical and/or mental health needs are dynamically affected by their long-term social roles and relationships (Lewis, 2011; Ron, 2009).

According to Role theory (eg, Biddle, 1986), a "role" relates to a person's activities and identity within a social context. Gender role, among other issues, impacts the many different roles that women occupy into later life. Quéniart and Charpentier (2013) purported the idea that women over a life span have an interesting "transmission" role within a family system and broader culture, involving the processes of "initiating," "bequeathing," and "remembering" over time. Within Role theory, there are related concepts that are important for understanding the nature of roles with women in later life (Biddle, 1986, 2013): "Role demand" pertains to the expectations of responsibilities within a designated role, "role overload" occurs when the demands of the role exceed the capabilities of the person occupying the role, "role conflict" is when a person has more than one role to occupy and multiple roles conflict in one or more ways (eg, time conflict, physical space conflict, value conflict), and, finally, a "role stressor" manifests itself when a person experiences negative psychological tension in response to the one or more roles occupied.

Using Carstensen's concept of a social optimization with compensation strategy with social roles (Young, Baltes, & Pratt, 2007), it may be most adaptive for aging women to choose social roles that best support personal aging needs such as a strong social support system and social status. Maintaining long-term social connections is a socio-motivational need, whether intrinsic or socialized from early childhood, which is associated more with women over the course of a life span (Wallston, 1987).

EXPANDED ROLE DURATION

Expansion and change of women's roles in societies across the world are in response to the social and economic changes of the communities in which they live. For example, multiple cohorts of aging women are currently, and will continue to be, faced with working longer than ever before due to declining economies and increasingly scarce financial resources accumulated over time (eg, concept of "feminization of poverty;" Minkler & Stone, 1985). This elongation of workforce participation translates into the elongation of life roles for aging women.

QUOTES FROM FAMOUS, POSITIVELY AGING WOMEN

If you age with somebody, you go through so many roles –
you're lovers, friends, enemies, colleagues, strangers;
you're brother and sister.
That's what intimacy is, if you're with your soulmate.
—*Cate Blanchett, Actress*

Women's multiple roles of being a caregiver, an employee, significant other/companion, and social roles may certainly impact their aging trajectories into later adulthood but this experience may be quite beneficial if women's experience of stress is relatively positive in nature (ie, a motivational feeling of "eustress;" Iida & Oguma, 2014), and positively engages the aging woman's mind and body in daily activities. Paggi and Hayslip (1999), among other researchers, emphasized the role of "mental aerobics" in an adult's successful aging. The active engagement of women across multiple social roles that entail appropriate levels of physical and cognitive engagement with others in immediate social environment would be beneficial for all involved. Thus, it is important for communities to encourage the active mental and physical engagement of women as they age. Older women have much to contribute to society, and this extended social participation may be of mutual benefit if engagement activities are appropriate in levels of activity.

CHECK IT OUT!

Search the Internet to find resources related to supporting the many different role responsibilities of women in later life, from extended working role to on-going caregiving/eldercare duties. What are some "role support" programs and resources that aging women can participate in on a daily basis? What are emergent roles for aging women in different cultures based on your Internet search? As you are examining these factors, think about the following questions:

1. What are the cultural "messages" about women and later-life roles?
2. Are there apparent stereotypes about women's roles in later life?
3. Are there motivational factors to consider when understanding the evolution and expansion of women's roles across their life span?

TIPS FOR WOMEN'S BALANCING OF MULTIPLE LIFE ROLES

1. Find a "balance" of roles that you enjoy.
2. Only do what you can do and rely on others.
3. Establish a daily routine and set goals for activities.
4. Anticipate the "unanticipated" and be flexible.
5. Forgive yourself if not everything gets done as planned.

MULTIPLE SOCIAL ROLES IN "BALANCE"

Related to women's roles over time is the concept of a "superwoman syndrome" (Shaevitz, 1984), which is the idea that women may feel compelled to occupy and fully accomplish more than one social role (eg, employee, caregiver, companion, mentor, and/or friend) when it may be that this circumstance is causing feelings of role-related stressors, task overload, and/or role conflict for women into later life. It is ironic that as women's social status has increased in many different societies across the world, the complexity of their lives has correspondingly increased. Why is this an aging issue that impacts women's later-life adjustment? The proceeding sections will explore this question and explain why women's current effort toward this standard has important implications toward the probability of achieving positive aging.

Elder caregiving role. Internationally, women typically are engaged in formal and/or informal (filial) caregiving roles. The challenges are often talked about and, yet, the rewards of these important caregiver–recipient relationships are not discussed as much as they should be as they impact a woman's positive aging trajectory. For example, Butler, Wardamasky, and Brennan-Ing (2012) investigated the positive benefits of caring for aging women clients among a sample of female home care aides. The researchers revealed that there was an unanticipated bonding on an emotional and social level that was a definite benefit and which may have a corresponding positive influence on the aging trajectory of both women involved.

An intriguing process within the eldercare relationship dynamic occurs when (some) women experience the feeling of a "role reversal" in caring for aging parents and other relatives/significant others. An ethnographic study conducted by Dubus (2010) examined the role-related adjustment issues of aging Southeast Asian refugees in the United States. Among other findings, results of the cultural investigation revealed difficult role transitions for some mothers in relinquishing the role of caregiver (mother) to become a dependent care recipient. Assuming the role of caregiver can be an equally challenging transition, if not anticipated and planned for by a woman across her life span. The experience of becoming a caregiver to aging parents can be a "universal" phenomenon for women across the world (Pope, Kolomer, & Glass, 2012) but the degree to which there are support resources and positive caregiving outcomes may be dependent upon the cultural context of the eldercare situation (Lahaie, Earle, & Heymann, 2013; Ron, 2009) and the nature of the care demand (eg, caring for parents with intellectual disabilities; Rowbotham, Cuskelly, & Carroll, 2011).

The caregiving role for women is best supported when community resources understand the changing capabilities of the aging woman as a caregiver. As the functioning ability of the aging woman changes, it is critical to have available community supports and educational programs to address the issue and resolve any "barriers" to access. As a "real world" example, if an aging woman's driving capability is limited due to sensory and/or physical changes over time, the nature of the regional location (urban versus rural) can definitely impact the ability of the aging woman to continue in the role of a responsive and responsible elder as well as the quality of care extended to her care recipients (Byles & Gallienne, 2012).

An interesting extension of this concept of aging women involved in the eldercare process is the nature of the family roles and family members involved. To illustrate this point, one such societal phenomenon on a national and international basis is the increasing number of grandmothers becoming part- or full-time caregivers of their grandchildren (ie, second parenthood), and this is becoming an increasingly normative role for women in many different races and ethnicities (eg, African-American women; Conway, Jones, & Speakes-Lewis, 2011) with care recipients of many different need levels (eg, grandchildren with special needs; Park, Hogan, & D'Ottavi, 2004). This certainly can be a challenging and unanticipated later-life responsibility for women but it may also be viewed as a way for aging women to socially and physically engage with younger generations and other social contacts. This situation may create an enhanced role for aging women within the family dynamic (Anderson, Liu, & Liao, 2013), as well as fulfilling their possible need to "give back" to others (Villar, Celdrn, & Triad, 2012).

Conversely, there is a growing number of cases related to childless aging women faced with a paucity of family members to care for and, thus, be cared for (De Medeiros et al., 2013). The social situation faced by older women without offspring is not necessarily an obstacle to achieving positive aging outcomes. Rather, the challenge for childless women is to develop long-lasting "nonbiological" social relationships with younger generations to compensate for a potential "care gap" in later life when dependency needs may arise.

Work and retirement roles. As with the caregiver role, the experience of women being in the role of worker and even retiree is longer than previous cohorts of women and will continue to expand over the coming decades. As "baby boomers" and other generations of women continue to live longer and healthier lives than previous generations, there is a need to reevaluate how to optimize the aging experience during what can be an extended period of life in both the workplace and retirement (Byles et al., 2013).

The "key" to working-related positive aging outcomes (eg, good mental health status) for women across their life spans is to have an absence of role conflicts with other life obligations and the presence of support resources to balance their work and nonwork roles (Opree &

Kalmijn, 2012; Van Putten, Vlasblom, Dykstra, & Schippers, 2010; Wong & Almeida, 2012). The social status of paid employment can certainly positively impact the social status and decision-making power of aging women in many different cultures across the world (eg, married women in Kashmir; Arooj et al., 2013).

The timing of retirement has many issues to consider for women across their lives. The decision of when to retire is influenced by many other nonwork-related factors but still significantly influence a woman's financial and social status (Price & Nesteruk, 2010). These factors may include, for example, becoming divorced and the associated need for many different economically vulnerable women to continue working past traditional retirement age (Butrica & Smith, 2012). Frieze, Olson, and Murrell (2011) examined the desired timing factors of retirement for women with MBAs. The researchers found that some aging women considered later-life retirement because of financial concerns but some also wanted to delay retirement because they may hold nontraditional gender role beliefs about working and wanted to engage in stimulating cognitive and social activities in the workplace.

Volunteer and other social activities. The role of volunteer within a community is a vital activity for aging women to make a meaningful social contribution; this is especially true if the activity is appropriately planned for and societally valued (Manning, 2010; Nesteruk & Price, 2011). Being active and civically engaged can be a mutual benefit to both the community receiving the volunteerism outcomes and active older women. Recent research suggests that community engagement can positively impact the mental health of women retirees in many different cultures (eg, sample of Australian retirees; Olesen & Berry, 2011). From an international perspective, women's social status and social support in times of personal transitions and loss (eg, widowhood) can be enhanced through these pro-active social engagement efforts (eg, Isherwood, King, & Luszcz, 2012).

Because women in most societies typically have longer life expectancies than their male peers, the nature of older women's social engagement activities and their maintenance of intimate relationships may be rather complex and involve multiple generations of social support. A woman becoming a widow in mid to later life may experience a meaningful fluctuation in her social networks and significant role-related transitions affecting her personal quality of life in many different ways (Bharati, 2011; Halleröd, 2013; Wilson & Supiano, 2011). Social engagement on a continual basis has the benefits of increasing older adults' physical and mental activity levels through communication and behavioral interactions (eg, McAuley et al., 2009).

A major benefit for aging women maintaining their social relationships and continuing their active social engagement within the community is that these pro-active behaviors help in reducing the risk of social isolation and depression while increasing older women's physical health, feelings of personal autonomy, and elevated social status within the cultural context (Bojorquez-Chapela, Manrique-Espinoza, Mejía-Arango, Solís, & Salinas-Rodríguez, 2012; Kim, Kim, & Kim, 2013; Ladin, Daniels, & Kawachi, 2010; Tintle, Bacon, Kostyuchenko, Gutkovich, & Bromet, 2011).

Recent studies of intergenerational support from within the community or family system for aging adults in Indonesia, Bangladesh, and England have concluded that maintaining social relationships is a universal factor which predicts positive aging results for older adults (Frankenberg & Kuhn, 2004; Grundy & Read, 2012). Societal expectations toward younger generations actively engaging older adults in social activities, however, vary by culture (eg, Israel; Lowenstein, Katz, & Daatland, 2004) but more education and community programs are needed to encourage intergenerational interactions.

WITHIN-ROLE TASK EXPANSION

Each social role has more than one context for women to balance. For example, a woman may find that she is a caregiver for many different people in her family system for decades of her life but the number of people she is caregiver for may fluctuate as their associated needs of dependency shift. Brody (1990) discussed the idea of "women in the middle" as it relates to women experiencing being a caregiver for multiple generations of both younger and older family members simultaneously. As much as this social and physical engagement as a caregiver may be beneficial to women, it is realistic to acknowledge that caregivers may experience feelings of physical and mental burden. The Wear and Tear theory (Park & Yeo, 2013), as one of many "programmed theories" of aging, might argue that being a caregiver may have a cumulative negative effect upon the physical aging of women, accelerating the physical deterioration of a woman's joints, bones, and/or muscular structure. Understanding and supporting the needs of women caregivers, as most caregivers in the world are traditionally women (Brody, 1990; Wootton, 1998), is an ethical imperative in many parts of the world (eg, industrialized nations) as the mean age of the population continues to rise in these countries and so will the role demands of women as caregivers.

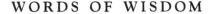

WORDS OF WISDOM

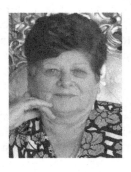

Paulina is a 71-year-old woman originally from Albania. Paulina, better known as Nina, came to the United States at the age of 51 with her husband and two sons. Before Nina moved to the United States she was a high school Math teacher in her hometown. Nina has always been dedicated to her family throughout her life. When she left Albanian to come to the United States with her husband, her role as a wife and mother motivated her to learn the English language and work hard to help support her family. Now that Nina is not only a wife and a mother but also a grandmother, she finds herself at the happiest point in her life. Nina believes that her evolving roles have only made her happier because to her they are accomplishments.

Nina believes that patience is one of the most important traits she has carried throughout her roles as a wife, mother, grandmother, and mother-in-law. Nina advises other women going through these roles to always remain patient, give unconditional care and love to their children, to always understand everything fully without jumping to conclusions, and to be a friend to everyone. Nina believes that her ability to ignore the negative and instead look at the positive has allowed her to successfully evolve through her roles as a wife, mother, grandmother, and mother-in-law. The strong relationships she has cultivated with her family members have helped to keep her strong, and the strength in turn has helped to keep those family members strong. Most importantly, always keep family as the number one priority and goal because that is where the strength lies.

The quality of women's aging is inextricably linked to the roles they occupy over a life span from childhood onward. What women learn about their roles in society and how they should feel about aging is guided through social role modeling according to Bandura (1977). Roles define who we are and how we perceive ourselves over time. Self-esteem and self-expectations toward goal accomplishments influence women's aging trajectory in very meaningful ways. Education, community outreach programs, and support programs can assist women's role-related development over time. How early should education and other societal interventions be implemented to assist in achieving women's quality of aging? Cultures and societies should consider communicating ways to optimize role-related activities for women as early as elementary education through stories and activities that promote positive aging role models for learners.

SUMMARY

As women in many industrialized nations across the world are typically living longer than ever before, it is important to understand the dynamic nature of roles lost, acquired, and maintained over time. The expansion of role responsibilities in the workplace and in the family, among other contexts, needs to be better understood and supported within communities in order to optimize women's aging trajectories into later life. For example, women might find themselves in the situation of "multitasking" in the role of caregiver, caring for multiple generations both in and beyond the family (biological) system. From a cross-cultural perspective, better understanding the emerging role-related support and educational needs of aging women will assist in creating improved quality-of-life outcomes for all involved.

DISCUSSION QUESTIONS

1. Are women's feelings of positive aging potentially related to role-related activities and accomplishments? How so?
2. Is the "superwoman syndrome" best understood as being a culture-specific or a universal experience for aging women?
3. What is the role of education in supporting women's role choices over a life span? Is this shaped by the cultural context in which the women live?
4. How does culture impact the range and longevity of women's roles as they age? Explain cultural factors potentially impacting women's positive aging outcomes.
5. Do you think peer pressure exists in women's lives and how can it be channeled to promote positive aging?
6. Does the media influence women's life role choices? If yes, how?
7. Who are the potential early role models in women's lives who influence their later-life activities and role responsibilities?
8. Are women's roles going to expand further as life expectancies are projected to continue to increase for many countries across the world through the year 2050? Will aging men's roles also show an expansion in parallel?
9. For positive aging to be achieved, is it important for aging women to be selective about the roles to continue in their lives (eg, Baltes' concept of selective optimization with compensation)? What issues should determine this role selection (eg, health)?

10. One might argue that it is an ethical responsibility of societies to help an aging population be productive and contributory within the community. In what ways can communities better educate and support older women's multiple roles?

T E S T   Y O U R   K N O W L E D G E !

Take the following quiz about your personal attitudes about women's lifespan roles:

http://testyourself.psychtests.com/testid/2435

SUPPLEMENTAL BOOK READINGS

Over the past decades, there have been many books written on the topic of the many roles of aging women across a life span. Here are some recommended *additional readings*:

Bertini, K. (2011). *Strength for the sandwich generation: Help to thrive while simultaneously caring for our kids and our aging parents*. Westport, CT: Praeger.

This book raises an important social issue of middle-aged women increasingly faced with the multifocused role of caregiver for multiple generations within a family system. The book takes a positive perspective on this role for aging women, suggesting that this is a life-growth opportunity ("thrive") rather than a negative role obligation. The message behind the book reflects the need for aging women (and men) to meaningfully examine their life circumstances and to reevaluate the true life-learning value of such experiences for positive aging to occur.

Turner, B. F., & Troll, L. E. (Editors). (1993). *Women growing older: Psychological perspectives*. Thousand Oaks, CA: Sage Publications, Inc.

The authors acknowledge that women's lives are complex and entail occupying multiple roles, balancing parenthood, work, marriage, and all other social roles. There is no a typical "pattern" to an aging woman and many psychological theories are presented to explain the ego ("self") and social development into later life.

Morris, V. (2014). *How to care for aging parents* (3rd edition).
New York, NY: Workman Publishing Company.
   This is a wonderful guidebook for all people faced with the life-changing step of switching roles to become the caregiver of their parents. The book's chapters offer comprehensive information related to this complex process of care and suggests very helpful points in how best to optimize this care situation for all involved. Aging women caregivers would appreciate the positive, pro-active nature of the book which could assist them to be better caregivers as well as help with their own role transitions to become care recipients.

Winston, L., Kaplan, M., Perlstein, S., Tietze, R., & Greene, M. (2001). *Grandpartners: Intergenerational learning and civic renewal, K-6.* Chicago, IL: Heinemann.
   Becoming a grandparent and the associated role responsibilities for aging women is a well-known role but has interesting implications toward later-life caregiving, intergenerational relationships, and personal growth for all involved. The role dynamics within this grandparent–grandchild relationship bond creates wonderful opportunities for physical and mental activities for aging women which further enhance their positive aging.

SUPPLEMENTAL AGING VIDEOS

For learning purposes, the video can be used by both instructors and readers. Here are some recommended *supplemental videos*:

Generations United: http://www.gu.org/SearchResults.aspx?Search=videos (Format: Website)
   This is a great website that offers short videos on intergenerational learning.

Edutopia: http://www.edutopia.org/blog/intergenerational-learning-brendan-okeefe (Format: Website)
   This is a great website that offers YouTube videos on intergenerational learning processes and outcomes.

i2i Intergenerational Society: http://www.intergenerational.ca/index.php?option=com_content&view=article&id=50:whose-grandma-are-you&catid=39:20-minute-version (Format: Website)
   This is a great website that offers a 20 min video about intergenerational learning in a classroom setting.

When Your Parent Needs You: A Guide to Positive Growth When Caring for Aging Parents (Format: DVD)

> *Description*: This is a great video for giving advice on how to optimize the caregiving experience for an aging woman and those she cares for in her life.

ADDITIONAL INFORMATION LINKS

The following are some recommended *supplemental Internet links*:

American Federation for Aging Research website: http://www.afar.org/infoaging/

NIA Demography Centers website: http://agingcenters.org/

World Health Organization website: http://www.who.int/ageing/about/facts/en/index.html

Centers for Disease Control and Prevention website: http://www.cdc.gov/mmwr/preview/mmwrhtml/mm5206a2.htm

United Nations website: http://www.un.org/esa/population/publications/Worldageing19502050/

U.S. Census Bureau website: http://www.census.gov/newsroom/releases/archives/2010_census/ cb12-239.html

References

Anderson, S. G., Liu, M., & Liao, M. (2013). Subsidized child care by grandparents: Profiles of caregivers in an emerging public service context. *Journal of Women & Aging, 25*(3), 242–259. http://dx.doi.org/10.1080/08952841.2013.791599.

Arooj, S., Hussain, W., Arooj, A., Iqbal, A., Hameed, S., & Abbasi, A. (2013). Paid work and decision making power of married women cross sectional survey of Muzaffarabad Azad state of Jammu & Kashmir. *Advances in Applied Sociology, 3*(3), 165–171.

Bandura, A. (1977). *Social learning theory*. Englewood Cliffs, NJ: Prentice Hall.

Bharati, K. (2011). Being old and widow: Understanding their social realities. *Indian Journal of Gerontology, 25*(3), 415–437.

Biddle, B. J. (1986). Recent development in role theory. *Annual Review of Sociology, 12*, 67–92.

Biddle, B. J. (2013). *Role theory: Expectations, identities, and behaviors*. Waltham, MA: Academic Press.

Bojorquez-Chapela, I., Manrique-Espinoza, B., Mejía-Arango, S., Solís, M., & Salinas-Rodríguez, A. (2012). Effect of social capital and personal autonomy on the incidence of depressive symptoms in the elderly: Evidence from a longitudinal study in Mexico. *Aging & Mental Health, 16*(4), 462–471. http://dx.doi.org/10.1080/13607863.2011.651432.

Brody, E. M. (1990). *Women in the middle: Their parent-care years*. New York, NY: Springer Publishing, Co.

Butler, S. S., Wardamasky, S., & Brennan-Ing, M. (2012). Older women caring for older women: The rewards and challenges of the home care aide job. *Journal of Women & Aging, 24*(3), 194–215. http://dx.doi.org/10.1080/08952841.2012.639667.

Butrica, B. A., & Smith, K. E. (2012). Racial and ethnic differences in the retirement prospects of divorced women in the baby boom and generation x cohorts. *Social Security Bulletin, 72*(1), 23–36.

Byles, J., & Gallienne, L. (2012). Driving in older age: A longitudinal study of women in urban, regional, and remote areas and the impact of caregiving. *Journal of Women & Aging, 24*(2), 113–125. http://dx.doi.org/10.1080/08952841.2012.639661.

Byles, J., Tavener, M., Robinson, I., Parkinson, L., Smith, P. W., Stevenson, D., et al. (2013). Transforming retirement: New definitions of life after work. *Journal of Women & Aging, 25*(1), 24–44. http://dx.doi.org/10.1080/08952841.2012.717855.

Cicirelli, V. G. (2011). Elders' attitudes toward extending the healthy life span. *Journal of Aging Studies, 25*(2), 84–93. http://dx.doi.org/10.1016/j.jaging.2010.08.011.

Conway, F., Jones, S., & Speakes-Lewis, A. (2011). Emotional strain in caregiving among African American grandmothers raising their grandchildren. *Journal of Women & Aging, 23*(2), 113–128. http://dx.doi.org/10.1080/08952841.2011.561142.

De Medeiros, K., Rubinstein, R. L., Onyike, C. U., Johnston, D. M., Baker, A., Mcnabney, M., et al. (2013). Childless elders in assisted living: Findings from the Maryland assisted living study. *Journal of Housing for the Elderly, 27*(1/2), 206–220. http://dx.doi.org/10.1080/-02763893.2012.754823.

Dubus, N. (2010). "I feel like her daughter not her mother:" Ethnographic trans-cultural perspective of the experiences of aging for a group of Southeast Asian refugees in the United States. *Journal of Aging Studies, 24*(3), 204–211. http://dx.doi.org/10.1016/j.jaging.2010.2.002.

Evers, A., Klusmann, V., Schwarzer, R., & Heuser, I. (2011). Improving cognition by adherence to physical or mental exercise: A moderated mediation analysis. *Aging & Mental Health, 15*(4), 446–455.

Ferrucci, L., Schrack, J. A., Knuth, N. D., & Simonsick, E. M. (2012). Aging and the energetic cost of life. *Journal of the American Geriatrics Society, 60*(9), 1768–1769. http://dx.doi.org/10.1111/-j.1532-5415.2012.04102.x.

Frankenberg, E., & Kuhn, R. S. (2004). The role of social context in shaping intergenerational relations in Indonesia and Bangladesh. *Annual Review of Gerontology & Geriatrics, 24,* 177–199.

Frieze, I. H., Olson, J. E., & Murrell, A. J. (2011). Working beyond 65: Predictors of late retirement for women and men MBAs. *Journal of Women & Aging, 23*(1), 40–57. http://dx.doi.org/10.1080/08952841.2011.540485.

Global Aging. (2001). The ageing of the world's population. Retrieved from: <http://www.globalaging.org/waa2/documents/theagingoftheworld.htm>.

Grundy, E., & Read, S. (2012). Social contacts and receipt of help among older people in England: Are there benefits of having more children? *Journals of Gerontology Series B: Psychological Sciences & Social Sciences, 67*(6), 742–754.

Halleröd, B. (2013). Gender inequality from beyond the grave: Intrahousehold distribution and well-being after spousal loss. *Ageing and Society, 33,* 783–803. http://dx.doi.org/10.1017/S01446-86X12000268.

Iida, K., & Oguma, Y. (2014). The relationship between flow experience and sense of coherence: A 1-year follow-up study. *Holistic Nursing Practice, 28*(2), 91–97.

Isherwood, L. M., King, D. S., & Luszcz, M. A. (2012). A longitudinal analysis of social engagement in late-life widowhood. *International Journal of Aging & Human Development, 74*(3), 211–229.

Kim, J., Kim, M., & Kim, J. (2013). Social activities and health of Korean elderly women by age groups. *Educational Gerontology, 39*(9), 640–654. http://dx.doi.org/10.1080/03601277.-2012.730454.

Ladin, K., Daniels, N., & Kawachi, I. (2010). Exploring the relationship between absolute and relative position and late-life depression: Evidence from 10 European countries. *Gerontologist, 50*(1), 48–59.

Lahaie, C., Earle, A., & Heymann, J. (2013). An uneven burden: Social disparities in adult caregiving responsibilities, working conditions, and caregiver outcomes. *Research on Aging, 35*(3), 243–274. http://dx.doi.org/10.1177/0164027512446028.

Lewis, L. M. (2011). Medication adherence and spiritual perspectives among African American older women with hypertension. *Journal of Gerontological Nursing, 37*(6), 34–41. http://dx.doi.org/10.3928/00989134-20100201-02.

Lowenstein, A., Katz, R., & Daatland, S. O. (2004). Filial norms and intergenerational support in Europe and Israel: A comparative perspective. *Annual Review of Gerontology & Geriatrics, 24*, 200–223.

Manning, L. K. (2010). Gender and religious differences associated with volunteering in later life. *Journal of Women & Aging, 22*(2), 125–135. http://dx.doi.org/10.1080/08952841003719224.

McAuley, E., Hall, K. S., Motl, R. W., White, S. M., Wójcicki, T. R., Hu, L., et al. (2009). Trajectory of declines in physical activity in community-dwelling older women: Social cognitive influences. *Journal of Gerontology: Psychological Sciences, 64B*(5), 543–550. http://dx.doi.org/10.1093/geronb/gbp049.

Minkler, M., & Stone, R. (1985). The feminization of poverty and older women. *The Gerontologist, 25*(4), 351–357. http://dx.doi.org/10.1093/geront/25.4.351.

Nesteruk, O., & Price, C. A. (2011). Retired women and volunteering: The good, the bad, and the unrecognized. *Journal of Women & Aging, 23*(2), 99–112. http://dx.doi.org/10.1080/08952841-.2011.561138.

Olesen, S. C., & Berry, H. L. (2011). Community participation and mental health during retirement in community sample of Australians. *Aging & Mental Health, 15*(2), 186–197. http://dx.doi.org/10.1080/13607863.2010.501053.

Opree, S. J., & Kalmijn, M. (2012). Exploring causal effects of combining work and intergenerational support on depressive symptoms among middle aged women. *Ageing and Society, 32*, 130–146. http://dx.doi.org/10.1017/S0144686X11000171.

Paggi, K., & Hayslip, B. J. (1999). Mental aerobics: Exercises for the mind in later life. *Educational Gerontology, 25*(1), 1–12.

Pakarinen, M., Raitanen, J., Kaaja, R., & Luoto, R. (2010). Secular trend in the menopausal age in Finland 1997–2007 and correlation with socioeconomic, reproductive and lifestyle factors. *Maturitas, 66*(4), 417–422. http://dx.doi.org/10.1016/j.maturitas.2010.04.005.

Park, J. M., Hogan, D. P., & D'Ottavi, M. (2004). Grandparenting children with special needs. *Annual Review of Gerontology & Geriatrics, 24*, 120–149.

Pope, N. D., Kolomer, S., & Glass, A. P. (2012). How women in late midlife become caregivers for their aging parents. *Journal of Women & Aging, 24*(3), 242–261. http://dx.doi.org/10.1080/08952841.2012.639676.

Price, C. A., & Nesteruk, O. (2010). Creating retirement paths: Examples from the lives of women. *Journal of Women & Aging, 22*(2), 136–149. http://dx.doi.org/10.1080/08952841003719240.

Quéniart, A., & Charpentier, M. (2013). Initiate, bequeath, and remember: Older women's transmission role within the family. *Journal of Women & Aging, 25*(1), 45–65. http://dx.doi.org/10.1080/08952841.2012.720181.

Ron, P. (2009). Daughters as caregivers of aging parents: The shattering myth. *Journal of Gerontological Social Work, 52*(2), 135–153.

Rowbotham, M., Cuskelly, M., & Carroll, A. (2011). Sustainable caregiving? Demands upon and resources of female carers of adults with intellectual disability. *Journal of Women & Aging, 23*(2), 129–148. http://dx.doi.org/10.1080/08952841.2011.561141.

Shaevitz, M. H. (1984). *The superwoman syndrome* (pp. 6–12). New York, NY: Warner Books.

Tintle, N., Bacon, B., Kostyuchenko, S., Gutkovich, Z., & Bromet, E. J. (2011). Depression and its correlates in older adults in Ukraine. *International Journal of Geriatric Psychiatry, 26*, 1292–1299.

Van Putten, A. E., Vlasblom, J. D., Dykstra, P. A., & Schippers, J. J. (2010). The absence of conflict between paid work hours and the provision of instrumental support to elderly parents among middle aged women and men. *Ageing and Society, 30,* 923–948. http://dx.doi.org/10.1017/S0144686X10000127.

Villar, F., Celdrn, M., & Triad, C. (2012). Grandmothers offering regular auxiliary care for their grandchildren: An expression of generativity in later life? *Journal of Women & Aging, 24*(4), 292–312. http://dx.doi.org/10.1080/08952841.2012.708576.

Wallston, B. S. (1987). Social psychology of women and gender. *Journal of Applied Social Psychology, 17*(12), 1025–1050.

Wiggs, C. M. (2010). Creating the self: Exploring the life journey of late-midlife women. *Journal of Women & Aging, 22*(3), 218–233. http://dx.doi.org/10.1080/08952841.2010.495574.

Wilson, S. C., & Supiano, K. P. (2011). Experiences of veterans' widows following conjugal bereavement: A qualitative analysis. *Journal of Women & Aging, 23*(1), 77–93. http://dx.doi.org/10.1080/08952841.2011.540479.

Wong, J. D., & Almeida, D. M. (2012). The effects of employment status and daily stressors on time spent on daily household chores in middle-aged and older adults. *The Gerontologist, 53*(1), 81–91. http://dx.doi.org/10.1093/geront/gns047.

Wootton, J. C. (1998). Women as caregivers. *Journal of Women's Health, 7*(5), 597–599.

Young, L., Baltes, B., & Pratt, A. (2007). Using selection, optimization, and compensation to reduce job/family stressors: Effective when it matters. *Journal of Business and Psychology, 21*(4), 511–539.

10

The Role of Social Relationships for Aging Women

Global Fact: *...Older women are also less likely to be married than older men, are less likely to remarry than older men, and are less likely to be outlived by their male spouses.*
—**United Nations, Women Coordination Division report (2012)**

There is much research about the benefits of maintaining social ties for women across their life span (Lubben, 1988; Lubben & Gironda, 2004). This section will review research on the benefits of social relationships for older women's aging adjustment and self-growth.

THE IMPORTANCE OF A STRONG SOCIAL SUPPORT SYSTEM

Older women who live alone are considered to be at high risk for loneliness and depression (Aday, Kehoe, & Farney, 2005; de Jong Gierveld, Keating, & Fast, 2015). However, many research studies have demonstrated how a strong social network may alleviate the negative feelings associated with loneliness and depression (Norris & Murrell, 1990; Norwood, 2009). Therefore, this chapter will address the research on social relationships for aging women and suggest ways to help foster relationships in an effort to combat negative adjustment and promote self-growth. Social support is generally thought of as "information leading the subject to believe that he is cared for and loved, esteemed, and a member of a network of mutual obligation" (Cobb, 1976, p. 300).

As women age they often lose important relationships in their life, as both friends and partners may have died, as a result of "residential relocation" (eg, Litwak & Longino, 1987; Perkins, Ball, Whittington, & Hollingsworth, 2012) and/or gaps in the support system because the social network cannot meet the "intensifying support needs" of aging

Women and Positive Aging.
DOI: http://dx.doi.org/10.1016/B978-0-12-420136-1.00010-4

adults (eg, Rook, 2009) subsequently social networks often decline (eg, Field & Minkler, 1988). However, friends throughout the life span help to promote self-growth and ease difficulties associated with transition into older adulthood (eg, Lewittes, 1989). Several theories have been tested regarding the relative importance of the breadth and depth of social support for aging adults.

THEORIES ABOUT SOCIAL RELATIONSHIPS IN AGING ADULTS

Two prominent theories have been put forth to explain social networks among aging adults: the Activity theory and the Disengagement theory. These two theories make somewhat contradictory predictions about relationships in the aging population. The Activity theory asserts that challenges with personal health and/or the death of friends are a barrier to social contact. Proponents of the Activity theory posit that the maintenance of social relationships and remaining active is key to satisfaction in later life (Havighurst, 1961). Further, most scholars who study gerontology believe that one of the key components to "positive aging" is engagement in social activities (eg, Rowe & Kahn, 1997). Interestingly, Pavela (2015) utilizing data from just shy of 10,000 noninstitutional adults, found a relationship between those who had the greatest functional limitations (ie, lack of activity) and the amount of contact with their friends. Specifically decreased functional states were associated with decreased social contact. Active older adults also reported an increase in their interpersonal relationships (Aranceta, Perez-Rodrigo, Gondra, & Orduna, 2001). Similarly, Menec (2003) found that social activities were related to longevity, happiness, and functionality. Volunteering and participation often increase with age and older adults have more free time due to a decrease in work obligations, as a result these adults feel more engaged (Cornwell, Laumann, & Schumm, 2008). Social engagement can help to explain, in part, how adults age successfully even in the face of deteriorating health and/or the many changes to life circumstances (Minkler & Fadem, 2002).

Although not without criticism, Disengagement theory maintains that older adults may withdraw from social contact in "symbolic" preparation for their deaths and that social relationships are more impaired as people age (Cumming & Henry, 1961). Furthermore, advocates of this theory agree that the process of disengagement differs for men and women as men have a more instrumental role in society and women a more socioemotional one. Despite the limited support and controversy surrounding this theory, the theory is important as it is one of the first attempts to formulate a conceptual and theoretical framework specifically applied to gerontology (eg, Hochschild, 1975).

The concepts of a "convoy" and engaging in "socioemotional selectivity" offer a relatively optimistic view of the state of interpersonal relationships among aging adults. "Convoy" is a social term borrowed from the field of anthropology and describes a social group which provides a variety of social support (eg, protection) and, subsequently, positively impacts a person's health and well-being (Antonucci, 2009; Kahn & Antonucci, 1980). Because older adults are more likely to experience loss of friends and/or residential relocation, this social idea argues that social attachments may vary over time in response to aging changes (Antonucci & Akiyama, 1987a) but individuals with the most intimate interpersonal ties (eg, spouses, siblings, best friends) will remain fairly stable over the life span (Khan & Antonucci, 1980). Socioemotional selectivity theory (Carstensen, Isaacowitz, & Charles, 1999) suggests that, as a person ages, she/he invests more time in relationships (and activities/goals) that are rewarding and maximize their positive social relationships through this process. In a study conducted by Fredrickson and Carstensen (1990), it was found that older adults preferred familiar partners more often than younger adults; however, when end of life was made more salient, younger people and older adults' preferences were similar (for familiar partners). In a sample that includes adults between the ages of 70–104, adults in the "very old" age group had nearly half the number of friends as those adults in the "old" age group; however, the number of "very close relationships" did not differ as a function of age (Lang & Carstensen, 1994).

QUOTE FROM FAMOUS, POSITIVELY AGING WOMEN

The human heart, at whatever age,
opens only to the heart that opens in return.

—*Maria Edgeworth, Novelist*

Furthermore, older adults express more satisfaction (eg, Lansford, Sherman, & Antonucci, 1998; Luong, Charles, & Fingerman, 2011) and more positive emotions (Charles & Piazza, 2007) with the friendships that they do have. Older adults also express fewer conflicts in their interpersonal relationships than do younger adults (eg, Birditt & Fingerman, 2003; Fingerman, Miller, & Charles, 2008) and are more likely to employ avoidance strategies in response to conflict (Charles, Piazza, Luong, & Almeida, 2009). Because of role transitions such as retirement, older adults often have more opportunities to select whom they would like as social partners and with whom they would like to spend their leisure time (Rosenkoetter, Garris, & Engdahl, 2001). Finally, Gillespie, Lever, Frederick, and Royce (2014) found that satisfaction with one's friends did a better job at predicting life satisfaction than did the actual number of friends.

THE QUALITY AND FUNCTION OF SOCIAL SUPPORT

Members of the *Red Hat Society*, a social group for older women whose mission is to "celebrate the silliness of life," were asked a number of open-ended questions about their involvement with the group and the most frequently reported benefit was that their friends in the society provided social support (eg, providing food for funerals, accompanying someone to a doctor's appointment) (Hutchinson, Yarnal, Staffordson, & Kerstetter, 2008). Interestingly, Thomas (2009) reported that the well-being of older adults is often related more strongly to support that is given rather than received, especially for friends and children. The nature of this association was different for support received from spouses and siblings. Women who live alone (versus with a spouse) were more likely to participate in senior center activities and thus widen their social circle (Aday, Kehoe, & Farney 2006). Brown, Nesse, Vinokur, and Smith (2003) examined mortality differences among older married adults, via a longitudinal study, and found that rates of mortality were less among individuals who provided support to those in their network (ie, friends, spouse, neighbors) and that being the recipient of support did not have a relationship to mortality rates once support provided was taken into account. Antonucci and Akiyama (1987b) suggested that aging women typically had more nonfilial social support (eg, a larger social network of friends) while older men relied primarily on their spouses. Social class disparities appear to exist among aging adults as a function of amount of contact with friends and the amount of support given to others and the level of satisfaction with the support received (Krause & Borawski-Clark, 1995).

An interesting line of research investigating the role of social support in later life demonstrates the influential role of genetics on social support networks and one study has found a link between genetics and social support, specifically as it related to the "perceived adequacy" of support received (Bergeman, Plomin, Pedersen, McClearn, & Nesselroads, 1990). Boomsma, Willemsen, Dolan, Hawkley, and Cacioppo (2005) reported that just under 50% of variation in loneliness can be explained by genetic contribution.

TIPS FOR AGING WOMEN'S SOCIAL SUPPORT NETWORKS

1. Get socially connected online (eg, Pinterest, Facebook).
2. Take an exercise or instructional class.
3. Phone friends or drop by their house.
4. Volunteer in your community.

CHECK IT OUT!

Conduct an interview with an aging adult woman. As you conduct your interview try to think how the respondent's answers might fit in with some of the theories of social support with respect to the aging adult (eg, socioemotional selectivity theory). Here are some potential questions to ask:

1. Has the person' social network changed (ie, diminished) over time?
2. Has the quality of friendships changed over time?
3. In which social activities, if any, does the person regularly participate? What function does it serve for this person?
4. Does this person have any advice to offer other aging women in terms of maintaining social relationships?

THE IMPORTANCE OF SOCIAL SUPPORT ON PHYSICAL AND MENTAL/COGNITIVE HEALTH

Physical health. Many researchers have demonstrated how maintaining social networks can lead to better mental and physical health relative to older adults who do not maintain social networks (eg, Krause, 2001). Social support has consistently been linked to lower rates of mortality (eg, Uchino, 2006). The benefits include a decreased risk of heart disease, such that individuals with lower levels of support have higher mortality rates specifically from cardiovascular disease (eg, Berkman, Leo-Summers, & Horwitz, 1992; Janevic et al., 2004). Social support is also associated with lower mortality rates from cancer (eg, Hibbard & Pope, 1993; Shannon & Bourque, 2005). The perceived quality of social support (eg, a sense of belonging) was related to lower cortisol levels in the saliva of women with breast cancer (Turner-Cobb, Sephton, Koopman, Blake-Mortimer, & Spiegel, 2000).

Patients who report being from cohesive families show more adherence to medical treatment than families in conflict (DiMatteo, 2004). Finally, social support has been demonstrated to positively affect the outlook and recovery of individuals who are diagnosed with serious illnesses (Hurdle, 2001).

Mental health and cognitive vitality. Wildes, Harkness, and Simons (2002) found that insufficient social support was a stronger predictor of depression than were life events, although both were related to depressive symptomatology. Using multiple regression, Norris and Murrell (1990) found that depression and poor health nine months after the death of a spouse could be predicted, in part, by poor social support. Seeman, Lusigolo, Albert, and Berkman (2001) conducted a longitudinal study and demonstrated that stronger emotional support at baseline predicted better cognitive functioning almost eight years later. Aging adults who were engaged with their community demonstrated greater cognitive vitality than their "disengaged" counterparts (Fillit et al., 2002).

The definition of a positively aging woman often includes the idea of "aging in place" and maintaining one's autonomy in daily activities (Bookman, 2008). Some researchers (eg, Thomas & Blanchard, 2009), however, have suggested that such efforts can often lead to perceived social isolation and boredom, limiting opportunities for meaningful social interactions. Norwood (2009) described the experience as being "social death" for many adults who live alone, are physically limited, and potentially miss out on opportunities for social engagement with others.

WORDS OF WISDOM

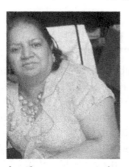

Soledad is a 59-year-old woman who believes that her friendships and social relationships have changed drastically, for the better, over the years. Soledad is from Mexico and she stated that her friendships over there were humble and caring. She expressed how everyone was from the same socioeconomic status which made it easier to get along. Once she came to the United States, she noticed her friendships were quite different. She recalls having social relationships for the purposes of parties and other social events throughout the year. Soledad has formed some strong friendships in the United States and the friendship is based on the fact that the other women were from the same country and share the same cultural values.

continued

In addition, Soledad truly believes that social relationships affect her emotional state in positive ways. She feels blessed to be surrounded by friends who do not give her any problems and make her feel at ease. An example of a friendship that makes her feel at ease is the one she shares with her best friend. This friendship started when they met at work more than 25 years ago. She values this friendship greatly because she knows she can count on her best friend for both the simple and complicated things in life. They communicate effectively by talking on the phone while they are both watching the same Spanish soap opera each night.

Once a positive friendship has been made, Soledad suggests that younger women should find ways to communicate effectively in order to sustain a long-lasting friendship. Soledad understands that as you get older it becomes difficult to keep in touch with others because of work and other factors, therefore it is important to find a way of communication that works whether it be phone calls, texts, or e-mails.

Of course, there are a number of positive aspects of remaining in one's home and/or community such as fewer reports of depression and better cognition functioning relative to older adults in nursing homes (eg, Marek et al., 2005). While the literature suggests that aging in place may not always be the best option for all older adults, aging adults are also reluctant to be placed in long-term assisted living or nursing home. In fact, many older adults expressed more fear at being placed in a nursing home (13%) than they did of death (3%) (Clarity, 2007). On the surface it would seem that assisted living/nursing homes would provide many opportunities to engage at a social level; however, research has suggested that these relationships tend to be superficial in nature and are not particularly meaningful (eg, Bear, 1990). There are some studies suggesting that some external factors to the living situation at a long-term facility may influence the level of connectedness. For example, Sugihara and Evans (2000) found a positive relationship between social support and the distance to the central/activity building in a retirement community, such that social support was greater the closer residents lived to the activity center.

Other alternatives to assisted living include adult day-care centers and senior citizen centers. These types of community-based centers can help aging adults to connect with other people in their community through exercise classes, bereavement group therapy, meal programs, and educational classes. Research has shown that older adults who engage in such programs have stronger friendships and corresponding overall well-being (eg, Aday et al., 2006) and fewer depressive symptoms (Choi & McDougall, 2007).

"Aging-in-community" might be one way in which to provide a balance between aging in place and residential/assisted living. The crux of aging in community is that older adults will provide support for one another and that they rely on social interdependence and social connected (eg, McWhinney-Morse, 2013; Thomas & Blanchard, 2009). The notion of aging within a community environment is still considered a relatively new movement but is slowly gaining momentum as a means to increase self-sufficiency and interconnectedness among older adults.

SOCIAL NETWORK INTERVENTIONS

Many social support interventions are targeted toward aging adults who are "at-risk," or those adults who are already experiencing physical and psychological problems (Birditt & Fingerman, 2003; Uchino, 2009).

A significant number of studies have demonstrated that support is associated with better long-term health status (eg, Hogan, Linden, & Najarian, 2002). Kaplan (2000) argued that interventions should focus on "primary prevention" which helps to prevent health problems from occurring in the first place (as opposed to secondary prevention that focuses primarily on the treatment of a disease or condition). Furthermore, social needs differ across the life span and aging adults also have highly distinction and diverse social needs and the differentiation of their needs should be kept in mind when social programs are designed for this group (Rook, 1984).

Friendship enrichment programs are based on theories of positive aging which suggest that aging adults set goals, attempt to achieve them, and select resources that allow one to adapt to changes that occur with age (eg, Schultz & Heckhausen, 1996). Martina and Stevens (2006) designed a friendship enrichment program which had the aim of improving friendships and reducing loneliness among aging women. The program was relatively successful, especially in older women's self-reported outcomes in both quantity and quality of friendships. In a one-year follow up, there was still a significant decrease in loneliness after the intervention was initiated (Stevens, Martina, & Westerhof, 2006).

Some researchers have purported that it might be more effective to focus on "kin ties" versus "peer ties" when attempting to increase the well-being of aging adults (eg, Rook, 1991), as family support is critical because of the emotional support involved in these relationships (Yeung & Fung, 2007). Perkins, Ball, Kemp, and Hollingsworth (2012) found that a high proportion of family members in a person's network was the strongest predictor of well-being; however, research also suggests that self-reported well-being is more related to relationships with friends than it is with family (Antonucci & Akiyama, 1995). Therefore, those researchers who design and implement social support network interventions may need to consider the nature of the support (eg, friend versus family) when designing a program as well-being and emotional support may differ as a function of who is providing the support.

In a review of published studies that evaluated interventions over the course of about 30 years, the results suggested that group (as opposed to one-on-one social) interventions did a better job of reducing social isolation and loneliness among aging adults (Cattan, White, Bond, & Learmouth, 2005). Finally, Hogan et al. (2002) cautioned that interventions are difficult to implement and test because of the large amount of different "treatment" protocols and the different contexts in which an intervention can be administered. Thus, not enough evidence exits to determine which intervention will work best in which environments and under which conditions.

SUMMARY

Early research on social support and aging had a pessimistic attitude regarding older adults' need to remain socially engaged (eg, Disengagement theory); however, more recent research has found that aging adults are satisfied with their relationships in later life and that aging adults tend to experience fewer conflicts in the relationships that they do have. These findings may be due, in part, to conflict resolution strategies that are employed by older (but not younger) adults, an increased "say" in how leisurely time is spent, and with greater selectivity in terms of whom an aging person chooses to spend time with (eg, preference for those who provide a rewarding relationship). There is a robust body of literature showing that social support has repeatedly been linked to better health and cognitive/mental outcomes. Interventions designed to increase social ties among "at risk" older adults have been met with some success. Overall, the research suggests that social systems do not necessary diminish with time, in fact, relationships appear to be more rewarding and satisfactory as adults age.

DISCUSSION QUESTIONS

1. What benefits do women receive from their social relationships over time?
2. Do aging women differ from their male peers in terms of their need for social connections with others?
3. What is the role of culture on the nature of a woman's social relationships?

4. Do you think that different cohorts of women have different social relationship needs? Why or why not?
5. Can early education assist in the establishment of better social support systems in communities for aging women? How so?
6. Across different cultures, what could be the intergenerational activities that would mutually benefit both older and younger cohorts of women?
7. Can the use of technology assist women in maintaining their social relationships into later life? If so, in what ways?
8. How can community-based programs assist in this process of creating and/or maintaining social support relationships for women?
9. Older adults can become socially isolated in neighborhoods. What are some ways that communities can effectively outreach to older women?
10. Does social networking benefit older women in terms of physical and mental aging? How so? Please give examples.

TEST YOUR KNOWLEDGE!

Take the following quiz about your attitude toward healthy social relationships:

http://medicine.yale.edu/spiitualselfschema/training/hhrp/566_160680_HHRP%Plusgrp12_handouts.pdf

---

SUPPLEMENTAL BOOK READINGS

Over the past decades, there have been many books written on the topic of the significance of social relationships in older women's lives. Here are some recommended *additional readings*:

Hofsess, R., & Hofsess, C. (2014). *Emerging from the shadows: The needs of older women and the benefits of supporting them.* Plantation, FL: Llumina Press.

An interesting social support model in communities and broader societies, referred to as "Trust in the Lives of Older Women (TLOW)," is suggested by the authors. The book's content presents ideas about the need for communities to support the needs of aging women. The perspective taken is that there is an ethical, social responsibility for individuals and countries to reach out and help women as they get older and who may increase in their dependency needs over time.

Kaye, L. W. (1997). *Self-help support groups for older women: Rebuilding elder networks through personal empowerment.* New York, NY: Taylor & Francis.
This book is a great resource for both aging women and the counseling professionals who may be working with aging female clients. The author presents an empowering message of self-healing and social engagement to help in adapting to the many adjustments related to later life, from aging changes of the body to losses within one's social network.

Allen, K. R. (1989). *Single women/family ties: Life histories of older women.* Thousand Oaks, CA: Sage Publications, Inc.
This book examines an important aspect of women and aging, when women are single in later life and the many different ramifications for their personal aging and associated family relationships (eg, eldercare expectations). It is important for this lifestyle factor to be examined across many different cultures and regions across the world as there are potentially significant meanings toward positive aging outcomes for women.

Krause, N. M. (2008). *Aging in the church: How social relationships affect health.* West Conshocken, PA: Templeton Press.
The author presents one aspect of social relationships for aging women, being the role of the church as an on-going socialization and social support resource. The factors of personal spirituality and broader community outreach through spiritual institutions to otherwise disenfranchised, isolated older adults in communities cannot be minimized as important quality-of-life determinants for many aging women.

van den Hoonaard, D. K. (2001). *The widowed self: The older woman's journey through widowhood.* Waterloo, ON: Wilfrid Laurier University Press.
Because most women have longer life expectancies than the aging men in their lives, the likelihood that they may enter widowhood exists. The social, emotional, and psychological role transition to becoming a widow can be a significant experience which dramatically affects a woman's aging trajectory in multiple ways.

Glicken, M. D. (2010). *Mature friendships, love, and romance: A practical guide to intimacy for older adults.* Westport, CT: Praeger.
This book offers a very empowering statement to aging adults: your sexual life does not stop when you turn 60. The book reviews the many different issues of intimacy in later life, from getting adult children to accept the nonplatonic relationships in the

adult's life to adjusting to the changing physical and psychological nature of sex in later adulthood. Aging women would benefit from the supportive ideas regarding their evolving sexual "self" identity and how society responds presented in this practical guide.

Matthews, S. (1986). *Friendships through the life course: Oral biographies in old age*. Thousand Oaks, CA: Sage Publications, Inc.
The power of friendship is a key part of an on-going social support network as individuals age. Sixty-three older adults are interviewed and tell their life histories related to sustained friendship ties from childhood into adulthood. The positive influence of these long-term, platonic relationships on the adults' aging underlies the importance of this book for women of all ages as they traverse the sometimes rocky path of getting older in a society that may not fully understand their needs.

SUPPLEMENTAL AGING VIDEOS

For learning purposes, the use of videos can be very beneficial for both instructors and readers. Here are some recommended *supplemental videos*:

Sunset Story (Format: DVD)
Sunset Story tells an engaging documentary drama about two friends in later life. Irja, age 81, and Lucille, age 95, show how you can be activists and civically engaged in the time of life when society might stereotypically believe that older retirees become docile and stagnant in their activities. The film shows the humor and heartache of aging that is shared between these two good friends.

ADDITIONAL INFORMATION LINKS

The following are some recommended *supplemental Internet links*:

Generations Working Together website: http://generationsworkingtogether .org/

Intergeneration Foundation website: http://intergenerationmonth.org/ participating_organizations.htm

Older Women's League website: http://www.owl-national.org/

Red Hat Society website: http://redhatsociety.com/

Supportive Older Women's Network website: http://www.sown.org/

Temple University's Intergenerational Center website: http://templeigc.org/

References

Aday, R. H., Kehoe, J. C., & Farney, L. E. (2006). Impact of senior center friendships on aging women who live alone. *Journal of Women Aging, 18*, 57–73.

Antonucci, T. (2009). Convoy model of social relations. In H. Reis & S. Sprecher (Eds.), *Encyclopedia of human relationships* (pp. 327–329). Thousand Oaks, CA: Sage Publications, Inc.

Antonucci, T. C., & Akiyama, H. (1987a). An examination of sex differences in social support among older men and women. *Sex Roles, 17*, 737–749.

Antonucci, T. C., & Akiyama, H. (1987b). Social networks in adult life and a preliminary examination of the convoy model. *Journal of Gerontology, 42*, 519–527.

Antonucci, T. C., & Akiyama, H. (1995). Convoys of social relations: Family and friendship within a lifespan context. In R. Bleizner & V. H. Bedford (Eds.), *Handbook of aging and the family* (pp. 355–371). Westport, CT: Greenwood Press.

Aranceta, J., Perez-Rodrigo, C., Gondra, J., & Orduna, J. (2001). Community-based programme to promote physical activity among elderly people: The Gerobilbo study. *Journal of Nutritional Health Aging, 5*, 238–242.

Bear, M. (1990). Social network characteristics and the duration of primary relationships after entry into long-term care. *Journal of Gerontology: Social Sciences, 45*(4), 156–162.

Bergeman, C., Plomin, R., Pedersen, N., McClearn, G., & Nesselroads, J. (1990). Genetic and environmental influences on social support: The Swedish adoption/twin study of aging. *Journal of Gerontology, 45*(3), 101–106.

Berkman, L. F., Leo-Summers, L., & Horwitz, R. I. (1992). Emotional support and survival after Myocardial infarction: A perspective population-based study of the elderly. *Annals of Internal Medicine, 117*(12), 1003–1009.

Birditt, K. S., & Fingerman, K. L. (2003). Age and gender differences in adults' emotional reactions to interpersonal tensions. *Journals of Gerontology: Psychological Sciences, 58B*, 237–245.

Bookman, A. (2008). Innovative models of aging in place: Transforming our communities for an aging population. *Community, Work & Family, 11*(4), 419–438.

Boomsma, D., Willemsen, G., Dolan, C., Hawkley, L., & Cacioppo, J. (2005). Genetic and environmental contributions to loneliness in adults: The Netherlands twin registry study. *Behavior Genetic, 35*(6), 745–752.

Brown, S. L., Nesse, R. M., Vinokur, A. D., & Smith, D. M. (2003). Providing social support may be more beneficial than receiving it: Results from a prospective study of mortality. *Psychological Science, 14*(4), 320–327.

Carstensen, L. L., Isaacowitz, D. M., & Charles, S. T. (1999). Taking time seriously: A theory of socioemotional selectivity. *American Psychologist, 54*, 165–181.

Cattan, M., White, M., Bond, J., & Learmouth, A. (2005). Preventing social isolation and loneliness among older people: A systematic review of health promotion interventions. *Aging and Society, 25*(1), 41–67.

Charles, S. T., Piazza, J., Luong, G., & Almeida, D. M. (2009). Now you see it, now you don't: Age differences in affective reactivity to social tensions. *Psychological Aging, 24*(3), 645–653.

Charles, S. T., & Piazza, J. R. (2007). Memories of social interactions: Age differences in emotional intensity. *Psychology and Aging, 22*, 300–309.

Choi, N., & McDougall, G. (2007). Comparison of depressive symptoms between homebound older adults and ambulatory older adults. *Aging Mental Health, 11*(3), 310–322.

Clarity. (2007). Attitudes of seniors and baby boomers on aging in place. Retrieved from: <http://www.clarityproducts.com/research/Clarity_Aging_in_Place_2007.pdf>.

Cobb, S. (1976). Social support as a moderator of life stress. *Psychosomatic Medicine, 5*, 300–314.

Cornwell, B., Laumann, E. O., & Schumm, L. P. (2008). The social connectedness of older adults: A national profile. *American Sociological Review, 73*(2), 185–203.

Cumming, E., & Henry, W. (1961). *Growing old.* New York, NY: Basic Books.

de Jong Gierveld, J., Keating, N., & Fast, J. E. (2015). Determinants of loneliness among older adults in Canada. *Canadian Journal on Aging/La Revue Canadienne Du Vieillissement, 34*(02), 125–136.

DiMatteo, R. M. (2004). Social support and patient adherence to medical treatment: A meta-analysis. *Health Psychology, 23*(2), 207–218.

Field, D., & Minkler, M. (1988). Continuity and change in social support between young-old, old-old, and very-old adults. *Journal of Gerontology, 43*(4), 100–106.

Fillit, H. M., Butler, R. N., O'Connell, A. W., Albert, M. S., Birren, J. E., Cotman, C. W., et al. (2002). Achieving and maintaining cognitive vitality with aging. *Mayo Clinical Proceedings, 77*, 681–696.

Fingerman, K. L., Miller, L., & Charles, S. T. (2008). Saving the best for last: How adults treat social partners of different ages. *Psychology and Aging, 23*, 399–409.

Fredrickson, B., & Carstensen, L. (1990). Choosing social partners: How old age and antici-pated endings make people more selective. *Psychology of Aging, 5*(3), 335–347.

Gillespie, B., Lever, J., Frederick, D., & Royce, T. (2014). Close adult friendships, gender, and lifecycle. *Journal of Social and Personal Relationships, 26*, 1–28.

Havighurst, R. J. (1961). Successful aging. *The Gerontologist, 1*, 8–13.

Hibbard, J. H., & Pope, C. R. (1993). The quality of social roles as predictors of morbidity and mortality. *Social Science Med, 36*, 217–225.

Hochschild, A. R. (1975). Disengagement theory: A critique and proposal. *American Sociological Review, 40*(5), 553–569.

Hogan, B. E., Linden, W., & Najarian, B. (2002). Social support interventions: Do they work? *Clinical Psychology Review, 22*(3), 383–442.

Hurdle, D. E. (2001). Social support: A critical factor in women's health and health promo-tion. *Health Social Work, 26*(2), 72–79.

Hutchinson, S., Yarnal, C., Staffordson, J., & Kerstetter, D. (2008). Beyond fun and friendship: The red hat society as a coping resource for older women. *Aging & Society, 28*(7), 979–999.

Janevic, M. R., Janz, N. K., Dodge, J. A., Lin, X., Wang, Y., Sinco, B. R., et al. (2004). Longitudinal effects of social support on the health and functioning of older women with heart dis-ease. *International Journal of Aging and Human Development, 7*(2), 205–215.

Kahn, R. L., & Antonucci, T. C. (1980). Convoys over the life course: Attachment, roles, and social support. In P. B. Baltes & O. G. Brim (Eds.), *Life-span development and behavior* (pp. 253–286). New York: Academic Press.

Kaplan, R. M. (2000). Two pathways to prevention. *American Psychologist, 55*, 383–396..

Krause, N. (2001). Social support. In R. H. Binstock & L. K. George (Eds.), *Handbook of aging and the social sciences* (pp. 272–294). San Diego, CA: Academic Press.

Krause, N., & Borawski-Clark, E. (1995). Social class differences in social support among older adults. *The Gerontologist, 35*(4), 498–508.

Lang, F. R., & Carstensen, L. L. (1994). Close emotional relationships in later life: Further support for proactive aging in the social domain. *Psychological Aging, 9*, 315–324.

Lansford, J. E., Sherman, A. M., & Antonucci, T. C. (1998). Satisfaction with social networks: An examination of socioemotional selectivity theory across cohorts. *Psychology of Aging, 13*(4), 544–552.

Lewittes, H. (1989). Just being friendly means a lot: Women, friendship, and aging. *Women and Health, 14*(3-4), 139–159.

Litwak, E., & Longino, C. F. (1987). Migration patterns among the elderly: A developmental perspective. *The Gerontologist, 27*, 266–272.

Lubben, J. E. (1988). Assessing social networks among elderly populations. *Family and Community Health, 11*, 42–52.

Lubben, J. E., & Gironda, M. (2004). Measuring social networks and assessing their benefits. In C. Phillipson, G. Allan, & D. Morgan (Eds.), *Social networks and exclusion: Sociological and policy perspectives* (pp. 20–35). Hampshire, UK: Ashgate.

Luong, G., Charles, S., & Fingerman, K. (2011). Better with age: Social relationships across adulthood. *Journal of Social and Personal Relationships, 28*(1), 9–23.

Marek, K., Popejoy, L., Petroski, G., Mehr, D., Rantz, M., & Lin, W. (2005). Clinical outcomes aging in place. *Nursing Research, 54*(3), 202–211.

Martina, C. M. S., & Stevens, N. L. (2006). Breaking the cycle of loneliness? Psychological effects of a friendship enrichment program for older women. *Aging & Mental Health, 10*(5), 467–475.

McWhinney-Morse, S. (2013). Life at Beacon Hill Village. In J. M. Blanchard (Ed.), *Aging in community*. Chapel Hill, NC: Second Journey.

Menec, V. (2003). The relation between everyday activities and successful aging: A 6-year longitudinal study. *Journal of Gerontology, 58*(2), 74–82.

Minkler, M., & Fadem, P. (2002). Successful aging: A disability perspective. *Journal of Disability Policy Studies, 12*(4), 229–235.

Norris, F. H., & Murrell, S. A. (1990). Social support, life events, and stress as modifiers of adjustment to bereavement by older adults. *Psychology and Aging, 5*(3), 429–436.

Norwood, F. (2009). *The maintenance of life: Preventing social death through euthanasia talk and end-of-life care-lessons from the Netherlands*. Durham, NC: Carolina Academic Press.

Pavela, G. (2015). Functional status and social contact among older adults. *Research on Aging* Online publication. doi:10.1177/0164027514566091.

Perkins, M., Ball, M. M., Kemp, C. L., & Hollingsworth, C. (2012). Social relations and resident health in assisted living: An application of the convoy model. *The Gerontologist, 53*(3), 495–507.

Perkins, M., Ball, M. M., Whittington, F. J., & Hollingsworth, C. (2012). Relational autonomy in assisted living: A focus on diverse care settings for older adults. *Journal of Aging Studies, 26*(2), 214–225.

Rook, K. (1984). The negative side of social interaction: Impact on psychological well-being. *Journal of Personality and Social Psychology, 46*(5), 1097–1108.

Rook, K. (1991). Facilitating friendship formation in later life: Puzzles and challenges. *American Journal of Community Psychology, 19*, 103–110.

Rook, K. (2009). Gaps in social support resources later in life: An adaptation challenge in need of further research. *Journal of Social and Personal Relationships, 26*(1), 103–112.

Rosenkoetter, M. M., Garris, J. M., & Engdahl, R. A. (2001). Postretirement use of time: Implications for preretirement planning and post retirement management. *Activities, Adaptations, & Aging, 25*, 1–18.

Rowe, J., & Kahn, R. (1997). Successful aging. *The Gerontologist, 37*(4), 433–440.

Schultz, R., & Heckhausen, J. (1996). A lifespan model of successful aging. *American Psychologist, 51*, 702–714.

Seeman, T., Lusigolo, T., Albert, M., & Berkman, L. (2001). Social relationships, social support, and patterns of cognitive aging in healthy, high-functioning older adults: MacArthur studies of successful aging. *Health Psychology, 20*(4), 243–255.

Shannon, C. S., & Bourque, D. (2005). Overlooked and underutilized: The critical role of leisure interventions in social support throughout breast cancer treatment and recovery. *Social Work in Health Care, 42*(1), 73–92.

Stevens, N., Martina, C., & Westerhof, G. (2006). Meeting the need to belong: Predicting effects of a friendship enrichment program for older women. *The Gerontologist, 46*(4), 495–502.

Sugihara, S., & Evans, G. (2000). Place attachment and social support at continuing care retirement communities. *Environment and Behavior, 32*(3), 400–409.

Thomas, P. (2009). Is it better to give or to receive? Social support and the well-being of older adults. *Journal of Gerontology, 65*(3), 351–357.

Thomas, W., & Blanchard, J. (2009). Moving beyond place: Aging in community. *Generations-Journal of the American Society on Aging, 33*(2), 12–17.

Turner-Cobb, J., Sephton, S., Koopman, C., Blake-Mortimer, J., & Spiegel, D. (2000). Social support and salivary cortisol in women with metastatic breast cancer. *Psychosomatic Medicine, 62*(3), 337–345.

Uchino, B. (2006). Social support and health: A review of physiological processes potentially underlying links to disease outcomes. *Journal of Behavioral Medicine, 29*(4), 377–387.

Uchino, B. (2009). Understanding the links between social support and physical health: A life-span perspective with emphasis on the reparability of perceived and received support. *Perspectives on Psychological Science, 4*(3), 236–255.

United Nations, Women Coordination Division. (2012). Between gender and ageing: The status of the world's older women and progress since the Madrid International Plan of Action on Ageing. Retrieved from: <http://www.un.org/womenwatch/osagi/ianwge2012/-Between-Gender-Ageing-Report-Executive-Summary-2012.pdf>.

Wildes, J., Harkness, K., & Simons, A. (2002). Life events, number of social relationships, and twelve-month naturalistic course of major depression in a community sample of women. *Depression and Anxiety, 16*, 104–113.

Yeung, G., & Fung, H. (2007). Social support and life satisfaction among Hong Kong Chinese older adults: Family first? *European Journal of Aging, 4*, 219–227.

Women's Sexuality in Later Life

Global Fact: *Results show that the sexual revolution continues in the older population as Boomers continue to age. Opposition to sex among those who are not married is down by half over the past 10 years, and belief that there is too much emphasis on sex in our culture today is down since 2004.*

—AARP (2010)

In addition to maintaining platonic social relationships, it is equally important to understand factors supporting diverse women's experiences of positive intimate relationships in later life. Emotional, social, physical, and other health-related factors impacting older women's positive sexuality outcomes in both attitude and behavior are vital to understand for both education and community support from an international perspective (eg, older Australian women; Fileborn et al., 2015). This chapter will explore the different factors that contribute to supporting women's positive sexual aging.

OLDER WOMEN AND SEXUAL ENGAGEMENT

Researchers have found that one of the strongest predictors of sexual interest in women is chronological age (eg, DeLamater & Sill, 2005; Tomic et al., 2006), along with other factors like sexual need and the presence of a partner (eg, Basson, Brotto, Laan, Redmond, & Utian, 2005; Howard, O'Neill, & Travers, 2006). Sexual disinterest is commonly reported by women as they age and women are more likely than men to report a lack of interest in sexual activity (Kontula & Haavio-Mannila, 2009). A study conducted by Chao et al. (2011) found that approximately 40% of older adult respondents to a survey reported having sex a minimum of one time a month. Among women who were not sexually active, most did not have a desire to resume sexual activity; however, the desire for sexual activity for aging men remained high (Smith, Mulhall, Deveci, Monaghan,

& Reid, 2007). Trompeter, Bettencourt, and Barrett-Connor (2012) investigated the prevalence of sexual activity and satisfaction among women.
Questionnaires were mailed to women over the age of 40 (mean age of a
respondent was 67 years) that inquired about sexual activity, satisfaction,
and included the Female Sexual Function Index (a measure designed to
assess sexual dysfunction). Over half of the respondents reported that
they had engaged in sexual activity within the past month and well over
half of those women indicated arousal.

Thus, there appears to be a wide range of sexual engagement as women
age. There are several situational factors that may explain, in part, the disparity of engagement levels among aging women. For example, cultural
attitudes regarding sex, such as reproductive fitness and the association
between youth and "sexiness," likely contribute to the feeling that aging
women should be asexual and this pattern is more common among older
women who reside in Western cultures (Deacon, Minichiello, & Plummer,
1995). Stimson, Wase, and Stimson (1981) have suggested that women are
socialized to believe that youth equates to desirability and the concept of
"beauty" is more restrictive for aging women than for their male peers.
Personal changes in appearance due to aging (eg, wrinkles) may have an
influence on women's self-perceptions and sexuality (Graziottin, 1996).
However, more than 35 years ago, Roff and Klemmack (1979) found that
respondents to a survey did not perceive sexual activity between older
persons to be less appropriate than sexual activity between younger adults.

The loss of a sexual partner is more common for aging women as women
typically live longer than men and are often younger than their male sexual
partners (eg, Howard, O'Neill, & Travers, 2006; Kalra, Subramanyam, &
Pinto, 2011; Wilkins & Warnock, 2009). The trend of women outliving
their male partners holds true across cultures and countries. For example,
Howard et al. (2006) found that women without a sexual partner rose from
15% for women in their 40s to about 54% for women in their 70s.

CHECK IT OUT!

Check out this online informational resource (review different sub-
links) for older women to assist in adjusting to later-life changes in personal sexual functioning and related sexuality issues: https://www.nia.
nih.gov/health/publication/sexuality-later-life

In reviewing this online content, answer the following questions:

1. What are some important support resources that aging women may
   need to help in maintaining positive sexual relationships?
2. What role does culture play in how this information is
   communicated to older women?

3. What are the cultural "messages" about women and later-life sexuality?
4. Are there motivational factors to consider when creating community education programs for aging women?

Even when aging adults reenter into an intimate relationship, they may experience "widower's syndrome," which describes sexual difficulties following a period of sexual inactivity due to the death of an intimate partner (Meston, 1997). Greendale, Hogan, and Shumaker (1996) developed a "sexual functioning" questionnaire, and were able to gather data from a large sample of approximately 900 adults aged 45–64 years. Their study revealed that the leading cause (ie, 64% of respondents) of sexual inactivity in postmenopausal women was the absence of an intimate partner.

BARRIERS TO OLDER WOMEN'S SEXUAL ACTIVITY

Institutional barriers may also discourage sexual activity/expression between aging adults. This may be especially evident for nursing home residents who indicate that they have a lack of privacy and feel restrained by the culture of the nursing home (eg, Ehrenfeld, Bronner, Tabak, Alpert, & Bergman, 1999; Hillman, 2000). In fact, Roach (2004) argues that a change of culture should occur so that staff can become comfortable with issues of older adults' sexuality. Furthermore, those concerned with the expression of older adults' sexuality (eg, Mulligan & Palguta, 1991) suggest that home visits should be arranged if a nursing home resident has an intimate sexual partner at home. Walker and Ephross (1999) developed a survey to address older adults' attitudes toward sexual expression, knowledge toward sexuality issues, and staff practices in residential care facilities. The researchers found that respondents, as a whole, were knowledgeable about sex; had a positive attitude toward sex throughout their life span; and were in favor of a pro-active staff.

Reingold and Burros (2004) discussed initiatives for nursing home staff that frame sexual expression as a normal act between consenting adults. This includes, for example, the development of a training video for nursing home staff that sought to promotes sexual expression as a natural part of consenting adults. Somewhat counterintuitively, Glass, Mustian, and Carter (1986) found that the staff members with the most knowledge about sexuality held more conservative views toward older adults' sexuality than staff members who possessed less knowledge.

QUOTES FROM FAMOUS, POSITIVELY AGING WOMEN

Age does not protect you from love. But love, to some extent, protects you from age.

—*Anais Nin, Author*

Life is short. Break the rules, forgive quickly, kiss slowly, love truly, laugh uncontrollably, and never regret anything that made you smile.

—*Mae West, Comedienne and Actress*

Loving someone liberates the lover as well as the beloved. And that kind of love comes with age.

—*Maya Angelou, National Poet Laureate*

Staff training is needed regarding later-life sexuality (Bouman, Arcelus, & Benbow, 2007). Bauer, McAuliffe, Nay, and Chenco (2013) educated residential care nurses on aging adults' sexuality in a residential setting, and found nurses' attitudes were more accepting of older people expressing their sexuality in nursing homes. The issues of maintaining intimate relationships in nursing homes may be a more pronounced issue in Western cultures as many non-Western cultures do not rely on residential support to help care for older adults. Indeed, even within the United Sates, certain (minority) segments of the population do not reliably use residential care facilities compared to other (majority) segments, psychosocial factors and cultural expectations can, in part, predict residential care utilization (eg, Bradley et al., 2002).

Although sexual activity levels decline with age, Kalra et al. (2011) found that love and intimacy levels remain the same in later life. Malatesta (2007) argues that many of the treatments for sexual disengagement/ dysfunction in older adult women place too much emphasis on "genital function" (ie, Viagra) and fail to appreciate the importance of intimate interpersonal relationships. Intimate personal relationships, like sexual activity, are associated with positive health indicators (Antonucci, Birditt, & Webster, 2010). Traupmann, Eckels, and Hatfield (1982) concluded that there is a significant association between intimate relationships (among married women) and life satisfaction, passionate and companionate love.

"Companionate love" is defined by Sternberg's (1986) as the intersection between intimacy, commitment, and sexual satisfaction. However, in subsequent research, Hatfield, Traupmann, and Sprecher (1984) found that over time passionate and companionate love both declined. Why does this happen, and how can different societies better support aging women in maintaining healthy sexuality?

BIOLOGY OF WOMEN'S LATER-LIFE SEXUAL DESIRE

In addition to some of the social factors that contribute to a decrease in sexual activity, many biological factors or health issues (eg, cancer; Sacerdoti, Lagana, & Koopman, 2010) also contribute to a wane in sexual interest; however, the most compelling factor is arguably menopausal status. Menopause influences sexual interest and women invariably indicate their concern that menopause has an adverse relationship with sexuality (eg, Dennerstein, Alexander, & Kotz, 2003; Dennerstein, Dudley, & Burger, 2001). In a large-scale study with over 3000 women, Avis et al. (2009) found that perimenopausal (ie, "around menopause") women reported a decrease in sexual desire and an increase in how painful the women rated their sexual experience. Scores of low sexual function, as measured by the *McCoy Female Sexuality Questionnaire*, began at about 42% in early menopause and increased to 88% during late menopause (Ambler, Bieber, & Diamond, 2012).

However, many women do not express any concerns about sexual activity postmenopause, in fact, some women report the opposite in that they find sexual activity to be a more rewarding experience after menopause. Kingsberg (2000) reported that sex after menopause is more pleasurable because anxiety levels associated with birth control and pregnancy are no longer relevant issues. Furthermore, Hartmann, Philippsohn, Heiser, and Ruffer-Hesse (2004) argued that women are not "victims" to their hormones and that sociocultural factors (eg, stress, past life events) are better predictors of sexual engagement than menopause status. Research by Dennerstein, Lehert, and Dudley (1999) demonstrated in a large-scale observational study, and employing Structural Equation Modeling (SEM), that hormonal effects have a weak effect on women's sexuality and that stronger predictors of women's sexuality include her feelings toward her partner. Importantly, a woman's sexual satisfaction is related to her later-life quality of life (Chao et al., 2011).

WORDS OF WISDOM

Lin has been a midwife for many years. When asked about stereotypes regarding women and intimate relationships, Lin said that older women are facing a lot of stereotypes regarding their sexual lives. Women go through hormonal changes during menopause and it might affect their sex life. Some women might need a little coaching or help to be able to enjoy sex; it is great when a woman has a partner who is willing to be part of it, or she can even be her own partner.

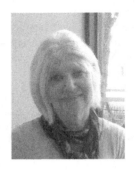

It is important that a woman feels comfortable with her partner, someone who will help her enjoy sex. Intimate relationships are not only sexual but also they can be stimulating intellectually as well as emotionally. Being in an intimate relationship is about companionship and having someone to share experiences with and enjoy things together. Women should not feel left out because they are single; according to Lin women should think, "I am enough, just me is enough." Being in an intimate relationship might also affect health; for example, people tend to take better care of themselves; nevertheless, being in a bad unhealthy relationship will result in more stress and negativity.

What advice would Lin give to younger women? She said it is never too late to find ways to maintain a healthy relationship; it is about intimacy and connection. Hormonal changes during menopause might change women and it is important that partners change together. It is important to keep relationships positive; if a woman is not feeling happy in a relationship it is important to take a closer look at what might be missing and what she might need—every woman should realize that she deserves her own happiness. "Listen to your heart, your soul and do not put up with something that is not worth it."

Using a longitudinal research design, Dennerstein, Lehert, and Burger (2005) concluded that a woman's prior sexual functioning and relationship variables are more significant predictors of sexual function than are hormonal determinants. With this in mind, education for women in many different parts of the world regarding potential changes in their sexual functioning is vital. There are a number of sexual disorders that may lead to a decrease in sexual desire or the ability to engage in sexual activity with aging women. Among the disorders which may be part of an educational and/or support program, some of the more common include: hypoactive sexual desire disorder, female sexual arousal disorder, sexual pain disorder, and female orgasmic disorder (Wilkins & Warnock, 2009). Ratner, Erekson, Minkin, and Foran-Tuller (2011) discussed the relationship between gynecological pathology (eg, pelvic prolapse, urinary and fecal incontinence) and sexual activity. The likelihood of having a gynecological pathology increases with age and women who have a pathology report being "worried" and "distressed" about sexual activity. The following are additional sexuality behavior issues that women should be aware of as they age over time.

Sexual drive and desire. The desire to have sexual contact is both physical and psychological in nature, and any complication in satisfying this drive is the focus of sex therapy (eg, Wilkins & Warnock, 2009). The underlying societal and/or personal developmental factors restricting an older woman's positive, healthy sexuality would need to be discussed. One such issue would be a lack of desire to have sexual contact. There are psychological disorders related to a lack of desire to have sexual contact with others. *Hypoactive Sexual Desire Disorder* (HSDD) and *Sexual Aversion Disorder* (SAD) are mental health disorders related to a lack of desire to have sexual contact with others. These disorders have been examined with the global aging female population, but could be applied to any individual or people in relationship experiencing anxiety in having sexual contact (Diagnostic and Statistical Manual of Mental Disorders, 2013). Furthermore, cultural considerations need to be taken into account as some cultures strongly discourage sex for reasons other than for reproduction, therefore, sexual enjoyment and/or expression may not be viewed as appropriate behaviors as a woman ages (Deacon et al., 1995).

Sexual contact itself may not be the issue causing the anxiety but rather sexual difficulties might be due to debilitating social pressures and/or social reactions to one's sexual behavior (Avis et al., 2009; Trudel, Turgeon, & Piche, 2000). From a societal perspective, stereotyping and proliferating associated myths about an individual's sexuality in later life leading to inevitable sexual performance issues must be eradicated through education (Hinchliff & Gott, 2008). Past research examining sexual wellness in later-life relationships has identified personal factors creating potential sexual intimacy "barriers," such as mental depression, the presence of children in the family, and/or stressors due to career and/or financial stability. In addition, it is important to understand the interplay of sexual desires between people in a relationship (eg, incongruent sexual frequency needs).

Sexual arousal. To achieve and maintain sexual arousal can be influenced by a combination of physical and psychological factors impacting their sexual performance. The degree to which this is a physiological condition may be related to the effects of aging (ie, a decrease in testosterone level), other on-going health problems (eg, diabetes), and/or to prescribed medications. It is important for a person to consult his or her physician to identify potential health-related concerns impacting sexual performance.

The difficulty may equally be attributable to psychological issues. Working with a sex therapist can assist an aging woman in resolving any psychological stress reactions that may underlie and/or are in response to sexual performance complications (eg, Leiblum & Segraves, 1989). Sex therapy may focus on specific sexual behaviors within the relationship of the client which can assist in sexual excitement and satisfaction. Although there may be medical issues underlying these performance complications, a sex therapist may be very assistive in offering counseling and assigning sexual "homework" exercises to help the client to work through these performance complications (eg, Drench & Losee, 1996).

One important aim of the sex therapy process is to help a female client better understand her sexual history. Through sexual history narratives, women clients may reveal social, emotional, and/or other personal factors which shaped their current feelings of sexuality from early childhood through adolescence and adulthood. Societal processes of acculturation and socialization through clients' past relationships with family, friends, peers, and/or sexual partners can have a profound effect on their present conscious and/or unconscious perceptions of personal sexuality (eg, Kass, 1981). Through this discussion of their personal history, different societal factors are examined which may have shaped their present personal sexuality, relationship needs, and associated behaviors (eg, sexual behaviors). All of these insights during the sex therapy process should lead to a better understanding of a woman's sexual attitudes and sexual needs.

POSITIVE SUPPORTS FOR OLDER WOMEN'S SEXUALITY

The treatment for disorders that influence sexual functioning usually includes a lifestyle assessment (eg, exercise, stress reduction), and both biological (eg, estrogen deficiency) and psychosocial (eg, sex education, therapy) considerations (Wilkins & Warnock, 2009). Likewise, Walsh and Berman (2004) suggest that treatment options for sexual dysfunction can range from counseling to physical therapy to medication; however, Ambler et al. (2012) suggested that relationship and psychological determinants of the dysfunction should be addressed before medication is prescribed for sexual dysfunction.

TIPS FOR AGING WOMEN'S SEXUAL HEALTH

1. Be self-aware of your sexual needs and communicate your needs to a partner.
2. Use protection when engaging in sexual activities.
3. Be realistic about changing capabilities.
4. Consult with a physician about any physical performance concerns.

Research has reliably demonstrated that sexually activity among aging adults is associated with better physical, psychological, and social factors (Bach, Mortimer, VandeWeerd, & Corvin, 2011). Finding meaningful interventions to support women's positive sexuality and sexual behavior is an important endeavor for all cultures and countries. For example, it is important for aging women to discuss their changing feelings of sexuality with their healthcare provider (Lindau et al., 2007). Likewise, healthcare professionals need to better initiate discussions about sexual health with their aging clients (Sacerdoti et al., 2010). Healthcare professionals must be aware of the stereotypes associated with sexuality and aging but they need to balance the stereotypes with a discussion about the normative development of sexuality across the life span so that older women, for example, can engage in meaningful introspection about their sexuality, one that is grounded in research (eg, Watters & Boyd, 2009). Further, sex therapists who are working with older women should pay special attention to and/or receive additional training to work with women who identify themselves as an ethnic minority or as gay, lesbian, bisexual, or transgender as these factors result in different sociocultural pressures (eg, Muzacz & Akinsulure-Smith, 2013).

The most comprehensive intervention to improve the quality of a woman's sex life should take a "biopsychosocial" approach to treatment (Ratner et al., 2011). Trudel and colleagues (Trudel et al., 2008) noted that treatment for sexual disorders may include physical therapy, counseling, and supplements but that neither the biological or the psychological aspects of dysfunction occur in a vacuum, so researchers and healthcare professionals need to recognize the psychological, cultural, and physiological contributions to a woman's sexual functioning and the interaction between the two. Muliira and Muliira (2013) reviewed the literature and also found that the sexual functioning of older adults is determined by physical changes, changes to their intimate relationship, health problems, and psychosocial situations. Therefore, any interventions must include a range that addresses all or some of these factors (eg, relationship counseling, pharmaceuticals, and sexual health).

Carvalho and Nobre (2010) were interested in what factors (ie, psychopathology, disengaged sexual thought, dyadic cohesion and affection, menopausal status, age, and medical problems) were the best predictors of sexual desire. Their analysis suggested that disengaged thought during sexual activity was the strongest predictor of sexual desire suggesting that cognitive dimensions play a critical role in the treatment of sexual dysfunction. In a similar vein, evidence suggests (eg, Galinsky, 2012) that both older males and females may benefit from frequent sexual touching (during sex) as this leads to fewer reported difficulties with orgasm and sexual arousal, and more reported sexual pleasure. Reassuringly, both Meston (1997) and Deacon et al. (1995) concluded that physiological and psychological changes associated with aging do not mean that sexual relationships in older adults need to be difficult and, in the absence of negative cultural expectations through community-based education/training, a fulfilling sex life is attainable for aging women.

SUMMARY

This chapter examined the underlying issues of women's positive expression of sexuality in later life. Sexual satisfaction is one part of the quality-of-life needs for women into later life. A dominant theme in the available research indicates that as women age, they are less likely to be as sexually active as they were when they were younger; however, the loss of sexual functioning is not inevitable. As discussed in this chapter, there are many factors related to how women cope with biological changes and other issues in response to later-life relationships and intimacy. From a positive aging perspective, many interventions are in place to address female sexual functioning and these interventions are promising, particularly those interventions that focus on the intersection between biological and social considerations.

DISCUSSION QUESTIONS

1. How do women typically regard their personal sexuality as they age?
2. Are men different in this perception of personal sexuality in later life? Why or why not?
3. What role does society play in shaping women's attitudes about personal later-life sexuality? How?

4. To what degree does the media influence sexual behaviors and attitudes among aging women?
5. How can community education across a woman's life span create a more positive outcome?
6. Are older generations of women different than today's women in terms of attitudes toward personal sexuality?
7. Will future generations of women have different aging attitudes about sexuality than older generations? Why or why not?
8. Does the media promote positive images of older women's sexuality? If not, why?
9. Are family members a key part of the attitudes that older women hold regarding their own sexuality? If so, how?
10. Education regarding safe sexual practices in later life is part of optimizing sexual health and activity for aging women. How would you design such a program?

TEST YOUR KNOWLEDGE!

Take the following quiz about attitudes toward personality sexuality:
http://personality=testing.info?tests/MSSCQ.php

SUPPLEMENTAL BOOK READINGS

Over the past decades, there have been many books written on the topic of women's later-life sexuality. Here are some recommended *additional readings*:

Banner, L. W. (1993). *In full flower: Aging women, power, and sexuality.* London, UK: Vintage.

The author examines many different sources of literature and cultural artifacts related to the topic of older women and younger men in romantic relationships. The book communicates the idea that older women are sexual beings and should be regarded as such, contradicting the stereotype that women lose their sexual desires and become asexual as they age. Many different cultures have different beliefs about the sexuality of aging women, and is certainly a quality-of-life issue for women across their lifetime.

Price, J. (2011). *Naked at our age: Talking out loud about senior sex.* Berkeley, CA: Seal Press.

    This is a great book for aging women (and men) who are dealing with issues of aging and how this is influenced by personal and societal attitudes about sex in later life. Exploring different sexual orientations and sexual relationships, the author thoughtfully discusses the importance of self-acceptance and personal acknowledgment that sexual desire does not cease in later adulthood. This would be a good reference book both for sex therapists working with aging clients and laypeople interested in their own evolving sense of sexual identity. This would be a helpful guide for women as they continue on a path of self-understanding within their nonplatonic relationships.

Brayne, S. (2011). *Sex, meaning and the menopause.* New York, NY: Bloomsbury Academic.

    The book examines an important adjustment issue for aging women, entering into postmenopause and its effect on feelings of sexual desire toward others. There are certainly ramifications of intimacy in later-life relationships which need to be addressed. The emotional, psychological, and physiological changes experienced by the aging woman necessitate frank and honest discussions with intimate partners.

SUPPLEMENTAL AGING VIDEOS

For learning purposes, the use of videos can be very beneficial for both instructors and readers. Here are some recommended *supplemental videos*:

Sex and Aging: Overcoming the Obstacles to Maintaining a Vital Sex Life (Format: DVD)

    The video attempts to dispel myths about loss of libido and sexual desire in later life. Changing society's attitudes toward later-life sexual expression and experimentation in light of physical changes in functional capacity is discussed.

ADDITIONAL INFORMATION LINKS

The following are some recommended *supplemental Internet links*:

Aging in Action website: http://aginginaction.com/2010/12/gender-and-aging-what-do-we-know/

American Public Health Association website: http://www.apha.org/membergroups/sections/aphasections/a_ph/

Everyday Health website: http://www.everydayhealth.com/senior-health/enhancing-your-sexuality.aspx

NIH/NIAging website: http://www.nia.nih.gov/about/minority-aging-and-health-disparities

WebMD website: http://www.webmd.com/healthy-aging/guide/sex-aging

World Health Organization website: http://www.who.int/ageing/gender/en/index.html

References

AARP. (2010). Sex, romance, and relationships: AARP survey of midlife and older adults: <http://www.aarp.org/research/topics/life/info-2014/srr_09.html>.

Ambler, D., Bieber, E., & Diamond, M. (2012). Sexual function in older adult women: A review of current literature. *Review of Obstetrics and Gynecology, 5*(1), 16–27.

Antonucci, T., Birditt, K., & Webster, N. (2010). Social relations and mortality: A more nuanced approach. *Journal of Health Psychology, 15*(5), 649–659.

Avis, N., Brockwell, S., Randolph, J., Shen, S., Cain, V., Ory, M., et al. (2009). Longitudinal changes in sexual functioning as women transition through menopause: Results from the study of women's health across the nation (SWAN). *Menopause, 16*(3), 442–452.

Bach, L. E., Mortimer, J. A., VandeWeerd, C., & Corvin, J. (2011). The association of physical and mental health with sexual activity in older adults in a retirement community. *Journal of Sex Medicine, 11*, 2671–2678.

Basson, R., Brotto, L., Laan, E., Redmond, G., & Utian, W. (2005). Assessment and management of women's sexual dysfunctions: Problematic desire and arousal. *Journal of Sex Medicine, 2*, 291–300.

Bauer, M., McAuliffe, L., Nay, R., & Chenco, C. (2013). Sexuality in older adults: Effect of an education intervention on attitudes and beliefs of residential aged care staff. *Educational Gerontology, 39*(2), 82–91.

Bouman, W., Arcelus, J., & Benbow, S. (2007). Nottingham study of sexuality and ageing (NoSSA II). Attitudes of care staff regarding sexuality and residents: A study in residential and nursing homes. *Sexual and Relationship Therapy, 22*(1), 45–61.

Bradley, E., McGraw, S. A., Curry, L., Buckser, A., King, K. L., Kasl, S. V., et al. (2002). Expanding the Andersen model: The role of psychosocial factors in long-term care use. *Health Services Research, 35*(5), 1221–1242.

Carvalho, J., & Nobre, P. (2010). Predictors of women's sexual desire: The role of psychopathology, cognitive-emotional determinants, relationship dimensions, and medical factors. *Journal of Sex Medicine, 7*, 928–937.

Chao, J., Lin, Y., Ma, M., Lai, C., Kuo, W., & Chao, I. (2011). Relationship among sexual desire, sexual satisfaction, and quality of life in middle-aged and older adults. *Sex and Marital Therapy, 37*(5), 386–403.

Deacon, S., Minichiello, V., & Plummer, D. (1995). Sexuality and older people: Revisiting the assumptions. *Educational Gerontology, 21*, 497–513.

DeLamater, J., & Sill, M. (2005). Sexual desire in later life. *The Journal of Sex Research, 42*, 138–149.

Dennerstein, L., Alexander, J., & Kotz, K. (2003). The menopause and sexual functioning: A review of the population-based studies. *Annual Review of Sex Research, 14*, 64–82.

Dennerstein, L., Dudley, E., & Burger, H. (2001). Are changes in sexual functioning during midlife due to aging or menopause? *Fertility and Sterility, 76*(3), 456–460.

Dennerstein, L., Lehert, P., & Burger, H. (2005). The relative effects of hormones and relationship factors on sexual function of women through the natural menopausal transition. *Fertility and Sterility, 84*(1), 174–180.

Dennerstein, L., Lehert, P., & Dudley, E. (1999). Factors affecting sexual functioning of women in the mid-life years. *Climacteric, 2*, 254–262.

Diagnostic and Statistical Manual of Mental Disorders, (2013). Washington, D.C.: American Psychiatric Association.

Drench, M. E., & Losee, R. H. (1996). Sexuality and sexual capacities of elderly people. *Rehabilitation Nursing, 21*(3), 118–123.

Ehrenfeld, M., Bronner, G., Tabak, N., Alpert, R., & Bergman, R. (1999). Sexuality among institutionalized older adult patients with dementia. *Nursing Ethics, 6*, 144–149.

Fileborn, B., Thorpe, R., Hawkes, G., Minichiello, V., Pitts, M., & Dune, T. (2015). Sex, desire and pleasure: Considering the experiences of older Australian women. *Sexual and Relationship Therapy, 30*(1), 117–130.

Galinsky, A. (2012). Sexual touching and difficulties with sexual arousal and orgasm among U.S. older adults. *Archives of Sexual Behavior, 41*(4), 875–890.

Glass, J., Mustian, D., & Carter, L. (1986). Knowledge and attitudes of healthcare providers toward sexuality in the institutionalized elderly. *Educational Gerontology, 12*(5), 465–475.

Graziottin, A. (1996). HRT: The women's perspective. *International Journal of Gynecological Obstetrics, 52*, 11–16.

Greendale, G. A., Hogan, P., & Shumaker, S. (1996). Sexual functioning in postmenopausal women: The postmenopausal estrogen/progestin interventions (PEPI) trial. *Journal of Women's Health, 5*, 445–458.

Hartmann, U., Philippsohn, S., Heiser, K., & Ruffer-Hesse, C. (2004). Low sexual desire in midlife and older women: Personality factors, psychosocial development, present sexuality. *Menopause, 11*(6, part 2), 726–740.

Hatfield, E., Traupmann, J., & Sprecher, S. (1984). Older women's perceptions of their intimate relationships. *Journal of Social and Clinical Psychology, 2*(2), 108–124.

Hillman, J. (2000). *Clinical perspectives on older adults' sexuality*. New York, NY: Kluwer Academic/Plenum Publishers.

Hinchliff, S., & Gott, M. (2008). Challenging social myths and stereotypes of women and aging: Heterosexual women talk about sex. *Journal of Women and Aging, 20*(1-2), 65–81.

Howard, J. R., O'Neill, S., & Travers, C. (2006). Factors affecting sexuality in older Australian women: Sexual interest, sexual arousal, relationships and sexual distress in older Australian women. *Climacteric, 9*(5), 355–367.

Kalra, G., Subramanyam, A., & Pinto, C. (2011). Sexuality: Desire, activity, and intimacy in the elderly. *Indian Journal of Psychiatry, 53*(4), 300–306.

Kass, M. J. (1981). Geriatric sexuality breakdown syndrome. *International Journal of Aging and Human Development, 13*, 71–77.

Kingsberg, S. A. (2000). The psychological impact of aging on sexuality and relationships. *Journal of Women's Health Gender Based Medicine, 9*(1), S33–S38.

Kontula, O., & Haavio-Mannila, E. (2009). The impact of aging on human sexual activity and sexual desire. *The Journal of Sex Research, 46*(1), 46–56.

Leiblum, S. R., & Segraves, R. T. (1989). Sex therapy with aging adults. In S. R. Leiblum & R. C. Rosen (Eds.), *Principles and practice of sex therapy* (pp. 352–381). New York, NY: Guilford Press.

Lindau, S., Schumm, P., Laumann, E., Levinson, W., O'Muircheartaigh, C., & Waite, L. (2007). A study of sexuality and health among older adults in the United States. *New England Journal of Medicine, 357*(8), 762–774.

Malatesta, V. J. (2007). Sexual problems, women, and aging: An overview. *Journal of Women Aging, 19*(1), 139–154.

Meston, C. M. (1997). Aging and sexuality. *Successful Aging, 167*, 285–290.

Muliira, J., & Muliira, R. (2013). Sexual health for older women: Implications for nurses and other healthcare providers. *Sultan Qaboos University Medicine Journal, 13*(4), 469–476.

Mulligan, T., & Palguta, R. F. (1991). Sexual interest, activity, and satisfaction among male nursing home residents. *Archives of Sex Behavior, 20*, 199–204.

Muzacz, A. K., & Akinsulure-Smith, A. M. (2013). Older adults and sexuality: Implications for counseling ethnic and sexual minority clients. *Journal of Mental Health Counseling, 35*(1), 1–14.

Ratner, E. S., Erekson, E. A., Minkin, M. J., & Foran-Tuller, K. A. (2011). Sexual satisfaction in the elderly female population: A special focus on women with gynecologic pathology. *Maturitas, 70*(3), 210–215.

Reingold, D., & Burros, N. (2004). Sexuality in the nursing home. *Journal of Gerontological Social Work, 43*, 2–3.

Roach, S. M. (2004). Sexual behavior of nursing home residents: Staff perceptions and responses. *Journal of Advanced Nursing, 48*, 371–379.

Roff, L., & Klemmack, D. (1979). Sexuality activity among older persons: A comparative analysis of appropriateness. *Research on Aging, 1*(3), 389–399.

Sacerdoti, R. C., Lagana, L., & Koopman, C. (2010). Altered sexuality and body image after gynecological cancer treatment: How can psychologists help? *Professional Psychology, 41*(6), 533–540.

Smith, L., Mulhall, J., Deveci, S., Monaghan, N., & Reid, M. (2007). Sex after seventy: A pilot study of sexual function in older persons. *Journal of Sex Medicine, 4*(5), 1247–1253.

Sternberg, R. (1986). A triangular theory of love. *Psychological Review, 93*(2), 119–135.

Stimson, A., Wase, J., & Stimson, J. (1981). Sexuality and self-esteem among the aged. *Research on Aging, 3*(2), 228–239.

Tomic, D., Gallicchio, L., Whiteman, M. K., Lewis, L. M., Lagenberg, P., & Flaws, J. A. (2006). Factors associated with determinants of sexual functioning in midlife women. *Maturitas, 53*(2), 155–157.

Traupmann, J., Eckels, E., & Hatfield, E. (1982). Intimacy in older women's lives. *The Gerontologist, 22*(6), 493–498.

Trompeter, S., Bettencourt, R., & Barrett-Connor, E. (2012). Sexual activity and satisfaction in healthy community-dwelling older women. *American Journal of Medicine, 125*(1), 37–43.

Trudel, G., Boyer, R., Villeneuve, V., Anderson, A., Pilon, G., & Bounader, J. (2008). The marital life and aging well program: Effects of a group preventive intervention on the marital and sexual functioning of retired couples. *Sexual and Relationship Therapy, 23*(1), 5–23.

Trudel, G., Turgeon, L., & Piche, L. (2000). Marital and sexual aspects of old age. *Sexual and Relationship Therapy, 15*(4), 381–406.

Walker, B. L., & Ephross, P. H. (1999). Knowledge and attitudes toward sexuality of a group of older adults. *Journal of Gerontological Social Work, 31*, 85–107.

Walsh, K. E., & Berman, J. R. (2004). Sexual dysfunction in the older woman: An overview of the current understanding and management. *Drugs Aging, 21*(10), 655–657.

Watters, Y., & Boyd, T. (2009). Sexuality in later life: Opportunity for reflections for health care providers. *Sexual and Relationship Therapy, 24*(3-4), 307–315.

Wilkins, K., & Warnock, J. (2009). Sexual dysfunction in older women. *Primary Psychiatry, 16*(3), 59–65.

AGING WOMEN'S ROLES IN SOCIETY

Relevant chapters

12 *Women's Economic Health and Work/Retirement in Later Life* *219*

13 *Breaking Stereotypes of Aging Women* *237*

14 *Civic Engagement and the Power of Older Women* *251*

15 *Public Policies and the Next Steps in the Evolution of Women's Aging* *269*

The fourth section of the book examines in many different ways the involvement of women in society into later adulthood. Issues related to aging women's social status and power, skill development/training opportunities, empowerment needs, and economic resources in society will be examined throughout the chapters in this section. The roles and contributions of older women in communities and broader societies will grow in significance in correspondence with their growing demographic numbers. The purpose of this section is to introduce emerging ideas related to the current and future impact of a growing world population of older women. Across sections of the world, women are living longer than ever before and increasingly are in need of a "voice" in public policies and programs affecting their daily existence. As with other sections of the book, a cross-cultural examination of aging women's issues is conducted to identify both the "universal" and unique experiences of women aging that can then be applied to public policies and related societal practices. Across chapters in this section, the social status and associated social power of older women is examined in order to best identify practices supporting positive aging outcomes for women into later life.

Women's Economic Health and Work/Retirement in Later Life

Global Fact: *Women's participation in the labour market is lower than men's at every stage, and the gender gap is greatest between ages 50 and 64 years.*
—**United Nations, Women Coordination Division report (2012)**

As women live longer and healthier lives than ever before, their desire to explore new career options and progress within existing careers will become more evident. Take the *Can You Spot Age Discrimination in the Workplace* and the *Experienced Workforce* quizzes from AARP in Appendix A to better understand potential topics to consider for aging female workers across the world.

ISSUES RELATED TO RETIREMENT

In a survey of male and female MBAs, 20% indicated that they planned to continue to work after the age of 65 (Frieze, Olson, & Murrell, 2011). The rate of older adults remaining in the workforce is at an all-time high (AARP, 2008). Many older adults are instead remaining at their job or exploring the notion of an "encore career" (ie, a second, professional job that may be more financially secure and/or may be more personally rewarding than the first job). Furthermore, many adults also have "bridge jobs" or a transitional job (eg, part-time work) between one's career and complete retirement (Quinn & Kozy, 1996).

While many mature workers indicate that they would like to remain in their job, many also indicate that they desire more flexibility with their work schedule. Older adults may wish to have fewer hours on the job so that they can care for a loved one, a grandchild, or take more control over their own health and well-being (eg, Koc-Menard, 2009). And, caregivers are more likely to be women and the demands of caregiving seem to play a large role around the middle of life (ages 45–65) (Moen, Robison, & Fields, 1994).

Women and Positive Aging.
DOI: http://dx.doi.org/10.1016/B978-0-12-420136-1.00012-8 **219**

While fewer hours on the job are one way to achieve this, older workers may also explore the option of "job sharing" and/or working from home (Eyster, Johnson, & Toder, 2008).

Many variables influence whether an individual will remain retired (eg, Schlosser, Zinni, & Armstrong, 2012). Armstrong-Stassen, Schlosser, and Zinni (2012) conducted a survey of retired adults in an attempt to predict what variables have the greatest impact of who will return to work ("unretire") and found that those retirees who indicate the greatest desire to return to work also experienced a role loss and/or financial loss as a function of leaving their job. Interestingly, retired women expressed a more positive sense of well-being than retired men (Mandal & Roe, 2008) but investment in a woman's role at work influenced how well she transitioned into retirement (Price, 2002). And, in particular, professional women may need to actively take steps to ease the transition from "work life" to "retirement life" by remaining active and utilizing her work-related skill set (eg, by volunteering time) (Price, 2003). Also of interest is the notion of the "healthy worker effect" or the idea that older adults who work have lower morbidity rates than same-age adults who do not work, this may be due; however, to self-selection into (or out of) the work environment (eg, Nuyts, Elseviers, & DeBroe, 1993).

TRY IT OUT!

Conduct an interview with an employed aging adult woman. Here are some potential questions to ask:

1. Has your experience changed over time?
2. Do you feel you are taken more or less seriously at work as you have gotten older? Why?
3. What has been the biggest advantage of getting older for your work career? Disadvantage?
4. Do you look forward to retirement? What is the most appealing aspect of retirement? What concerns you the most about retiring?

THE PSYCHOLOGICAL FUNCTION OF WORK

The importance of work differs for individuals, some view work as a way to make money and little more; whereas others perceive work as a way to derive meaning from their life (eg, Wrzesniewski, McCauley, Rozin, & Schwartz, 1997). Clearly, the level of *job involvement* (ie, engagement and concern with one's job) and *job centrality* (ie, the importance of work to one's life) (Paullay, Alliger, Stone-Romero, 1994) will influence an aging adult's view of work. In general, *job centrality* is considered to be a fairly stable attitude toward the importance of one's work and is not necessarily sensitive to the particulars of a work environment (Hirschfeld & Feild, 2000). However, *job involvement* is expected to change as a function of the work environment, such as the demands of the job and/or available resources at the workplace. Not surprisingly, Armstrong-Stassen and Schlosser (2008) found an association between the degree of work centrality and the older adults' willingness to stay with an organization. Indeed, through a series of in-depth interviews with older women, there were a number of factors that contributed to a woman's desire to engage in paid work beyond the financial aspect, such as independence and involvement and engagement with her work (Altschuler, 2004).

Mor-Barak (1995) argued that work for older adults serves four major goals: social, personal, financial, and, perhaps most importantly, generativity. Generativity is a concept that is pitted against "stagnation" in Erikson's psychosocial stages of development (Erikson, 1959). The generativity versus stagnation stage is the seventh of eight stages proposed by Erickson and is said to take place in "adulthood," defined as being approximately 40 to 65 years old. Generativity, as it applies to the workplace, can be thought of as teaching or passing along one's skill set to the younger generation. Dendinger, Adams, and Jacobson (2005) found evidence of this in that older adults indicate that they wish to remain at work in order to share their knowledge with others. Finch and Robinson (2003) indicated that older adults were interested in mentoring their younger coworkers, and 60% of the employed older adults indicated that since turning 50 they felt like more of their colleagues came to them for work-related advice (Benz, Sedensky, Tompson, & Agiesta, 2013). Further, as Pitt-Catsouphes and Matz-Costa (2009) noted, companies run the risk of "brain drain" when older workers leave the workforce without being able to properly pass along their knowledge to younger workers. This line of research supports the notion that older women have a clear and important role within an organizational setting.

Most research investigating the relationship between job satisfaction and age has found that older workers are more satisfied with various aspects of their jobs (eg, tasks, supervisors, etc.) than younger workers (eg, Dendinger et al., 2005; Janson & Martin, 1982; Ng & Feldman, 2010; Wright & Hamilton, 1978) but Clark, Oswald, and Warr (1996) provided evidence that the relationship might be more nuanced than a strictly linear relationship and provide data that demonstrate an "U-shaped" relationship between age and job satisfaction, in that satisfaction decreases after an initial hire and into the middle years but then rises steadily until retirement. Relatedly, Magee (2014) showed that in the early stages of a career, men report more pride with their jobs; however, from about midlife until the age of retirement, women report more pride in their jobs.

Globally, work life is also related to the issue of aging women's self-esteem. Women in autonomous jobs report higher levels of self-esteem than women in less autonomous jobs (Mutran, Reitzes, Bratton, & Fernandez, 1997). Further, cognitively complex work improves intellectual function, and this is true for all ages; however, this relationship is the greatest for older workers (Schooler, Mulatu, & Oates, 1999). Thus, working women, especially older women, are best served by jobs that offer a certain level of independence and that are also cognitively engaging. Workplaces can be designed to support such aims for aging workers (eg, human factors; Smith, 1990).

POSITIVELY AGING AT THE WORKPLACE

Many researchers and practitioners have applied the concept of positive aging to the work environment (eg, generativity; Mor-Barak, 1995). From a broad perspective, positive aging at work is reflected by any positive outcome on the job by older employees (eg, Zacher & Frese, 2009); however, a more exacting definition also takes into account health, work, and family balance, and on-the-job development and training (Shultz & Adams, 2007). Robson, Hansson, Abalos, and Booth (2006) developed an inventory and found five dimensions that related to positive aging at work. These dimensions include health and adaptability, interpersonal relationships, opportunities for workplace growth, individual security, and achievement of individual goals. Of these different areas, an opportunity for workplace growth was the only domain that was inversely related to age. As workers age, there is a negative relationship with seeking out new opportunities and achieving new goals at work (Zacher & Frese, 2009).

TIPS FOR AGING WOMEN WORKERS

1. Keep your work and interview skills updated (avoid skill obsolescence).
2. Have a career succession plan (ie, where you want to work next).
3. "Know yourself" in terms of valuable work skills and knowledge.
4. Be pro-active and pursue career advancement opportunities.
5. Join a career networking group.

ADVANTAGES OF A MATURE WORKER

There is a great deal of evidence supporting the notions that an increase in age does not equate to a decline in work-related performance (eg, McEvoy & Cascio, 1989; Ng & Feldman, 2008; Smith, 1990). One study using field research over the course of half a decade found that older employees were rated more positively on both subjective and objective measures of performance than were younger employees (Liden, Stilwell, & Ferris, 1996). Older adults are also more likely than younger adults to remain with an organization (ie, less turnover on the job) (Strebler, 2006) in part because they indicate that they are "engaged" with their work and committed to the organization (Galinsky, 2007). Commitment to a job usually translates into less expenses for an organization (ie, fewer costs associated with recruitment and training) and the age group 55 (plus) is more likely than younger workers to indicate that they plan to remain with an organization (American Psychological Association, 2012). In a survey conducted by the Society for Human Resource Management (2015), it was discovered that Human Resource professionals believed that older workers offered more work experience/knowledge/ skills and professionalism, and stronger work ethics compared to other workers.

STEREOTYPES OF THE MATURE WORKER

Despite the growing evidence that older workers are productive and satisfied workers, aging adults are still often viewed in a negative fashion (eg, Brownell & Kelly, 2013; Kite, Stockdale, Whitley, & Johnson, 2005), and that managers often hold stereotypical views of their older workers on dimensions of "productivity," "adaptability," and "reliability" (Henkins, 2005). In fact, Malinen and Johnston (2013) demonstrated that workers showed a negative and stable implicit attitude toward older workers and that their explicitly expressed attitudes were not negative toward older workers suggesting that these negative views of older workers may be unconscious or may not be expressed explicitly given that they may be perceived as a socially undesirable position to hold. In response to the way the older adults are often characterized and to protect older adult workers, the Equal Employment Opportunity Commission was enacted and prohibits discrimination against workers who are of age 40 or over; the Age Discrimination Act protects aging adults in all aspects of the job process from hiring, firing, promotions, and training (*Age Discrimination and Employment Act*, 1967). Such on-the-job protection is especially important to older women as they face both age and gender bias, and the reality of double discrimination; however, it is important to note that the law currently only provides protection against one form of discrimination (Porter, 2003). The United States has a long history of age discrimination policies, relative to other countries, and some studies suggest that older Americans consequently fare better in the workplace than older adults employed in countries that only offer limited age protection rights (eg, Lain, 2012).

There is evidence suggesting that age-related stereotypes can lead to diminished on-the-job performance and a decrease in job satisfaction (Shiu, Hassan, & Parry, 2015). Conversely, Kirchner, Volker, and Otmar (2015) primed older adults with either a positive age word (eg, "wisdom") or, in the control condition, did not present the group with any words and then asked workers to complete a task. Older adults in the experimental (ie, positive prime condition) group completed the task significantly faster than did the older adults in the control condition. Human Resource Departments should, therefore, make efforts to thwart age-related discrimination and to make company policies in this regard explicit (Chui, Chan, Snape, & Redman, 2001). Human Resources practices that are "age-inclusive" have been shown to be related to an age-diverse culture and low turnover intentions (Boehm, Kunze, & Bruch, 2014) thus such practices should be implemented not only to be compliant with the law but also to increase productivity among aging workers. Finally, Armstrong-Stassen (2006) found that mature workers indicated that an organization showing respect for their contribution and recognition of their work were the most important elements for deciding to remain with the company.

Employment practices can be put into place that help aging adults remain at their jobs longer and help to ensure financial security after retirement. For example, any type of employability enhancing practice (eg, targeted training, workplace flexibility) will benefit all age groups at work but specific efforts should be directed toward older adults to maintain and enhance their work performance (Fleischmann, Koster, & Schippers, 2013). However, most of the research in this area (eg, Arulampalam, Bryan, & Booth 2004) reveals that older workers have lower participation rates in work-related training activities relative to younger workers. Also, organizations are more willing to make changes to the workplace (eg, making office items more ergonomically friendly) that are inexpensive but are more concerned about implementing expensive changes (eg, educational resources/training) (Fleischmann, et al., 2013). And, several researchers have demonstrated that Human Resource *development* practices (ie, a focus on growth and accomplishing new goals and challenges) are better associated with positive attitudes for younger workers (eg, Innocenti, Profili, & Sammarra, 2013; Kooij et al., 2013) but that some human resources practices that focus on *maintenance* (ie, practices which focus on retaining older workers, such as team work and information sharing) are positively related to favorable attitudes toward work and that this relationship is stronger as workers age (Kooij, Jansen, Dikkers, & DeLange, 2010). In short, in organization settings, developmental Human Resources practices seem to be implemented more often than maintenance practices (Veth, Emans, Van der Heijden, Korzilius, & DeLange, 2015). Hursh, Lui, and Pransky (2006) suggested that Human Resource departments can rely on some of the following strategies to minimize decline that may be associated with mature workers: health promotion activities, ergonomic designs, and technology that can assist an older worker on the job.

ON-THE-JOB FACTORS THAT INFLUENCE THE AGING WORKER

Age-related injury may also be an issue for older workers especially because some jobs are quite physically demanding (eg, a nurse who has to transfer patients from a bed to a wheelchair). In physically demanding jobs, the demand may not change over time; however, the physical capability of the person performing the job is expected to decline as a function of age. In fact, there is a positive association between the age of workers and the rates of disability (Kampfe, Wadsworth, Mamboleo, & Schonbrun, 2008). Some research has concluded that the physical demands of a job can be attenuated by having employees participate in regular physical activity (Kenny, Yardley, Martineau, & Jay, 2008).

Further, the cognitive demands of the job may influence which workers will age successfully at work. For example, jobs that rely on more experience-based knowledge may be better suited to older adults than are jobs that require the rapid processing of information (Kanfer & Ackerman, 2004). Research has also found that "old-older" adults (55–64) report significant less on-the job stress than "young-older" adults (45–54) and that older adults may be better prepared to manage and/or avoid stressors and have better life management skills (Aldwin, Sutton, Chiara, & Siro, 1996).

EXTENDING CAREER WORK LIFE EXPECTANCY

The global population is experiencing a growing aging segment who is living longer and healthier than previous generations, and this is impacting the nature of the workplace in Europe and other locations (Arulampalam et al., 2004). This same population trend is occurring in many different industrialized and developing nations (Ilmarinen, 2009). Thus, the issue of working past traditional retirement age becomes an increasingly normative issue for many middle-aged and older adults in response to increased life expectancies and the associated need to afford these added years of life. "Traditional retirement age" has typically been defined as being age 65 to 67. Over the coming decades, population longevity trends suggest that most individuals who are normatively aging will live 15 to 20 or more years past traditional retirement age. Many older adults are faced with the decision of when to retire in light of financial, health, and other factors. It is, however, important to realize that one's ability to maintain workforce involvement is reflective of one's aging trajectory.

QUOTES FROM FAMOUS, POSITIVELY AGING WOMEN

I have enjoyed greatly the second blooming that comes
when you finish the life of the emotions and
of personal relations; and suddenly you find
at the age of fifty, say—

that a whole new life has opened before you,
filled with things you can think about,
study, or read about.... It is as if a fresh sap of ideas
and thoughts was rising in you.

—*Agatha Christie, Mystery Writer*

Have regular hours for work and play; make each day both useful and pleasant,
and prove that you understand the worth of time by employing it well.
Then youth will be delightful, old age will bring few regrets,
and life will become a beautiful success.

—*Louise May Alcott, Novelist*

Working into later life past traditional retirement age may be realistic for most workers initially, but continued participation may be increasingly challenging over time as advanced aging changes, and potentially non-normative changes, impact mental and physical performance capabilities (eg, cognitive slowing) on the job. Furthermore, it is crucial to examine how regional, national, and international differences affect the life course trajectory of older adults and therefore the transition from "working life" to "retirement life" (Green, 2009).

It is vital for older workers to be cognizant of these age-related changes in order to potentially compensate or adapt on the job without compromising job performance outcomes. Education and training related to developing pro-active compensatory strategies on the job would help assist the maintenance of older workers' workplace participation, and it may be argued that they are more effective performance strategies that benefit all ages and workers within an organization.

FACTORS TO CONSIDER

The affordability of retirement is a major factor in motivating older adults to remain in the workforce. The cost of healthcare, eldercare responsibilities, and support of younger generations within the family system are just a few financial factors to consider when choosing to remain in the workforce. Certainly personal longevity is important to consider when thinking about a number of years one may be in retirement without an income. People are living longer than ever before, but they are also living with chronic conditions. The need for sustained healthcare coverage and financial resources to address extended healthcare needs is a motivating factor for qualified older workers to stay in their jobs past traditional retirement age (eg, Disney, 1996). In addition to personal health concerns, increasingly aging workers are faced with financial concerns and otherwise supporting the eldercare needs of one or more parents over an extended period of time.

Regarding quality-of-life considerations, the workplace is an important environment for social support and engagement for older adults. "Hobby poor" individuals who did not plan for roles outside of work may consciously or unconsciously delay retirement concern about losing the social connections through coworkers in the workplace (eg, Davies & Cartwright, 2011).

Self-concept is a related subjective issue in how an older adult perceives his/her meaningful roles in society. Maybe significantly based upon maintaining a work role identity. To retire may threaten, potentially, some retirees' positive self-concept and associated feelings of self-esteem. Society may contribute to this working-related self-esteem issue by reinforcing ideas of working and being active as defining what it means to successfully age. Activity theory (eg, Havighurst, 1961), among other successful aging paradigms, suggests that being mentally and physically active on the job assists maintaining cognitive and physical competency in later life. Job-related tasks and interacting with others on the job can create a stimulating social environment for older adults who may not be equivalent in nature within a retirement role for some individuals (eg, Cheung & Wu, 2013).

Some occupations are more amenable to extended workforce participation for older adults than others. A distinction can be made between occupations which require predominantly more physical labor (ie, blue-collar occupations) and occupations which predominantly entail more cognitive related activities (ie, white-collar occupations). White-collar jobs typically offer more opportunities for career work life extension, with continued skill updating training and reasonable accommodation in job duties among qualified older workers. Inherently, blue-collar jobs have workers who retire near traditional retirement age because of the stress and strain related to doing ongoing physical work (eg, construction work). Certain industries are more "aging friendly" than others. Industries valuing knowledge and experience may be more amenable to experienced older workers who can contribute years of job experience to the workplace (eg, higher-level management, college-level education). Further, the motivation to remain in a job differs as a function of the job and education level required (ie, sensitivity to stock market vs labor market conditions; Coile & Levine, 2010). With the continued growth of aging workers remaining in the workforce in the coming decades, it behooves employers to examine ways to support qualified, experienced older workers. Employers should focus on utilizing older workers' vast areas of knowledge and expertise within the design of jobs and specific work-related tasks. Further, employers would benefit from retaining qualified aging employees through pro-actively anticipating their training needs in light of changing job and/or organizational trends. The benefits of retaining qualified older workers relate to their contributions of relatively higher job, commitment, organizational commitment, and workplace attendance in comparison to younger workers. It is widely assumed that it costs more to maintain an aging workforce, but in actuality their contributions to the organization far outweigh the cost to train and generally support these employees.

REMAINING UPDATED

Avoidance of skill obsolescence is a critical factor in one's ability to continue participating in the workforce for sustained time into later life. The responsibility of engaging in continual skill updating is on both the older worker and his/her employer. More public policies and programs regarding workplace training for an aging workforce need to be instituted to avoid the possibility of age discrimination and to promote greater access to skill updating opportunities (eg, Taylor & Walker, 1997). Workplace education regarding these rights and responsibilities involving older workers is needed to ensure that this process is conducted fairly and correctly. Employers should actively encourage older workers to participate in workplace learning opportunities on a continual basis. Legal age limitation in certain occupations (ie, a "safety force" occupational classification) is another factor to be considered when examining long-term career planning past traditional retirement age. To remain active in the workforce over an extended period of time past traditional retirement age, older workers need to engage in long-term career succession planning in which they anticipate needing to transition from one career to the next in light of age limitations, skill updating opportunities, and personal career interests. For example, an aging pilot may be faced with the decision of transitioning to a more administrative position within an organization because of age-related restrictions of job activities past traditional retirement age. Increasingly, as the baby boomers continue trends in workforce participation beyond age 65, employers and broader employment policy may need to evaluate aging-related restrictions on certain public safety occupations. The need for skill assessments related to occupying certain job positions may become more prevalent in practice as the proportion of experienced older workers increases in many different industries and countries (eg, Martin, Dymock, Billett, & Johnson, 2014).

The issue of creating effective and meaningful workplace assessments for older workers is important to consider. Assessments regarding training needs and associated career trajectory decisions are an integral part of decision-making in light of the person-job "fit" determinations of qualified older workers in the workforce (eg, AARP, 2008). Employment decisions involving older workers pertaining to hiring, promotion, training needs assessment, and other work-related decisions should be guided by well-designed and continual organizational assessments of employees. Effective assessments require careful consideration and design, implementation, and scoring/interpretation to best determine the degree to which an older worker is qualified to remain in the workforce. Objective assessments with appropriate follow-up interventions will best support the maintenance of a qualified aging workforce in the decades to come. Understanding the associated needs of qualified older workers to more effectively accomplish job duties translates into more effective job and training design. Taking into consideration the on-going workplace needs of aging workers in redesigning the physical workplace and/or reconceptualizing the nature of cognitive tasks (eg, self-paced training materials) will both better support the sustained workplace attendance of older adults and enhance overall organizational effectiveness for all employees (eg, "universal design" outcomes).

SUMMARY

It is projected that the aging population will grow in number through the 2050s, and many older women within this growing segment will both desire and need to maintain workforce participation. This aging population trend in many industrialized nations will necessitate a paradigm change among employers, policymakers, and even older adults in how workplaces must support qualified aging workers. Working is a major factor in maintaining quality-of-life standards in a society and, thus, should be the focus of public policies in the coming decades.

With an unprecedented number of mature women in the workforce issues of retirement and the transition to retirement (eg, flexible scheduling) need to be explored. Further, psychological factors, such as the centrality of one's work to a person's self-concept and how that affects retirement-related issues must be understood. Given that older women are productive and loyal workers, efforts must be made to recruit and retain older adults in the workplace. Other dimensions of aging adults workers in the field deal with issues of generativity and mentoring younger workers, and focusing on the unique characteristics that mature workers can bring to the workforce.

DISCUSSION QUESTIONS

1. In today's workplace, what might be two beneficial experiences for an aging woman working past traditional retirement age?
2. Conversely, what might be two challenges that an older woman will need to overcome when working past traditional retirement age?
3. Erikson proposed that middle-aged and older adults may be motivated to mentor others in the workplace. This notion is referred to as "generativity." Why is it important to understand this concept for older women as they continue to work or transition to the retirement phase of their lives?
4. Age discrimination is an unfortunate reality. What are some actions that a Human Resource Department can take to "protect" their qualified aging women workers?
5. Skill updating, or the avoidance of skill obsolescence, is key for women to remain in the workforce if they need or desire to do so. How can aging women workers be pro-active in their skill updating process?
6. Would it help for older women workers to establish an onsite social support group to share strategies for positive "aging in place" in their careers?
7. What are the physical aging benefits of working across the life span?
8. What are the cognitive aging benefits of working past traditional retirement age?
9. What are the psychosocial benefits of working for women as they age?
10. If you were hired to create a workplace program to help older women think about ways to remain in the workforce, what topics would you cover in your training program?

TEST YOUR KNOWLEDGE!

Take the following quiz about attitudes retirement:

http://www.yourlifechoices.com.au/news/are-you-ready-to-retire-quiz

---

SUPPLEMENTAL BOOK READINGS

Over the past decades, there have been many books written on the topics of women's involvement in later life and their retirement experiences. Here are some recommended *additional readings*:

Fideler, E. F. (2012). *Women still at work: Professionals over sixty and on the job*. Lanham, MD: Rowman & Littlefield Publishers.

Based on the results on both national survey data and interviews with older women workers, the book presents information regarding workforce participation trends, work-related behaviors across regions, and working women's motivational attitudes toward working past traditional retirement age. Older women workers share their employment experiences and the reasons why they continue to work, ranging from having a financial need in order to support others as a caregiver to wanting to work as a women's rights issue across their life spans. This book offers a supportive, positive picture of aging women workers as a national (and international) resource to be appreciated and valued by all.

Watson, E. A., & Mears, J. (1999). *Women, work and care of the elderly*. Farnham, UK: Ashgate Pub Ltd.

This book focuses on the very important issue of women attempting to balance full-time workforce participation and full-time caregiving. The authors recommend that workplace and governmental policies need to better support the needs of this growing segment of employed women for the coming decades through 2050. Organizational cultures need to also shift to legitimize the dual-role obligations faced by aging women workers in order to best support their workplace attendance and career trajectories.

Cappelli, P., & Novelli, B. (2010). *Managing the older worker: How to prepare for the new organizational order*. Boston, MA: Harvard Business Review Press.

Organizations must better prepare for the changing workplace with the impact of a continuing graying workforce. The authors suggest that there are many benefits to retaining older employees who are experienced, have higher organizational commitment, and other positive characteristics. Aging women would gain valuable information regarding the rights and responsibilities of older workers if working past traditional retirement age is a necessity or a desire.

Bal, P. M., Kooij, D., & Rousseau, D. M. (2014). *Aging workers and the employee-employer relationship*. New York, NY: Springer Publishing Co. The relationship of the aging employee with the organization (eg, human resource manager) is examined. The responsibility of maintaining sustained workforce participation is on both the employer and the older employee. The employer needs to offer supportive resources and training for qualified older employees while aging employees need to avoid skill obsolescence and adapt to the changing workplace demands in light of changing physical functioning.

Price, R. K. (2009). *The successful retirement guide: Hundreds of suggestions on how to stay intellectually, socially and physically engaged for the best years of your life*. Lake Zurich, IL: Rainbow Books, Inc. This is an interesting guide which compels older adults to remain active on a social, physical, and mental level. The "key" to success in retirement according to the author is to anticipate your needs (eg, financial planning) but avoid the stereotypes that the concept of "retirement" might suggest.

SUPPLEMENTAL AGING VIDEOS

For learning purposes, the use of videos can be very beneficial for both instructors and readers. Here are some recommended *supplemental videos*:

Human Tech website: http://www.humantech.com/blog/new-video-ergonomics-and-the-aging-workforce/ (Format: Website)
This is a great website that offers information and a video on designing the workplace to support an aging workforce.

Daily Motion website: http://www.dailymotion.com/video/xiz7a4_the-advantages-of-hiring-older-workers_shortfilms/ (Format: Website)
This is a great video about the advantages of hiring older workers.

CNN website: http://money.cnn.com/video/news/2012/02/21/n_no_desire_retire_harlow.cnnmoney/ (Format: Website)
This is a great video about the advantages of hiring and retaining older workers.

Open Road—America Looks at Aging (Format: DVD)
This documentary film examines the impact of approximately 77 million baby boomers retiring for both the retirees themselves and society on a social, economic, and cultural basis.

ADDITIONAL INFORMATION LINKS

The Internet can be a good source of supplemental information for both instructors and readers of this textbook. The following are some recommended *supplemental Internet links*:

AARP website: http://www.aarp.org/

Age Workforce News website: http://www.agingworkforcenews.com/

Bureau of Labor Statistics website: http://www.bls.gov/spotlight/2008/older_workers/

National Older Worker Career Center website: http://www.nowcc.org/

Senior Community Service Employment Program website: https://olderworkers.workforce3one.org/

United States Senate Special Committee on Aging website: http://www.aging.senate.gov/issues/olderworkers/index.cfm

References

AARP. (2008). Investing in training 50+ workers: A talent management strategy. Retrieved from <http://assets.aarp.org/rgcenter/econ/invest_training.pdf>.

Age Discrimination and Employment Act. (1967) (29 U.S. Code § 623).

Aldwin, C. M., Sutton, K. J., Chiara, G., & Siro, A., III (1996). Age differences in stress, coping, and appraisal: Findings from the normative aging study. *Journal of Gerontology: Psychological Sciences, 51B*(4), P179–P188.

Altschuler, J. (2004). Beyond money and survival: The meaning of paid work among older women. *International Journal of Aging & Human Development, 58*(3), 223–239.

American Psychological Association. (2012). Work-life fit and enjoying what they do top the reasons why employees stay on the job. Retrieved from: <http://www.apaexcellence.org/-resources/goodcompany/newsletter/article/391>.

Armstrong-Stassen, M. (2006). Encouraging retirees to return to the workforce. *Human Resource Planning, 29*(4), 38–44.

Armstrong-Stassen, M., & Schlosser, F. K. (2008). Benefits of a supportive development climate for older workers. *Journal of Managerial Psychology, 23*, 419–443.

Armstrong-Stassen, M., Schlosser, F. K., & Zinni, D. (2012). Seeking resources: Predicting retirees' return to their workplace. *Journal of Managerial Psychology, 27*(6), 615–635.

Arulampalam, W., Bryan, M. L., & Booth, A. L. (2004). Training in Europe. *Journal of the European Economic Association, 2*, 346–360.

Benz, J., Sedensky, M., Tompson, T., & Agiesta, J. (2013). *Working longer: Older Americans' attitudes on work and retirement*. The Associated Press and NORC. Retrieved from: <http://www.apnorc.org/projects/Pages/working-longer-older-americans-attitudes-on-work-and-retirement.aspx>.

Boehm, S., Kunze, F., & Bruch, H. (2014). Spotlight on age-diversity climate: The impact of age-inclusive practices on firm-level outcomes. *Personnel Psychology, 67*(3), 667–704.

Brownell, P. J., & Kelly, J. J. (2013). *Ageism and mistreatment of older workers: Current reality, future solutions*. Dordrecht, NY: Springer.

Cheung, F., & Wu, A. (2013). Older workers' successful aging and intention to stay. *Journal of Managerial Psychology, 28*, 645–660. http://dx.doi.org/10.1108/JPM-09-2011-0062.

Chui, W. C. K., Chan, A. W., Snape, E., & Redman, T. (2001). Age stereotypes and discriminatory attitudes towards older workers: An east-west comparison. *Human Relations, 54*, 629–661.

Clark, A., Oswald, A., & Warr, P. (1996). Is job satisfaction U shaped in age? *Journal of Occupation and Organizational Psychology, 69*(1), 57–81.

Coile, C., & Levine, P. B. (2010). *Reconsidering retirement: How losses and layoffs affect older workers*. Washington, DC: Brookings Institution Press.

Davies, E., & Cartwright, S. (2011). Psychological and psychosocial predictors of attitudes to working past normal retirement age. *Employee Relations, 33*, 249–268. http://dx.doi.org/10.1108/01425451111121768.

Dendinger, V. M., Adams, G. A., & Jacobson, J. D. (2005). Reasons for working and their relationship to retirement attitudes, job satisfaction and occupational self-efficiency of bridge employees. *International Journal of Aging and Human Development, 61*, 21–35.

Disney, R. (1996). *Can we afford to grow older? A perspective on the economics of aging*. Cambridge, MA: MIT Press.

Erikson, E. (1959). *Identity and the life cycle*. New York, NY: International Universities Press.

Eyster, L., Johnson, R., & Toder, E. (2008). *Current strategies to employ and retain older workers*. Washington D.C.: The Urban Institute. Retrieved from: <http://www.urba.org/publications/411626.html>.

Finch, J., & Robinson, M. (2003). Aging and late onset disability: Addressing workplace accommodation. *Journal of Rehabilitation, 69*(2), 38–42.

Fleischmann, M., Koster, F., & Schippers, J. (2013). Nothing ventured, nothing gained! How and under which conditions employers provide employability-enhancing practices to their older workers. *The International Journal of Human Resource Management* on line: http://dx.doi.org/10.1080/09585192.2015.1004100.

Frieze, I. H., Olson, J. E., & Murrell, A. J. (2011). Working beyond 65: Predictors of late retirement for women and men MBAs. *Journal of Women & Aging, 23*(1), 40–57.

Galinsky, E. (2007). The changing landscape of work. *Generations, 31*(1), 16–22.

Green, A. (2009). Older people and transitions from employment to non-employment: International perspectives and policy issues. *The Professional Geographer, 61*(1), 46–58.

Havighurst, R. J. (1961). Successful aging. *The Gerontologist, 1*, 8–13. http://dx.doi.org/10.1093/-geront/1.1.8.

Henkens, C. J. I. M. (2005). Stereotyping older workers and retirement: The managers' point of view. *Canadian Journal of Aging, 24*, 353–366.

Hirschfeld, R. R., & Feild, H. S. (2000). Work centrality and work alienation: Distinct aspects of a general commitment to work. *Journal of Organizational Behavior, 21*, 789–800.

Hursh, N., Lui, J., & Pransky, G. (2006). Maintaining and enhancing older worker productivity. *Journal of Vocational Rehabilitation, 25*, 45–55.

Ilmarinen, J. (2009). Aging and work: An international perspective. In S. J. Czaja & J. Sharit (Eds.), *Aging and work: Issues and implications in a changing landscape* (pp. 51–73). Baltimore, MD: Johns Hopkins University Press.

Innocenti, L., Profili, S., & Sammarra, A. (2013). Age as moderator in the relationship between HR development practices and employees' positive attitudes. *Personnel Review, 42*, 724–744.

Janson, P., & Martin, J. (1982). Job satisfaction and age: A test of two views. *Social Forces, 60*(4), 1089–1102.

Kampfe, C., Wadsworth, J., Mamboleo, G., & Schonbrun, S. (2008). Aging, disability, and employment. *Work, 31*, 337–344.

Kanfer, R., & Ackerman, P. L. (2004). Aging, adult development, and work motivation. *Academy of Management Review, 29*, 440–458.

Kenny, G., Yardley, J., Martineau, L., & Jay, O. (2008). Physical work capacity in older adults: Implications for the aging worker. *American Journal of Industrial Medicine, 51*(8), 610–625.

Kirchner, C., Volker, I., & Otmar, O. L. (2015). Priming with age stereotypes influences the performance of elderly workers. *Psychology, 6*, 133–137.

Kite, M. E., Stockdale, G. D., Whitley, B. E., & Johnson, B. T. (2005). Attitudes toward younger and older adults: An updated meta-analytic review. *Journal of Social Issues, 61*(2), 241–266.

Koc-Menard, S. (2009). Flexible work options for older workers. *Strategic Human Resource Review, 8*(2), 31–36.

Kooij, D. T. A. M., Guest, D. E., Clinton, M., Knight, T., Jansen, P. G., & Dikkers, J. S. (2013). How the impact of HR practices on employee well-being and performance changes with age. *Human Resource Management Journal, 23*, 18–35.

Kooij, D. T. A. M., Jansen, P. G., Dikkers, J. S., & DeLange, A. (2010). The influence of age on the association between HR practices and both affective commitment and job satisfaction: A meta-analysis. *Journal of Organizational Behavior, 31*(8), 1111–1136.

Lain, D. (2012). Working past 65 in the UK and the USA: Segregation into 'Lopaq' occupations? *Work, Employment and Society, 26*, 78–94. http://dx.doi.org/10.1177/0950017011426312.

Liden, R. C., Stilwell, D., & Ferris, G. (1996). The effects of supervisor and subordinate age on objective performance and subjective performance ratings. *Human Relations, 49*(3), 327–347.

Magee, W. (2014). Effects of gender and age on pride in work, and job satisfaction. *Journal of Happiness Studies* Online publication. http://dx.doi.org/10.1007/s10902-014-9548-x.

Malinen, S., & Johnston, L. (2013). Workplace ageism: Discovering hidden bias. *Experimental Aging Research: An International Journal, 39*(4), 445–465.

Mandal, B., & Roe, B. (2008). Job loss, retirement and the mental health of older Americans. *The Journal of Mental Health Policy and Economics, 11*(4), 167–176.

Martin, G., Dymock, D., Billett, S., & Johnson, G. (2014). In the name of meritocracy: Managers' perceptions of policies and practices for training older workers. *Ageing & Society, 34*, 992–1018. http://dx.doi.org/10.1017/S0144686X12001432.

McEvoy, G. M., & Cascio, W. F. (1989). Cumulative evidence of the relationship between employee age and job performance. *Journal of Applied Psychology, 74*, 11–17.

Moen, P., Robison, J., & Fields, V. (1994). Women's work and caregiving roles: A life course approach. *Journal of Gerontology: Social Sciences, 49*(4), S176–S186.

Mor-Barak, M. (1995). The meaning of work for older adults seeking employment: The generativity factor. *The International Journal of Aging & Human Development, 41*(4), 325–344.

Mutran, E. J., Reitzes, D. J., Bratton, K. A., & Fernandez, M. E. (1997). Self-esteem and subjective responses to work among mature workers: Similarities and differences by gender. *Journal of Gerontology, 52*(2), 89–96.

Ng, T. W. H., & Feldman, D. C. (2008). The relationship of age to ten dimensions of job performance. *Journal of Applied Psychology, 93*, 393–423.

Ng, T. W. H., & Feldman, D. C. (2010). The relationships of age with job attitudes: A meta-analysis. *Personnel Psychology, 63*(3), 677–718.

Nuyts, G. D., Elseviers, M. M., & DeBroe, M. E. (1993). Healthy worker effect in a cross-sectional study of lead workers. *Journal of Occupational Medicine, 35*(4), 387–391.

Paullay, I., Alliger, G., & Stone-Romero, E. (1994). Construct validation of two instruments designed to measure job involvement and work centrality. *Journal of Applied Psychology, 79*(2), 224–228.

Pitt-Catsouphes, M., & Matz-Costa, C. (2009). *Engaging the 21st century multi-generational workforce: Findings from the Age and Generations Study*. Boston: Sloan Center on Aging and Work, Boston College. Retrieved from: <http://www.bc.edu/content/dam/files/research_sites/agingandwork/pdf/publications/IB20_Engagement.pdf>.

Porter, N. B. (2003). Sex plus age discrimination: Protecting older women workers. *Denver University Law Review, 81*, 79–111.

Price, C. A. (2002). Retirement for women: The impact of employment. *Journal of Women & Aging, 14*(3–4), 41–57.

Price, C. A. (2003). Professional women's retirement adjustment: The experience of re-establishing order. *Journal of Aging Studies, 17*(3), 341–355.

Quinn, J. F., & Kozy, M. (1996). The role of bridge jobs in the retirement transition: Gender, race, and ethnicity. *Gerontologist, 36*(3), 363–372.

Robson, S., Hansson, R., Abalos, A., & Booth, M. (2006). Successful aging: Criteria for aging well in the workplace. *Journal for Career Development, 33*(2), 156–177.

Schlosser, F., Zinni, D., & Armstrong, M. (2012). Intention to unretire: HR and the boomerang effect. *Career Development International, 17*(2), 149–167.

Schooler, C., Mulatu, M. S., & Oates, G. (1999). The continuing effects of substantively complex work on the intellectual functioning of older workers. *Psychology and Aging, 14*(3), 483–506.

Shiu, E., Hassan, L., & Parry, S. (2015). The moderating effects of national age stereotyping on the relationships between job satisfaction and its determinants: A study of older workers across 26 countries. *British Journal of Management, 26*(2), 255–272.

Shultz, K. S., & Adams, G. A. (2007). *Aging and work in the 21st century.* Mahwah, NJ: Lawrence Erlbaum.

Smith, D. B. D. (1990). Human factors and aging: An overview of research needs and application opportunities. *Human Factors, 32*, 509–526.

Society for Human Resource Management. (2015). The aging workforce basic and applied skills. Washington DC. Retrieved from: <http://www.shrm.org/research/surveyfind-ings/articles/pages/shrm-older-workers-basic-and-applied-skills.aspx>.

Sok, E. (2010). Record unemployment of older workers does not keep them out of the job market. Retrieved from: <http://www.bls.gov/opub/ils/summary_10_04/older_workers.htm>.

Strebler, M. R. (2006). Why motivation holds the key to an age-diverse workforce. *People Management, 12*(23), 48–49.

Taylor, P., & Walker, A. (1997). Age discrimination and public policy. *Personnel Review, 26*(4), 307–318.

United Nations, Women Coordination Division. (2012). Between gender and ageing: The status of the world's older women and progress since the Madrid International Plan of Action on Ageing. Retrieved from: <http://www.un.org/womenwatch/osagi/ian-wge2012/Between-Gender-Ageing-Report-Executive-Summary-2012.pdf>.

Veth, K., Emans, B., Van der Heijden, B., Korzilius, H., & DeLange, A. H. (2015). Development (f)or maintenance? An empirical study on the use and need for HR practices to retain older workers in health care organizations. *Human Resource Development Quarterly, 26*(1), 53–80.

Wright, J., & Hamilton, R. (1978). Work satisfaction and age: Some evidence for the 'job change' hypothesis. *Social Forces, 56*(4), 1140–1158.

Wrzesniewski, A., McCauley, C., Rozin, P., & Schwartz, B. (1997). Jobs, careers, and callings: People's relations to their work. *Journal of Research in Personality, 31*, 21–33.

Zacher, H., & Frese, M. (2009). Remaining time and opportunities at work: The interplay between age, job complexity, work characteristics and occupational future time perspectives. *Psychology and Aging, 24*, 487–493.

Breaking Stereotypes of Aging Women

Global Fact: *Women face age discrimination earlier in life than men do, and the combination of age and gender is particularly difficult for women to overcome.*

— *Older Women's League (OWL) (2012)*

To optimize their aging experiences and opportunities, older women need to break the stereotypes that might exist in today's society. Test yourself with the *Aging Perceptions Questionnaire* in Appendix A to better understand. Current research regarding pervasive misconceptions about aging women and how they can be eradicated in society will be discussed.

STEREOTYPES IMPACTING POSITIVE AGING

Research has shown that pervasive misconceptions about older adults exist and that these misconceptions have a harmful effect on the self-perceptions of the older adults. This chapter will explore some of the more common stereotypes associated with the older adults, why such stereotypes are harmful, and finally strategies to combat the effects of these stereotypes. This chapter will investigate the role of stereotypes and aging women largely through the lens of social psychological concepts. Zebrowitz and Montepare (2000) argued that aging research can benefit from the application of social psychological principles.

A stereotype is a socially shared belief about a particular group of people (eg, Cardwell, 1996). Stereotypes abound regarding different races (racism), gender (sexism), and older adults (ageism; Butler, 1969). Ageism was denounced by the American Psychological Association (American Psychological Association, 2002) in a resolution encouraging people to recognize age as an important element of diversity. Although positive stereotypes do exist regarding the older adults, in Western cultures negative

Women and Positive Aging.
DOI: http://dx.doi.org/10.1016/B978-0-12-420136-1.00013-X

stereotypes tend to be much more widespread (eg, Levy, Kasl, & Gill, 2004). Interestingly, of the many stigmatized groups (eg, racial minorities, women), age is the only group designation with very few exceptions where the "out-group" member will eventually become a member of the "in-group."

Palmore (2001) conducted a survey to further explore the issue of ageism and found that more than half of his respondents (ie, 84 adults aged 60 or older) indicated that they had experienced ageism "more than once." In Palmore's survey, ageism might include telling a joke that made fun of older people; being ignored by a restaurant's wait staff because of age; being treated with less dignity/respect because of age; and being talked down to because of age. Interestingly, research has shown that individuals believe that their group (eg, older adults) is more likely to be discriminated against than they personally are (as individuals). This is known as "the personal-group discrimination discrepancy" (Taylor, Wright, Moghaddam, & Lalonde, 1990). Therefore, it is possible that older adults recognize that ageism and discrimination are a problem, but they may fail to recognize the level to which they are experiencing it.

Negative stereotypes and corresponding behaviors toward older adults start early in life and largely persist unchanged throughout the life span. Isaacs and Bearison (1986) have shown that children as young as six years of age can accurately report stereotypes of older adults associated with their culture.

WORDS OF WISDOM

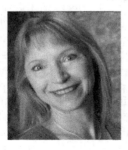

Toni is a 65-year-old Yoga Instructor who has broken the stereotype of an aging woman. As a healthy, physically active 65-year-old, Toni spends a lot of time helping others in addition to exercising daily. Toni volunteers at nursing homes teaching line dancing. She tutors children, utilizing her junior high school English Teacher skills, and she is a church volunteer helping older women tend their gardens.

Although Toni is aware that stereotypes do exist, she believes that instead of falling into those stereotypes, one has to break the stereotype.

continued

"You cannot let life happen to you, you have to happen to life," Toni states.

Toni believes there is no expiration date to feeling good at any age. In Toni's opinion, one of the leading misconceptions and stereotypes of an aging woman is that they suddenly fall apart physically. Toni oftentimes hears the middle-aged students in her yoga class say they are getting too old to be "fit." In Toni's opinion there is no magical age that says you cannot be healthy or fit. You can always grow to be better at any age.

The secrets to Toni's healthy attitude toward aging come from habits that Toni engages in daily and advises others to do. Eat healthy, drink a lot of water, pay attention to your body, and exercise daily. Always look at the positive side rather than the negative—do not center on your deficiencies, focus on your abilities and how they can be used. Volunteer—it is not all about you. Use your abilities to help others and you will feel fulfilled. Stay mentally active and utilize technology. In addition to this advice, Toni believes that one should always have confidence in one's self, because all women can be their best self at any age!

TIPS FOR WOMEN TO PROMOTE POSITIVE AGING ATTITUDES

1. Be a positive role model to other women.
2. Learn a new skill.
3. Be active in mind and body on a daily basis.
4. Choose a leadership role in an organization.
5. Volunteer and contribute to the community.

Many attitudes toward the older adults are the same for both young and older adults, that is "interage consensus" about the attributes associated with the older adults exists (Heckhausen, Dixon, & Baltes, 1989). For example, memory decline is associated with the older adults and is endorsed by both young and old adults (eg, Parr & Siegert, 1993; Ryan & See, 1992). Likewise, negative views of the older adults (eg, psychologically and physically impaired) do not differ substantially among young, middle-aged, and older adults (Hummert, Garstka, Shaner, & Strahm, 1994). What this means is that many aging adults hold negative views about aging and the older adults (Luszcz, 1983). Various studies have converged on the finding that older and younger adults have similar conceptions/ stereotypes of the older adults although the complexities of these stereotypes may differ as a function of age (eg, Hummert, 1990). Specifically, younger adults are more likely to associate negative stereotypes with the older adults and older adults are more likely to believe that positive and negative stereotypes are true of older adults (Hummert, Garstka, Shaner, & Strahm, 1995).

According to the stereotype content model, beliefs about individuals can be categorized along two dimensions: warmth and competency (Cuddy, Fiske, & Glick, 2008). When evaluating the older adults, the bag tends to be mixed in that the older adults may be perceived as "warm" (ie, grandmotherly) but also as "incompetent" (eg, Cuddy, Norton, & Fiske, 2005). For example, Nelson (2004) discussed how older adults are stereotyped as forgetful, slow, and weak (ie, negative and incompetent). When individuals are judged as being high in warmth but low in competence, the result is a "pitying stereotype" (Fiske, Cuddy, Glick, & Xu, 2002).

The older adults, along with the mentally challenged and disabled, are often grouped into this category and the result may be paternalistic attitudes toward the group. This is especially likely to be the case because old age is considered to be outside of one's control. Pity may result in "active facilitation" (ie, helping behavior) but it may also lead to "passive harm" whereas an individual avoids or is otherwise dismissive of the older adults (Cuddy et al., 2008). Most people will not explicitly recognize that they hold ageist beliefs. However, Levy and Banaji (2002) argue that people hold "implicit age stereotypes" and that these stereotypes operate automatically and outside of one's control.

Although Kite, Deaux, and Miele (1991) found that aging stereotypes "trumped" gender stereotypes, some stereotypes associated with the older adults are specific to women. For example, older woman are often categorized as "sexless" (Palmore, 1971). Although this notion of the sexless older woman was first described in 1971, 40 years later, the stereotype remains largely unchanged (see Chapter 11 for a more in-depth discussion of women's sexuality in later life). Depiction of older adult women in cartoons often depict women in a more negative light than older adult men (Palmore, 1971) with the "Maxine" comic strip illustrating this notion. Vernon, Williams, Phillips, and Wilson (1990) conducted a content analysis in an effort to determine how the older adults, and specifically older women, were portrayed on television.

QUOTES FROM FAMOUS, POSITIVELY AGING WOMEN

I didn't want to let women down.
One of the stereotypes I see breaking is
the idea of aging and older women not being beautiful.
                    —*Annie Lebowitz, Portrait Photographer*

Why do people talk of the horrors of old age? It's great.
I feel like a fine old car with the parts gradually wearing out,
but I'm not complaining, ...
Those who find growing old terrible are people
who haven't done what they wanted with their lives.
                    —*Martha Gelhorn, Journalist*

People who refuse to rest honorably on their laurels
when they reach retirement age seem very admirable to me.
                    —*Helen Hayes, Actress*

Both older adult men and women were stereotypically portrayed; however, their research suggested that television portrayal of men is more liberal than their portrayal of aging women.

Many researchers (eg, Wilcox, 1997) argue that women are subjected to a "double standard of aging" such that aging women are evaluated more negatively than aging men. Deutch, Zalenski, and Clarke (1986) found evidence for the double standard when participants evaluated photographs of males and females at three different ages. Participants rated both males and females more harshly as they aged; however, the decrease ratings were worse for aging women.

WHY ARE STEREOTYPES HARMFUL?

Steele and Aronson (1995) were the first researchers to describe and empirically investigate the notion of stereotype threat, and concluded that a person's behavior is influenced when she/he believes that her/his behavior might confirm a negative stereotype about the group to which she/he belongs. Stereotype threat has been shown to cause differences in test scores between African Americans and Caucasians (Steele & Aronson, 1995) and between males and females (Inzlicht & Ben-Zeev, 2000). Stereotype threat affects groups who are negatively stereotyped and can lead to decreased performance on task, especially if the stereotype is activated frequently and/or if the individual has a strong sense of identification with the stereotyped group.

Past research (eg, Inzlicht, McKay, & Aronson, 2006; Inzlicht & Schmader, 2012) has shown that after a threat, subsequent performance on tasks (even unrelated) is hindered and that self-control is also adversely affected. More specifically, Hess, Aumna, Colcombe, and Rahhal (2003) demonstrated differences in performance on a memory task when older adult participants were placed in a "threat" condition in which memory decline with aging is suggested. Meisner (2012) conducted a meta-analytic review and showed that negative views about older adults impaired behavioral outcomes (ie, memory, psychomotor, physiological, and social functioning) while positive views of old age encouraged those same behaviors.

Related to stereotype threat is the notion of stereotype embodiment: the idea that exposure, throughout the life span, to a culture's view of age, causes a person to internalize the constructs that are associated with ageist beliefs. A person begins to behave in a manner consistent to society's view of the "older adults" in a way that is similar to a self-fulfilling prophecy (Levy, 2009; Levy et al., 1999–2000; Levy, Slade, Kunkel, & Kasl, 2002; Nemmers, 2005). Media is thought to be a powerful influence in shaping a culture's beliefs and attitudes toward individuals (in terms of gender, age, and race), therefore, it is not particularly surprisingly to learn that older participants (60–92 years old) who watched the most television also held the most negative views of aging (Donlon, Ashman, & Levy, 2005). Internalizing ageist stereotypes has been associated with poor health outcomes. For example, individuals who held negative stereotypes about older age were more likely to experience a cardiovascular event earlier (in some case, decades earlier) than individuals who held more positive age stereotypes (Levy, Zonderman, Slade, & Ferrucci, 2009).

In Barg, Chen, and Burrow's (1996) seminal study, participants who were primed (ie, activating a link in memory prior to carrying out some type of task) with "older adults" words exhibited different behaviors than participants who were primed with neutral words. Half of the participants received words, in the form of scrambled sentences that were associated with the older adults (eg, "Florida," "rigid," "Bingo," "lonely") and half received neutral words (eg, "clean," "private," "thirsty"). After the participants viewed the words, their walking speed was measured. Participants who were exposed to the older adults' words walked the length of a corridor at a significantly slower speed than participants who were exposed to the neutral prime.

Giles and colleagues (eg, Giles, Fox, & Smith, 1993; Giles, Fox, Harwood, & Williams, 1994) found that older adults who have been spoken to in an "over accommodating manner" (ie, overly polite, slowly, and loudly) appeared to independent raters to "instantly age" in that the group began to act older than a control group of older adults who were not spoken to in an accommodating manner. Levy, Slade, and Kasl (2002) established that older adults who had a positive self-perception reported better health over the course of 18 years than did participants who held a more negative self-perception. Similarly, individuals with a positive self-perception were far more likely than those with negative self-perception to practice preventive health behaviors (Levy & Myers, 2004). Levy and colleague (2001B) found that participants (660, aged 50 and older) who had a negative self-perception lived, on average, almost eight years fewer than their positive self-perception counterparts. In an interesting experiment, Levy (2001) presented both younger and older participants with positive or negative stereotypes about old age and presented the groups with a vignette that required them to make a decision about a life-prolonging medical intervention. Older participants in the negative stereotype condition were more likely to refuse the intervention compared to those older adults in the positive stereotype condition prompting Levy to argue that stereotypes can influence an older adult's will to live.

WHAT CAN WE DO TO COMBAT THESE STEREOTYPES?

Dasgupta and Greenwald (2001) showed that "interventions" can be conducted that lead to more positive beliefs about age, in which students are shown pictures of admired older adults (eg, Mother Theresa) in contrast to pictures of controversial young adults (eg, Tona Harding). This was called the "pro-older adults" condition versus the "pro-young" condition. When students were presented with pictures of disliked older adults and admired younger ones, the students showed a decrease in their automatic age bias, as demonstrated by scores on the Implicit Association

CHECK IT OUT!

Search the Internet to find information that relates to attitudes toward older women. As you collect information, please analyze whether there are differences in attitudes by region of the world. As you examine these factors, think about the following questions:

1. What are some common stereotypes about aging women?
2. What role does culture have in the nature of these attitudes?
3. What are the cultural "messages" about aging and women?
4. If you found stereotypes about older women, are these erroneous beliefs similar to possible stereotypes about aging and men? Why or why not?
5. Are there motivational factors to consider when understanding why people may develop stereotypes about older women?

Test (Greenwald, McGhee, & Schwartz, 1998), although this change was only temporary. Snyder and Miene (1994) developed an intervention to help alleviate stereotyping of the older adults and concluded that women were less likely to engage in stereotypes related to ego protection. Cohen, Garcia, Apfel, and Master (2006) found that a self-affirmation exercise made their participants less susceptible to stereotype threat.

The contact hypothesis (Allport, 1954) has received empirical support for decreasing intergroup conflict and increasing positive attitudes toward out-group members (Pettigrew & Tropp, 2006). Several researchers have demonstrated success when implementing programs that focused on intergenerational contact (Aday, Aday, Arnold, & Bendix, 1996). Aday and colleagues found improved attitudes toward the older adults before and after "age-integrated friendships." Aday, Rice, and Evans (1991) found fourth graders who were paired with older adult participants had fewer misconceptions about aging. Additional research (Bales, Eklund, & Siffin, 2000) established that children used more positive words to describe older adults after intergenerational contact and Caspi (1984) showed that children who had daily contact with older adults held more positive attitudes toward that group. Hale (1998) conducted a study and found that both younger and older participants scored lower on a stereotype measure of the older adults when they had frequent contact with older adults.

According to Allport's original conceptualization of the "contact hypothesis," the quality of the interaction and not the frequency of the interaction is a better predictor of positive out-group attitudes. Schwartz and Simmons (2001) found support for the quality of intergenerational contact when they asked college-aged participants to self-report on both the quality and the frequency of their interaction with older adults. The quality of the interaction (but not frequency) was associated with positive attitudes toward older adults. Work by Tam, Hewstone, Harwood, Voci, and Kenworthy (2006) showed that both implicit and explicit attitudes toward the older adults may be predicted by quality and quantity of inter-generational contact. Specifically, the frequency of interaction was associated with more positive implicit attitudes, whereas, quality of interaction was associated with more positive explicit attitudes.

SUMMARY

Stereotypes about the older adults and older women, specifically, are pervasive and even if a person does not endorse a particular stereotype he/she is still aware of them. Not surprisingly, stereotypes are perpetuated through the depiction of the older adults in movies, television shows, and other forms of media. Furthermore, older women may be at risk for "double jeopardy" as they may be subject to sexist and ageist beliefs. Negative stereotypes have serious implications including poorer health outcomes, reduced memory performance, worse preventive health behaviors, and even a shorter life span.

Encouragingly, there is research suggesting suitable "interventions" for both the aging adult (eg, self-affirmations) and mechanisms for improving the attitudes of younger people toward older people (eg, intergenerational contact). In a broader sense, this is truly a quality-of-life concern for all women as they age across a life span. In many societies across the world, it is vital for young women as they mature to embrace the process of aging and understand that their beliefs about personal aging and others' aging can have a dramatic impact upon positive aging outcomes for all generations of women. For women to more realistically understand their own aging will potentially produce a more healthy future cohort of aging women, from both a mental and physical perspective. For all people in any culture, aging must not be feared or misunderstood, but rather fully integrated into a positive self-perspective.

DISCUSSION QUESTIONS

1. What are some common stereotypes about older women?
2. Do different cultures have different stereotypes about women or are there "universal" stereotypes? Give examples to support your answer.
3. Are stereotypes about older women predominantly negative or positive in nature? Give examples.
4. Negative aging stereotypes can create social barriers and restrictive biases for women across their life span. Give an example of a possible ageist barrier for women.
5. Is a positive stereotype about older women as concerning as a negative stereotype? Why or why not?
6. What is the best ways to eradicate stereotypes and improve understanding of realistic issues in getting older within a community? What would you suggest?
7. How early should societies educate people about realistic aging? What should be the content of this education and how could it possibly impact positive aging outcomes for women?
8. What role does culture play in creating negative, positive, or more desirably realistic attitudes toward aging women?
9. Have you ever encountered aging stereotypes? What happened and how did you feel about the social situation?
10. If you were to develop an educational program for schools and community centers regarding avoiding aging-related stereotypes about women, what topics would you incorporate into the program?

TEST YOUR KNOWLEDGE!

Take the following quiz about your attitudes about aging:
http://www.oregon.gov/.../Myths%20and%20Stereotypes%20 of%20Aging.pdf

---

SUPPLEMENTAL BOOK READINGS

Over the past decades, there have been many books written on the topic of how to eradicate negative stereotypes about women's aging and, instead, promote positive beliefs about the aging process for them. Here are some recommended *additional readings*:

Cole, E., Rothblum, E. D., & Thone, R. R. (1992). *Women and aging: Celebrating ourselves.* New York, NY: Routledge.
This book is an empowering text for all aging women, and those who care for them, who wish to challenge negative perceptions of older women and their value to society. The authors do a wonderful job of presenting the multiple roles, contributions, and achievements which are possible within a growing female segment of the national and international population. The book celebrates the multifaceted capabilities of aging women in many different contexts and social situations.

Cole, E., Rothblum, E. D., & Davis, N. C. (1993). *Faces of women and aging.* New York, NY: Routledge.
The authors wrote the book to address the many different myths about aging. Older women are typically regarded as being destitute, weak, and asexual in society but the reality is that aging women are quite successful in later life and have a great life expectancy than their male counterparts. The book is empowering to older women because it suggests that getting older is simply a new stage of opportunity that can be optimized through a positive self-concept and an effort to succeed.

Furman, F. K. (1997). *Facing the mirror: Older women and beauty shop culture.* New York, NY: Routledge.
The author investigates issues of ageism and sexism toward older women which need to be confronted and eradicated. How society regards and treats older women impacts many different aspects of their social power and personal efficacy in making important life choices.

Erber, J. T., & Szuchman, L. T. (2014). *Great myths of aging*. Hoboken, NJ: Wiley-Blackwell.

The authors examine the roots of many different misconceptions and outright stereotypes about older adults. Both negative stereotypes (eg, older people are frail) and positive stereotypes (eg, getting older means getting wiser) are suggested as being equally harmful for older adults because it distracts from better understanding the true nature of the aging process.

SUPPLEMENTAL AGING VIDEOS

For learning purposes, the use of videos can be very beneficial for both instructors and readers. Here are some recommended *supplemental videos*:

Shattering the Myth of Aging: Senior Games Celebrate Healthy Lifestyles, Competition and Community (Format: DVD)

The DVD presents active adults in their 70s 80s, and 90s who are fully engaged in life and sports activities. The Senior Games is a great highlight of older adults who show both physical and psychological strength as they test the "boundaries" of their capabilities and shatter the myths of aging.

Age Is Nothing but a Number (Format: Instant Video)

This is a great video showcasing seven "shorts" across five continents (ie, United States, Japan, Denmark, England, and Burundi) detailing cases of older adults who resist cultural stereotypes and, instead, live life to the fullest.

ADDITIONAL INFORMATION LINKS

The following are some recommended *supplemental Internet links*:

Administration on Aging website: http://www.aoa.gov/AoARoot/Aging_Statistics/index.aspx

American Federation for Aging Research website: http://www.afar.org/infoaging/

NIA Demography Center website: http://agingcenters.org/

United Nations website: http://www.un.org/esa/population/publications/Worldageing19502050/

World Health Organization website: http://www.who.int/ageing/about/facts/en/index.html

References

Aday, R. H., Aday, K. L., Arnold, J. L., & Bendix, S. L. (1996). Changing children's perceptions of the elderly: The effects of intergenerational contact. *Gerontology & Geriatrics Education, 16*, 37–51.

Aday, R. H., Rice, C., & Evans, E. (1991). Intergenerational partners project: A model linking elementary students with senior center volunteers. *The Gerontologist, 31*, 263–266.

Allport, G. W. (1954). *The nature of prejudice.* Cambridge, MA: Perseus Books.

American Psychological Association. (2002). Resolution on ageism. Retrieved from <http://www.apa.org/about/policy/ageism.aspx>.

Bales, S. S., Eklund, S. J., & Siffin, C. F. (2000). Children's perceptions of elders before and after a school-based intergenerational program. *Educational Gerontology, 26*, 677–689.

Bargh, J., Chen, M., & Burrows, L. (1996). Automaticity of social behavior: Direct effects of trait construct and stereotype activation on action. *Journal of Personality and Social Psychology, 71*, 230–241.

Butler, R. N. (1969). Age-ism: Another form of bigotry. *The Gerontologist, 9*, 243–246.

Cardwell, M. (1996). *The complete A-Z psychology handbook.* London, UK: Hodder and Stoughton.

Caspi, A. (1984). Contact hypothesis and inter-age attitudes: A field study of cross-age contact. *Social Psychology Quarterly, 47*(1), 74–80.

Cohen, G. L., Garcia, J., Apfel, N., & Master, A. (2006). Reducing the racial achievement gap: A social psychological intervention. *Science, 313*, 1307–1310.

Cuddy, A. J. C., Fiske, S. T., & Glick, P. (2008). Warmth and competence as universal dimensions of social perception: The stereotype content model and the BIAS map. *Advances in Experimental Social Psychology, 40*, 61–149.

Cuddy, A. J. C., Norton, M. I., & Fiske, S. T. (2005). This old stereotype: The pervasiveness and persistence of the older adult's stereotype. *Journal of Social Issues, 61*, 267–285.

Dasgupta, N., & Greenwald, A. (2001). On the malleability of automatic attitudes: Combating automatic prejudice with images of admired and disliked individuals. *Journal of Personality and Social Psychology, 81*, 800–814.

Deutch, F., Zalenski, C. M., & Clarke, M. E. (1986). Is there a double standard of aging? *Journal of Applied Social Psychology, 16*, 771–785.

Donlon, M., Ashman, O., & Levy, B. R. (2005). Re-vision of older television characters: A stereotype-awareness intervention. *Journal of Social Issues, 61*, 307–319.

Fiske, S. T., Cuddy, A. J. C., Glick, P., & Xu, J. (2002). A model of (often mixed) stereotype content: Competence and warmth respectively follow from perceived status and competition. *Journal of Personality and Social Psychology, 82*, 878–902.

Giles, H., Fox, S., Harwood, J., & Williams, A. (1994). Talking age and aging talk: Communicating through the life span. In M. Hummert, J. Wiemann, & J. Nussbaum (Eds.), *Interpersonal communication in older adulthood: Interdisciplinary theory and research* (pp. 130–161). New York, NY: Sage.

Giles, H., Fox, S., & Smith, E. (1993). Patronizing the elderly: Intergenerational evaluations. *Research on Language and Social Interaction, 26*, 129–149.

Greenwald, A., McGhee, D., & Schwartz, J. (1998). Measuring individual differences in implicit cognition: The implicit association test. *Journal of Personality and Social Psychology, 74*(6), 1464–1480.

Hale, N. (1998). Effects of age and interpersonal contact on stereotyping of the elderly. *Current Psychology, 17*, 28–38.

Heckhausen, J., Dixon, R., & Baltes, P. (1989). Gains and losses in development throughout adulthood as perceived by different adult age groups. *Developmental Psychology, 25*, 109–121.

Hess, T. M., Aumna, C., Colcombe, S. J., & Rahhal, T. A. (2003). The impact of stereotype threat on age difference in memory performance. *The Journals of Gerontology: Series B: Psychological Sciences and Social Sciences, 58*, 3–11.

Hummert, M. L. (1990). Multiple stereotypes of older adults and young adults: A comparison of structure and evaluations. *Psychology and Aging, 5,* 182–193.

Hummert, M. L., Garstka, T. A., Shaner, J. L., & Strahm, S. (1994). Stereotypes of the elderly held by young, middle-aged and elderly adults. *Journals of Gerontology: Psychological Sciences, 49,* 240–249.

Hummert, M. L., Garstka, T. A., Shaner, J. L., & Strahm, S. (1995). Judgments about stereotypes of the elderly: Attitudes, age associations, and typicality ratings of young, middle-aged, and older adults. *Research on Aging, 17,* 168–189.

Inzlicht, M., & Ben-Zeev, T. (2000). A threatening intellectual environment: Why females are susceptible to experiencing problem solving deficits in the presence of males. *Psychological Science, 11*(5), 365–371.

Inzlicht, M., McKay, L., & Aronson, J. (2006). Stigma as ego depletion: How being the target of prejudice affects self-control. *Psychological Science, 17,* 262–269.

Inzlicht, M., & Schmader, T. (2012). *Stereotype threat: Theory, process, and application.* New York, NY: Oxford University Press.

Isaacs, L. W., & Bearison, D. J. (1986). Development of children's prejudice against the aged. *International Journal of Aging and Human Development, 23,* 175–194.

Kite, M. E., Deaux, K., & Miele, M. (1991). Stereotypes of young and old: Does age outweigh gender? *Psychology and Aging, 6,* 19–27.

Levy, B. R. (2001). Eradication of ageism requires addressing the enemy within. *The Gerontologist, 41,* 578–579.

Levy, B. R. (2009). Stereotype embodiment: A psychosocial approach to aging. *Current Directions in Psychological Science, 18,* 332–336.

Levy, B. R., Ashman, O., & Dror, I. (1999–2000). *To be or not to be: The effects of aging stereotypes on the will to live* (40). Omega: *Journal of Death and Dying.*409420

Levy, B. R., & Banaji, M. R. (2002). Implicit ageism. In T. D. Nelson (Ed.), *Ageism: Stereotypes and prejudice against older persons* (pp. 49–75). Cambridge, MA: MIT Press.

Levy, B. R., Kasl, S. V., & Gill, T. M. (2004). Image of aging scale. *Perceptual and Motor Skills, 99,* 208–210.

Levy, B. R., & Myers, L. M. (2004). Preventive health behaviors influenced by self-perceptions of aging. *Preventive Medicine, 39,* 625–629.

Levy, B. R., Slade, M. D., & Kasl, S. V. (2002). Longitudinal benefit of positive self-perceptions of aging on functional health. *The Journals of Gerontology, 57,* 409–417.

Levy, B. R., Slade, M. D., Kunkel, R. R., & Kasl, S. V. (2002). Longevity increased by positive self-perceptions of aging. *Journal of Personality and Social Psychology, 83,* 261–270.

Levy, B. R., Zonderman, A. B., Slade, M. D., & Ferrucci, L. (2009). Age stereotypes held earlier in life predict cardiovascular events in later life. *Psychological Science, 20,* 296–298.

Luszcz, M. A. (1983). An attitudinal assessment of perceived intergenerational affinities linking adolescence and old age. *International Journal of Behavioral Development, 6,* 221–231.

Meisner, B. A. (2012). A meta-analysis of positive and negative age stereotype priming effects on behavior among older adults. *The Journals of Gerontology: Series B: Psychological Sciences and Social Sciences, 67,* 13–17.

Nelson, T. D. (2004). *Ageism: Stereotyping and prejudice against older persons.* Cambridge, MA: MIT Press.

Nemmers, T. M. (2005). The influence of ageism and ageist stereotypes on the elderly. *Physical and Occupational Therapy in Geriatrics, 22,* 11–20.

Older Women's League. (2012). Women and the workforce: Challenges and opportunities facing women as they age. Retrieved from: <http://www.owl-national.org/Files/Women_and_the_Workforce-Challenges_and_Opportunities_Facing_Women_as_They_Age.pdf>.

Palmore, E. (1971). Attitudes toward aging as shown by humor. *The Gerontologist, 11*(3), 181–186. http://dx.doi.org/10.1093/geront/11.3_Part_1.181.

Palmore, E. (2001). The ageism survey: First findings. *The Gerontologist, 41,* 572–575.

Parr, W., & Siegert, R. (1993). Adults' conceptions of everyday memory failures in others: Factors that mediate the effects of target age. *Psychology and Aging, 8*, 599–605.

Pettigrew, T., & Tropp, L. (2006). A meta-analytic test of intergroup conflict theory. *Journal of Personality and Social Psychology, 90*(5), 751–783.

Ryan, E., & See, S. (1992). Age-based beliefs about memory changes for self and others across adulthood. *The Journal of Gerontology, 48*, 199–201.

Schwartz, L. K., & Simmons, J. P. (2001). Contact quality and attitudes toward the elderly. *Educational Gerontology, 27*, 127–137.

Snyder, M., & Miene, P. K. (1994). Stereotyping of the elderly: A functional approach. *British Journal of Social Psychology, 33*, 63–82.

Steele, C. M., & Aronson, J. (1995). Stereotype threat and the intellectual test performance of African Americans. *Journal of Personality and Social Psychology, 69*, 797–811.

Tam, T., Hewstone, M., Harwood, J., Voci, A., & Kenworthy, J. (2006). Intergroup contact and grandparent–grandchild communication: The effects of self-disclosure on implicit and explicit biases against older people. *Group Processes & Intergroup Relations, 9*, 413–429.

Taylor, D., Wright, S., Moghaddam, F., & Lalonde, R. (1990). The personal/group discrimination discrepancy: Perceiving my group, but not myself, to be a target for discrimination. *Personality and Social Psychology Bulletin, 16*, 254–262.

Vernon, J., Williams, J., Phillips, T., & Wilson, J. (1990). Media stereotyping: A comparison of the way elderly women and men are portrayed on prime-time television. *Journal of Women & Aging, 2*(4), 55–68.

Wilcox, S. (1997). Age and gender in relation to body attitude: Is there a double standard of aging? *Personality of Women Quarterly, 21*, 549–565.

Zebrowitz, L. A., & Montepare, J. M. (2000). Integrating social psychology and aging research: Toward a social-developmental theory of behavior. *Basic and Applied Social Psychology, 22*, 257–260.

14

Civic Engagement and the
Power of Older Women

Global Fact: *When communities are displaced by natural disasters or armed conflict, older people may be unable to flee or travel long distances and may be left behind. Yet, in many situations, they can also be a valuable resource for their communities as well as for the humanitarian aid process when they are involved as community leaders.*

—World Health Organization (2014)

As defined, "civic engagement" pertains the active involvement of individuals within the workings of society, and it has interesting implications toward the role of older adults in the broader society (Minkler & Holstein, 2008). Hinterlong (2008) emphasized the social issue of "productive engagement" among older Americans, suggesting that societal support among aging adults has important consequences for both the functioning of society and public policy processes. Societies across the world need to adapt to and accommodate the needs of the aging population (Warburton, Sik Hung, & Shardlow, 2013).

Institutions within communities must recognize the need to accommodate and support the civic engagement of aging women in society. Volunteerism can have many social benefits for all aspects of society (Tan et al., 2010; Tang, Choi, & Morrow-Howell, 2010). The issue of "environmental" volunteerism is both a practical and public policy initiative within aging-friendly communities and broader societies (Bushway, Dickinson, Stedman, Wagenet, & Weinstein, 2011). It is vital to acknowledge both the barriers and benefits presented in social context to older women as potential volunteers (Cutler & Hendricks, 2000; Enguidanos, Pynoos, Denton, Alexman, & Diepenbrock, 2010; Gonzales & Morrow-Howell, 2009; Mukherjee, 2011; Rozanova, Keating, & Eales, 2012). One might argue that civic engagement permits both a better social valuation of older women in terms of their role within society (eg, Martinez, Crooks, Kim, & Tanner, 2011; Morrow-Howell, 2010) across many different countries in the World, as well as assist in the transitioning between their later-life social roles (eg, transition from a woman's work role to a retirement role; Kaskie, Imhof, Cavanaugh, & Culp, 2008; Lancee & Radl, 2012).

Longitudinal factors predicting the degree to which older women are actively engaged in social activities is crucial to understand for program development and intervention purposes (eg, community participation at age 80; Holahan & Chapman, 2002). To ensure that their "voice" is heard regarding needs and motivations, aging women need to be socially and civically engaged in community activities and processes (eg, voting in politics; Turner, Shields, & Sharp, 2001).

Aging women's social resources and attitudes toward social involvement may be influenced by race (eg, Black–White differences; Barnes, Mendes de Leon, Bienias, & Evans, 2004), functional capability (Dabelko-Schoeny, Anderson, & Spinks, 2010), sexual orientation (Davis, Crothers, Grant, Young, & Smith, 2012; Hostetler, 2012), work/retirement status (Nesteruk & Price, 2011), marital status (eg, widowhood; Donnelly & Hinterlong, 2009; Isherwood, King, & Luszcz, 2012; Utz, Carr, Nesse, & Wortman, 2002), and cohort membership (eg, "baby boomers;" Hudson, 2008; MaloneBeach & Langeland, 2011).

To gain and/or maintain social status within a society, women must vote, volunteer, and otherwise engage in community programs and/or local government to ensure social influence and further social knowledge about the aging population's growing social, psychological, physical, and emotional needs. Cullinane (2008) purported that active social engagement assists in creating a "purposeful" life in later adulthood among diverse populations in countries like Tikkun Olam. This concept can be applied to aging women living in many global locations.

BENEFITS OF OLDER WOMEN'S CIVIC ENGAGEMENT TO AGING WOMEN

Benefit of Intergenerational Learning and Mentoring

One very important outcome of social engagement is increased exposure to other age groups and cohorts. This mutual learning and intergenerational sharing of ideas can be both beneficial to younger and older generations (Kleiber & Nimrod, 2008). Interacting with others and communicating ideas can be a productive form of cognitive stimulation that can help older women maintain cognitive competency over time, barring any nonnormative or genetic issues (Anderson & Dabelko-Schoeny, 2010; Chappell, 2005) as well as enhance relationships within many different contexts (eg, family context; Davey, Janke, & Savla, 2004).

Sharing of ideas, activities, and interests enhances the quality of life of all age groups involved, demystifying the aging process while increasing gerocompetencies for younger women (eg, Dauenhauer, Steitz, Aponte, &

Fromm Faria, 2010) and adding meaning to later life for older women through engaging in meaningful activities (Eakman, Carlson, & Clark, 2010). The benefits of civic engagement is really a life span issue for all age groups of women. Insights from such exposure to different cultures and people through service learning activities may benefit younger women in becoming more culturally sensitive when interacting with aging generations (Hegeman, Roodin, Gilliland, & Ó'Flathabháin, 2010; Jones, Ivanov, Wallace, & VonCannon, 2010; Horowitz, Wong, & Dechello, 2010; Zucchero, 2011), as well as possibly their own aging trajectories. For example, the physical health of younger generations can be positively impacted through a close positive mentoring relationship within the context of a health program involving older community mentors (Simson, Wilson, Ruben, & Thompson, 2008).

QUOTES FROM FAMOUS POSITIVELY AGING WOMEN

The process of maturing is an art to be learned, an effort to be sustained.
By the age of fifty you have made yourself what you are,
and if it is good, it is better than your youth.
—*Marya Mannes, Author from her book* **More in Anger** *(1958)*

There is a plan and a purpose, a value to every life,
no matter what its location, age, gender or disability.
—*Sharron Angle, Politician*

It is utterly false and cruelly arbitrary to put all the play and learning into childhood,
all the work into middle age, and all the regrets into old age.
—*Margaret Mead, Anthropologist and Social Researcher*

Benefit of Extended Social Support Resources

Being civically engaged in the community and broader cultural contexts benefits older women because they can become empowered to access and maintain social support and other resources to optimize adjustment to later life. For example, involvement in religious activities through a church or synagogue can be a wonderful opportunity for older women's active civic engagement and can expose them to different social support contacts which may positively impact their longevity (eg, Mexican American adults; Hill, Angel, Ellison, & Angel, 2005). Through volunteering, older women can better maintain social connections with different community groups. These groups will benefit from the experience and knowledge of this large aging subpopulation of women. In turn, these different community groups may share information and resources benefiting aging women in society. Social exchange theory (Emerson, 1976) suggests that it is advantageous to establish and maintain social relationships that offer "benefits" to us. The civic engagement and community involvement of older women would assist in optimizing the social exchange process for positive aging outcomes.

Benefit of Active Social Participation

Active involvement of older women in society is beneficial to all, but it is important to "tailor" social activities to best motivate and match the interests and attitudes of those involved to ensure that the positive benefits and usefulness of the activities are apparent (Leedahl, Koenig, & Ekerdt, 2011; Morrow-Howell, Song-lee, & Fengyan, 2009; Okamoto & Tanaka, 2004). Older women who participate as "Polar Bears" every cold winter in Martha's Vineyard do so because they perceive an inherent and meaningful benefit to engaging in this physical activity which may not appeal to other groups of older women. It is important for aging women to "know thyself" during the aging process and choose civic activities which have a deep meaning to their lives to support personal positive aging outcomes.

It is argued from an activity theory perspective (Kelly, 1993) that older women would benefit from the social civic engagement on the psychological, social, physical, and emotional level (Duke, Leventhal, Brownlee, & Leventhal, 2002; Gottlieb & Gillespie, 2008). Successful physical and psychological aging of women can be optimized through active engagement in daily tasks on a cognitive and physical basis (Menec, 2003; Piercy, Cheek, & Teemant, 2011; Pillemer, Fuller-Rowell, Reid, & Wells, 2010; Wahrendorf, Ribet, Zins, Goldberg, & Siegrist, 2010; Walter-Ginzburg, Blumstein, Chetrit, & Modan, 2002). For example, Zunzunegui, Alvarado, Del Ser, and Otero (2003) suggest that active civic engagement and associated maintenance of social support networks can assist with cognitive competency in later life. Civic involvement of older women would be mutually benefitial to both maintaining activity levels of aging women and disseminating older women's wisdom and expertise to the community (eg, social participation of the oldest old; Bukov, Maas, & Lampert, 2002). Civic engagement for older women can take many forms, from Internet use (Bo, 2008) to face-to-face neighborhood participation (Cagney & Cornwell, 2010). The proceeding will discuss the benefits of older women's civic engagement to both aging women themselves and society in many different countries across the world.

Benefit of Having a "Voice" in Politics and Community Activities

The cognitive, social, psychological, or physical benefits of active civic engagement has been discussed in broad-based terms. More specifically, active civic engagement for older women creates a "voice" in community and political activities. This can be an empowering outcome for the aging subpopulation which may not experience the social valuation and social power that is needed to acquire and maintain needed social resources. Being a visible part of society through participation in different community-based activities can benefit all concerned. To create a voice, however, necessitates older women becoming much more active in their roles and their input (eg, voting activity on a local or national level; Binstock, 2000). In many different cultures, this may be a shift in cultural role expectations for women, and especially older women, in society.

Benefit of Positive "Role Models" of Aging

One very important, but subtle, benefit to increased visibility through increased civic engagement is that older women are more likely to become positive role models for younger women in society. Girls and younger women can be exposed to within-gender examples who can demonstrate positive aging outcomes as a woman in the community. Civic engagement across a woman's life span into later life can produce positive psychosocial growth for both the aging woman and the lives that she touches through her efforts (Peters, 2012). This cultural exposure to civically engaged aging women can help guide the aging trajectory of younger generations of women. Bandura (1977) suggested in social learning theory that role models that we deem to be significant in our lives can significantly impact our learning and associated development. Aging women who are actively engaged in community and broader national activities can significantly and positively influence future cohorts of women.

Benefit of Mentoring from Experienced Older Adults

The mentoring activities by older generations to younger generations is a valuable social process. Through women's continued civic engagement into later life, women of different age levels can learn from each other about ways to optimize their development and achieve successful developmental outcomes over time. Older women in many different cultures across the world are needed mentors for younger women and girls needing guidance in finding "who" they are and, possibly, more importantly, "who" they can be in later life. Mentoring activities within the context of community involvement may focus on attaining and/or maintaining social support resources, establishing financial security and other adjustment issues. The concept of "womentoring" (Hetherington & Barcelo, 1985) is an organizational idea regarding the formal and/or informal communication and assistance that can occur between experienced and novice female employees in an organization. Applying this concept of womentoring to a broader context outside of the workplace, older women can certainly actively guide and shape the aging paths of younger female generations (eg, a co-mentoring intergenerational program; Zucchero, 2011).

CHECK IT OUT!

Search the Internet to find information about aging women actively engaged in the community. In conducting this research, identify specific issues related to being both a woman and an aging adult engaged in community activities across many different regions of the world. Are there common issues related to older women or are they culture specific? Are the sociocultural factors you find related to specific generations of aging working women (ie, cohort-specific experiences)? As you are examining these factors, think about the following questions:

1. Are the issues for aging women similar to the issues for aging men regarding civic engagement?
2. What are the societal "messages" about women and later-life civic engagement?
3. What can be done to create greater fairness in community policies and practices in response to a growing subpopulation of older women volunteers in the coming decades?

TEST YOURSELF!

Civic Engagement Scale

Source: Doolittle, A., & Faul, A. C. (2013). Civic engagement scale: A validation study. *SAGE Open (July–September)*, 1–7. doi: 10.1177/2158244013495542.

Attitudes: In this section, there are eight statements that are designed to measure an individual's civic attitudes. For the purpose of this study, civic attitudes have been defined as the personal beliefs and feelings that individuals have about their own involvement in their community and their perceived ability to make a difference in that community. Please indicate the level to which you *agree* or *disagree* with each statement.

continued

	Disagree/Agree						
1. I feel responsible for my community	1	2	3	4	5	6	7
2. I believe I should make a difference in my community	1	2	3	4	5	6	7
3. I believe that I have a responsibility to help the poor and the hungry	1	2	3	4	5	6	7
4. I am committed to serve in my community	1	2	3	4	5	6	7
5. I believe that all citizens have a responsibility to their community	1	2	3	4	5	6	7
6. I believe that it is important to be informed of community issues	1	2	3	4	5	6	7
7. I believe that it is important to volunteer	1	2	3	4	5	6	7
8. I believe that it is important to financially support charitable organizations	1	2	3	4	5	6	7

Behaviors: In this section, there are six statements that are designed to measure the behaviors that indicate a level of civic engagement. Civic behaviors have been defined as the actions that one takes to actively attempt to engage and make a difference in his or her community. Please indicate the level to which you have participated on a scale from *never* to *always*.

	Never/Always						
1. I am involved in structured volunteer position(s) in the community	1	2	3	4	5	6	7
2. When working with others, I make positive changes in the community	1	2	3	4	5	6	7
3. I help members of my community	1	2	3	4	5	6	7
4. I stay informed of events in my community	1	2	3	4	5	6	7

continued

	Never/Always						
5. I participate in discussions that raise issues of social responsibility	1	2	3	4	5	6	7
6. I contribute to charitable organizations within the community	1	2	3	4	5	6	7

Scoring: Add up the scores in each section and get a measure of attitude toward and behavioral frequency of civic engagement.

TIPS FOR CIVIC ENGAGEMENT WITH AGING WOMEN

In deciding to become civically engaged within the community, women should consider the following.

1. Personal skills to contribute
2. Personal motivational needs to be satisfied
3. Volunteer opportunities and community needs
4. Personal flexibility in time and task investment

This reciprocal process of sharing benefits derived from increased civic engagement of older women in different communities across the world should also discuss the benefits of receiving the expertise of the older adults involved. Older women, as volunteers, will share an invaluable resource related to decades of knowledge and expertise. Older women have much to share in personal skills, knowledge and abilities (eg, how to cook traditional food recipes), and their local involvement can have national impact (Miles, 2005). The workplace, for example, will experience a "brain drain" as experienced older workers retire and leave with their accumulated knowledge and experience. The underutilization of older women as valuable social resources in communities, who may not be fully valued and actively pursued as contributors to societal programs and activities, can negatively impact the social and economic functioning of communities (Stallmann, Deller, & Shields, 1999). The challenge is for society to help aging women optimally "age in place" within organizations, extending their contributions to the workplace as skilled volunteers with invaluable knowledge and skills to offer (Netting & Thibault, 2012; Resnick, Klinedinst, Dorsey, Holtzman, & Abuelhiga, 2013).

WORDS OF WISDOM

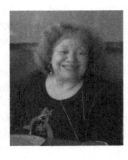

Lillian was born in Puerto Rico, and in 1981, she moved to the United States. She has been a teacher all her life; also she has volunteered her time with kids. She got involved in numerous after-school programs and others groups for children because she wanted to engage kids in something productive and useful, and help them stay away from negative activities. She plans to retire in two years and spend her time both volunteering in her church and with children.

Lillian has gained many emotional and physical benefits from volunteering her time with children. Lillian spent much time with children who were from immigrant families, and she helped them to assimilate to the new culture and learn necessary attitudes. Being able to help kids and become their support system was very rewarding emotionally; in addition to that, they always kept her physically active. Lillian's husband passed away long time ago and the children became her family.

What advice would Lillian give to younger women? Find time to volunteer and help others; it is not only very rewarding but it will also help you understand the needs of others. Spending time with children especially will teach you so much. It is very gratifying to see that you encouraged them to study, have fun, and to follow their dreams, or to helping them achieve whatever goals they might have. Lillian says that it is so important to share your time with kids, not only offer them knowledge and wisdom in terms of education but also help them be more mature, and the more mature they are the more they will be able to face life. "The impact I made in their lives, and that I have helped them achieve something—all these things keep me going and make me feel that I have accomplished something in life, and that it was all worth it!"

The recent "squaring" of the age pyramid (ie, change in the number of younger people to older people in a population demographic) combined with an international influx of older "baby boomers" (ie, people born between 1946 and 1964) has created a growing imbalance in financial (eg, Social Security) and social support ratios (eg, elder care) (Ingham, Chirijevskis, & Carmichael, 2009; United Nations, Department of Economic and Social Affairs, 2007). To counter this imbalance of support factors, increased social engagement in many different community-based contexts across different societies can only highlight and support the social, psychological, and physical care needs of a growing number of aging women (Cherry et al., 2013; Crooks, Lubben, Petitti, Little, & Chiu, 2008; Giles, Glonek, Luszcz, & Andrews, 2005; Zunzunegui et al., 2003). Church may be one of those important social contexts for such civic and social engagement for aging women (and men) in many different cultures and communities (Hendricks & Cutler, 2001).

Increased civic engagement and community political involvement can bring positive attention to the social issues, is occurring in many industrialized nations related to the many transitions in later life (eg, relocation to a new living situation; Dupuis-Blanchard, Neufeld, & Strang, 2009), and which directly impact women across a life span. Hopefully, increased attention and legislative action will assist in helping older women have equal access to civic engagement opportunities for many different purposes (Rozanova et al., 2012; Thomas, 2011).

EMPOWERMENT OF OLDER WOMEN

Encouraging older women to be a civically engaged, active part of communities can assist in their mental health outcomes, such as less susceptibility to possible social isolation and depression in later life (Saczynski et al., 2010). Their exposure to, and utilization of, social resources through their social involvement will create heightened social power, and independence which can empower older women within their living environments (Walker & Hiller, 2007).

Older women's impact upon the cultures they live within, for their own benefit and the benefit of future generations of aging women, will have positive ramifications for societies across the world. Giving a "voice" to segment of the population who may feel ignored and invisible is critical for the growth and development of the graying world population. As discussed previously, there are many mutual benefits to the empowerment and encouraged civic engagement of older women. As with other issues, this paradigm shift in valuing the contributions of women in later life must occur and grow in response to the proportional growth of this world population. This shift in perspective about the value of older women to society must occur through the implementation of community-based education in many different parts of the world. Both society and older women need to recognize their inherent value to each other to promote positive aging outcomes.

SUMMARY

As the number of older women increase in many countries across the world in the coming decades, it behooves societies to actively engage the knowledge, skills, and abilities of these older women with lifetimes of experience and wisdom. This active engagement of older women mutu-ally benefit all involved, creates opportunities for both multigenerational learning, and increases activity levels of this aging subpopulation within many diverse cultures and communities. Greater social and civic engage-ment for women will mean that they will be more physically and men-tally engaged on a daily basis, assisting in their positive aging over time. Understanding the cultural contexts in which older women can engage in such activities is important to understand from an interventionist per-spective in the design of community-based programs and supportive educational activities.

The valuation of older women's contributions to many aspects of social functioning (eg, political discourse) will help create ethical societies who help optimize positive aging outcomes for all societal members across their life span.

DISCUSSION QUESTIONS

1. What are the important ways that women can be taught to be civically engaged across their life spans?
2. In what ways can different cultures convey supportive "messages" to aging women about becoming civically engaged? Do you see the messages in today's society and in what ways?
3. How does greater civic engagement benefit older women's positive physical aging?
4. How does greater social involvement promote older women's positive cognitive aging?
5. How do older women psychosocially benefit from enhanced civic engagement in their communities?
6. Beyond the example in the chapter, who are some other women who changed history by being socially engaged into their later life? What are their personal qualities, and how did they break stereotypes about what it means to be an older woman in society?
7. What is the role of education within communities and creating opportunities for women to maintain active roles in society and be empowered throughout the life span?
8. How can societies better empower older women to volunteer for different roles within the community and take initiative in becoming involved in social activities on an ongoing basis?
9. Are there individual difference factors to consider when encouraging aging women to volunteer in the community?
10. How can communities promote aging women's civic engagement? What are cultural factors to be considered in such outreach efforts?

TEST YOUR KNOWLEDGE!

Take the following quiz about aging attitudes:
http:seniorhealthblog.wordpress.com/2014/04/11/healthy-aging-quiz/

SUPPLEMENTAL BOOK READINGS

Over the past decades, there have been many books written on the topic of older women and the positive benefits of engaging in volunteerism/civic engagement activities. Here are some *recommended additional readings*:

Wilson, L. (2006). *Civic engagement and the baby boomer generation: Research, policy, and practice perspectives.* New York, NY: Routledge.
  The book examines the role of the growing numbers of aging Baby Boomers and the implications of their civic engagement on social change within the United States, although this certainly could be an idea extrapolated to the impact in the world population. The author makes the assertion that the sheer numbers of this cohort can have a significant and positive impact on local, national, and global cultures and communities. The positive value of civic engagement by this generation of older adults is emphasized throughout the book, arguing that both older adults and their social environments would significantly benefit from such proactive activities. Older women from this generation, or other generations, would find this to be an informative and empowering resource text.

Morrow-Howell, M., & Mui, A. C. (2012). *Productive engagement in later life: A global perspective.* New York, NY: Routledge.
  The authors define "productive aging" as the active participation of older adults in all aspects of society, including working, volunteering and education. Older adults' contributions to society should be better acknowledged and valued. This book suggests that older adults' civic engagement yields important economic and social outcomes for their families, the community, and the broader society.

Delgado, M. (2008). *Older adult-led health promotion in urban communities: Models and interventions.* Lanham, MD: Rowman & Littlefield Publishers.
  The book presents topics related to older adults as agents of social change. Older adult-led health promotion efforts in regions of underserved aging populations represents a needed "grass roots" movement on a national and international level.

Gartner, C. (2013). *Biography, life transitions and social capital of seniors.* London, United Kingdom: Verlag.

The need to have societies promote later-life learning as a way to keep aging population from becoming withdrawn and isolated is discussed. The quality of life needs of vital and healthy older adults and their invaluable contributions to communities are two of many reasons why educational engagement is vital for people as they experience different phases of life transition (eg, postretirement).

CARE (2007). *Women empowered: Inspiring change in the emerging world.* New York, NY: Rizzoli.

CARE's program to empower women across the world highlights the struggles and successes of women in poor and war torn environments. The strength, endurance, and resiliency of women across the life span is celebrated through documented stories. This is an inspirational book that would be a great guidebook for women as they age and face many challenges of living plus the changes of aging.

SUPPLEMENTAL AGING VIDEOS

For learning purposes, the use of videos can be very beneficial for both instructors and readers. Here are some *recommended supplemental videos*:

Different video links on aging health: http://www.healthvideo.com/sitemap.php (Format: Website)

Different videos on human development: http://www.learner.org (Format: Website)

ADDITIONAL INFORMATION LINKS

The following are some *recommended supplemental Internet links*:

Aging Network's Volunteer Collaborative website: http://agingnetworkvolunteers.org/older-adult-volunteers/

Idealist website: http://www.idealist.org/info/Volunteer/Older

RetirementWeb.com website: http://www.retirementweb.com/articles/older_adult_volunteers.html

Urban Institute website: http://www.urban.org/publications/311325.html

US Administration on Aging website: http://www.aoa.gov/ AoAroot/Press_Room/Social_Media/Widget/Statistical_ Profile/2011/3.aspx

Volunteering and Civic Life in America website: http:// www.volunteeringinamerica.gov/*rankings/Large-Cities/ Older-Adult-Volunteer-Rates/2008*

VolunteerMatch website: http://blogs.volunteermatch.org/ engagingvolunteers/tag/older-adult-volunteering/

References

Anderson, K. A., & Dabelko-Schoeny, H. I. (2010). Civic engagement for nursing home residents: A call for social work action. *Journal of Gerontological Social Work, 53*(3), 270–282. http://dx.doi.org/10.1080/01634371003648323.

Bandura, A. (1977). *Social learning theory*. Englewood Cliffs, NJ: Prentice Hall.

Barnes, L. L., Mendes de Leon, C. F., Bienias, J. L., & Evans, D. A. (2004). A longitudinal study of Black–White differences in social resources. *The Journals of Gerontology Series B: Psychological Sciences and Social Sciences, 59*, S146–S153.

Binstock, R. H. (2000). Older people and voting participation: Past and future. *The Gerontologist, 40*(1), 18–31.

Bo, X. (2008). Civic engagement among older Chinese internet users. *Journal of Applied Gerontology, 27*(4), 424–445.

Bukov, A., Maas, I., & Lampert, T. (2002). Social participation in very old age: Cross-sectional and longitudinal findings from BASE. *The Journals of Gerontology Series B: Psychological Sciences and Social Sciences, 57*, P510–P517.

Bushway, L. J., Dickinson, J. L., Stedman, R. C., Wagenet, L. P., & Weinstein, D. A. (2011). Benefits, motivations, and barriers related to environmental volunteerism for older adults: Developing a research agenda. *International Journal of Aging & Human Development, 72*(3), 189–206. http://dx.doi.org/10.2190/AG.72.3.b.

Cagney, K. A., & Cornwell, E. Y. (2010). Neighborhoods and health in later life: The intersection of biology and community. *Annual Review of Gerontology & Geriatrics, 30*, 323–348.

Chappell, N. L. (2005). Perceived change in quality of life among Chinese Canadian seniors: The role of involvement in Chinese culture. *Journal of Happiness Studies, 6*, 69–91. http:// dx.doi.org/10.1007/s10902-004-1754-5.

Cherry, K. E., Walker, E. J., Brown, J. S., Volaufova, J., LaMotte, L. R., Welsh, D. A., et al. (2013). Social engagement and health in younger, older, and oldest-old adults in the Louisiana healthy aging study. *Journal of Applied Gerontology, 32*(1), 51–75.

Crooks, V. C., Lubben, J., Petitti, D. B., Little, D., & Chiu, V. (2008). Social network, cognitive function, and dementia incidence among elderly women. *American Journal of Public Health, 98*(7), 1221.

Cullinane, P. (2008). Purposeful lives, civic engagement, and Tikkun Olam. *Generations, 32*(2), 57–59.

Cutler, S. J., & Hendricks, J. (2000). Age differences in voluntary association memberships: Fact or artifact? *The Journals of Gerontology Series B: Psychological Sciences and Social Sciences, 55*, S98–S107.

Dabelko-Schoeny, H., Anderson, K. A., & Spinks, K. (2010). Civic engagement for elderly with functional limitations: Piloting an intervention for adult day health participants. *Gerontologist, 50*(5), 694–701.

Dauenhauer, J. A., Steitz, D. W., Aponte, C. I., & Fromm Faria, D. (2010). Enhancing student gerocompetencies: Evaluation of an intergenerational service learning course. *Journal of Gerontological Social Work, 53*(4), 319–335. http://dx.doi.org/10.1080/01634371003715577.

Davey, A., Janke, M., & Savla, J. (2004). Antecedents of intergenerational support: Families in context and families as context. *Annual Review of Gerontology &Geriatrics, 24,* 29–54.

Davis, S., Crothers, N., Grant, J., Young, S., & Smith, K. (2012). Being involved in the country: Productive ageing in different types of rural communities. *Journal of Rural Studies, 28*(4), 338–346. http://dx.doi.org/10.1016/j.jrurstud.2012.01.008.

Donnelly, E. A., & Hinterlong, J. E. (2009). Changes in social participation and volunteer activity among recently widowed older adults. *The Gerontologist, 50*(2), 158–169. http://dx.doi.org/10.1093/geront/gnp103.

Doolittle, A., & Faul, A. C. (2013). Civic engagement scale: A validation study. *SAGE Open (July–September),* 1–7. http://dx.doi.org/10.1177/2158244013495542.

Duke, J., Leventhal, H., Brownlee, S., & Leventhal, E. A. (2002). Giving up and replacing activities in response to illness. *The Journals of Gerontology Series B: Psychological Sciences and Social Sciences, 57,* P367–P376.

Dupuis-Blanchard, S., Neufeld, A., & Strang, V. R. (2009). The significance of social engagement in relocated older adults. *Qualitative Health Research, 19*(9), 1186–1195.

Eakman, A. M., Carlson, M. E., & Clark, F. A. (2010). The meaningful activity participation assessment: A measure of engagement in personally valued activities. *International Journal of Aging and Human Development, 70*(4), 299–317.

Emerson, R. M. (1976). Social exchange theory. *Annual Review of Sociology, 2*(1), 335–362.

Enguidanos, S., Pynoos, J., Denton, A., Alexman, S., & Diepenbrock, L. (2010). Comparison of barriers and facilitators in developing NORC programs: A tale of two communities. *Journal of Housing for the Elderly, 24*(3/4), 291–303. http://dx.doi.org/10.1080/02763893.-2010.522445.

Giles, L. C., Glonek, G. F., Luszcz, M. A., & Andrews, G. R. (2005). Effect of social networks on 10 year survival in very old Australians: The Australian longitudinal study of aging. *Journal of Epidemiology and Community Health, 59*(7), 574–579.

Gonzales, E., & Morrow-Howell, N. (2009). Productive engagement in aging-friendly communities. *Generations, 33*(2), 51–58.

Gottlieb, B. H., & Gillespie, A. A. (2008). Volunteerism, health, and civic engagement among older adults. *Canadian Journal on Aging, 27*(4), 399–406.

Hegeman, C. R., Roodin, P., Gilliland, K. A., & Ó'Flathabháin, K. (2010). Intergenerational service learning: Linking three generations: Concept, history, and outcome assessment. *Gerontology & Geriatrics Education, 31*(1), 37–54. http://dx.doi.org/10.1080/02701960903584418.

Hendricks, J., & Cutler, S. J. (2001). The effects of membership in church-related associations and labor unions on age differences in voluntary association affiliations. *The Gerontologist, 41,* 250–256.

Hetherington, C., & Barcelo, R. (1985). Womentoring: A cross-cultural perspective. *Journal of the National Association of Women Deans, Administrators, and Counselors, 49*(1), 12–15.

Hill, T. D., Angel, J. L., Ellison, C. G., & Angel, R. J. (2005). Religious attendance and mortality: An 8-year follow-up of older Mexican Americans. *The Journals of Gerontology Series B: Psychological Sciences and Social Sciences, 60,* S102–S109.

Hinterlong, J. E. (2008). Productive engagement among older Americans: Prevalence, patterns, and implications for public policy. *Journal of Aging & Social Policy, 20*(2), 141–164.

Holahan, C. K., & Chapman, J. R. (2002). Longitudinal predictors of proactive goals and activity participation at age 80. *The Journals of Gerontology Series B: Psychological Sciences and Social Sciences, 57,* P418–P425.

Horowitz, B. P., Wong, S., & Dechello, K. (2010). Intergenerational service learning: To promote active aging, and occupational therapy gerontology practice. *Gerontology & Geriatrics Education, 31*(1), 75–91. http://dx.doi.org/10.1080/02701960903578345.

Hostetler, A. J. (2012). Community involvement, perceived control, and attitudes toward aging among Lesbians and Gay men. *International Journal of Aging and Human Development*, 75(2), 141–167.

Hudson, R. B. (2008). Civic engagement and the baby boomer generation. *Gerontologist*, 48(1), 124–126.

Ingham, B., Chirijevskis, A., & Carmichael, F. (2009). Implications of an increasing old-age dependency ratio: The UK and Latvian experiences compared. *Pensions*, 14, 221–230. http://dx.doi.org/10.1057/pm.2009.16.

Isherwood, L. M., King, D. S., & Luszcz, M. A. (2012). A longitudinal analysis of social engagement in late-life widowhood. *International Journal of Aging and Human Development*, 74(3), 211–229.

Jones, E. D., Ivanov, L. L., Wallace, D., & VonCannon, L. (2010). Global service learning project influences culturally sensitive care. *Home Health Care Management & Practice*, 22(7), 464–469. http://dx.doi.org/10.1177/1084822310368657.

Kaskie, B., Imhof, S., Cavanaugh, J., & Culp, K. (2008). Civic engagement as a retirement role for aging Americans. *Gerontologist*, 48(3), 368–377.

Kelly, J. R. (1993). *Activity and aging: Staying involved in later life*. Newbury Park, CA: Sage Publications.

Kleiber, D., & Nimrod, G. (2008). Expressions of generativity and civic engagement in a 'learning in retirement' group. *Journal of Adult Development*, 15(2), 76–86. http://dx.doi.org/10.1007/-s10804-008-9038-7.

Lancee, B., & Radl, J. (2012). Social connectedness and the transition from work to retirement. *Journals of Gerontology Series B: Psychological Sciences & Social Sciences*, 67(4), 481–490.

Leedahl, S. N., Koenig, T. L., & Ekerdt, D. J. (2011). Perceived benefits of VFW Post participation for older adults. *Journal of Gerontological Social Work*, 54(7), 712–730. http://dx.doi.org/10.1080/01634372.2011.594149.

MaloneBeach, E. E., & Langeland, K. L. (2011). Boomers' prospective needs for senior centers and related services: A survey of persons 50–59. *Journal of Gerontological Social Work*, 54(1), 116–130. http://dx.doi.org/10.1080/01634372.2010.524283.

Martinez, I. L., Crooks, D., Kim, K. S., & Tanner, E. (2011). Invisible civic engagement among older adults: Valuing the contributions of informal volunteering. *Journal of Cross-Cultural Gerontology*, 26(1), 23–37. http://dx.doi.org/10.1007/s10823-011-9137-y.

Menec, V. H. (2003). The relation between everyday activities and successful aging: A 6-year longitudinal study. *The Journals of Gerontology Series B: Psychological Sciences and Social Sciences*, 58, S74–S82.

Miles, T. P. (2005). Think globally, act locally. *Annual Review of Gerontology &Geriatrics*, 25, R19–R29.

Minkler, M., & Holstein, M. B. (2008). From civil rights to … civic engagement? Concerns of two older critical gerontologists about a "new social movement" and what it portends. *Journal of Aging Studies*, 22(2), 196–204. http://dx.doi.org/10.1016/j.jaging.2007.-12.003.

Morrow-Howell, N. (2010). Volunteering in later life: Research frontiers. *Journals of Gerontology Series B: Psychological Sciences & Social Sciences*, 65B(4), 461–469.

Morrow-Howell, N., Song-lee, H., & Fengyan, T. (2009). Who benefits from volunteering? Variations in perceived benefits. *Gerontologist*, 49(1), 91–102. http://dx.doi.org/10.1093/geront/-gnp007.

Mukherjee, D. (2011). Participation of older adults in virtual volunteering: A qualitative analysis. *Ageing International*, 36(2), 253–266. http://dx.doi.org/10.1007/s12126-010-9088-6.

Nesteruk, O., & Price, C. A. (2011). Retired women and volunteering: The good, the bad, and the unrecognized. *Journal of Women & Aging*, 23(2), 99–112. http://dx.doi.org/10.1080/08952841.-2011.561138.

Netting, F., & Thibault, J. M. (2012). Challenges faced by staff in faith-related agencies when dedicated volunteers age in place. *Journal of Religion, Spirituality & Aging*, 24(3), 202–212. http://dx.doi.org/10.1080/15528030.2012.648846.

Okamoto, K., & Tanaka, Y. (2004). Subjective usefulness and 6-year mortality risks among elderly persons in Japan. *The Journals of Gerontology Series B: Psychological Sciences and Social Sciences, 59*, P246–P249.

Peters, D. (2012). "Take me to the water"—Community and renewal among aging women: A case study of social interaction and exercise among the "polar bears" of Martha's Vineyard. *Journal of Women & Aging, 24*(3), 216–226. http://dx.doi.org/10.1080/08952 8412012.639668.

Piercy, K. W., Cheek, C., & Teemant, B. (2011). Challenges and psychosocial growth for older volunteers giving intensive humanitarian Service. *Gerontologist, 51*(4), 550–560.

Pillemer, K., Fuller-Rowell, T. E., Reid, M. C., & Wells, N. M. (2010). Environmental volunteering and health outcomes over a 20-year period. *Gerontologist, 50*(5), 594–602.

Resnick, B., Klinedinst, J., Dorsey, S., Holtzman, L., & Abuelhiga, L. S. (2013). Volunteer behavior and factors that influence volunteering among residents in continuing care retirement communities. *Journal of Housing for the Elderly, 27*(1/2), 161–176. http://dx.doi.org/10.1080/02763893.-2012.75-I820.

Rozanova, J., Keating, N., & Eales, J. (2012). Unequal social engagement for older adults: Constraints on choice. *Canadian Journal on Aging, 31*(1), 25–36. http://dx.doi.org/10.1017/-S0714980811000675.

Saczynski, J. S., Beiser, A., Seshadri, S., Auerbach, S., Wolf, P. A., & Au, R. (2010). Depressive symptoms and risk of dementia: The Framingham Heart Study. *Neurology, 75*(1), 35–41.

Simson, S. P., Wilson, L. B., Ruben, K. A., & Thompson, L. M. (2008). Humor your way to good health: An intergenerational program to address a critical public health issue: The epidemic of overweight and obesity among children. *Journal of Intergenerational Relationships, 6*(1), 83–100. http://dx.doi.org/10.1300/J194v06n0106.

Stallmann, J. I., Deller, S. C., & Shields, M. (1999). The economic and fiscal impact of aging retirees on a small rural region. *The Gerontologist, 39*(5), 599–610.

Tan, E. J., Tanner, E. K., Seeman, T. E., Xue, Q., Rebok, G. W., Frick, K. D., et al. (2010). Marketing public health through older adult volunteering: Experience corps as a social marketing intervention. *American Journal of Public Health, 100*(4), 727–734.

Tang, F., Choi, E., & Morrow-Howell, N. (2010). Organizational support and volunteering benefits for older adults. *Gerontologist, 50*(5), 603–612.

Thomas, P. A. (2011). Gender, social engagement, and limitations in late life. *Social Science & Medicine, 73*(9), 1428–1435.

Turner, M. J., Shields, T. G., & Sharp, D. (2001). Changes and continuities in the determinants of older adults' voter turnout 1952–1996. *The Gerontologist, 41*, 805–818.

United Nations, Department of Economic and Social Affairs, (2007). *World population aging.* New York, NY: United Nations Population Division.

Utz, R. L., Carr, D., Nesse, R., & Wortman, C. B. (2002). The effect of widowhood on older adults' social participation: An evaluation of activity, disengagement, and continuity theories. *The Gerontologist, 42*, 522–533.

Wahrendorf, M., Ribet, C., Zins, M., Goldberg, M., & Siegrist, J. (2010). Perceived reciprocity in social exchange and health functioning in early old age: Prospective findings from the GAZEL study. *Aging & Mental Health, 14*(4), 425–432. http://dx.doi.org/10.1080/13607860903483102.

Walker, R. B., & Hiller, J. E. (2007). Places and health: A qualitative study to explore how older women living alone perceive the social and physical dimensions of their neighbourhoods. *Social Science & Medicine, 65*(6), 1154–1165.

Walter-Ginzburg, A., Blumstein, T., Chetrit, A., & Modan, B. (2002). Social factors and mortality in the old-old in Israel: The CALAS study. *The Journals of Gerontology Series B: Psychological Sciences and Social Sciences, 57*, S308–S318.

Warburton, J., Sik Hung, N., & Shardlow, S. M. (2013). Social inclusion in an ageing world: Introduction to the special issue. *Ageing & Society, 33*(1), 1–15. http://dx.doi.org/10.1017/S0144686-X12000980.

World Health Organization. (2014). Facts about ageing. Retrieved from: <http://www.who.int/ageing/about/facts/en/>.

Zucchero, R. A. (2011). A co-mentoring project: An intergenerational service-learning experience. *Educational Gerontology*, *37*(8), 687–702. http://dx.doi.org/10.1080/03601271003723487.

Zunzunegui, M. V., Alvarado, B. E., Del Ser, T., & Otero, A. (2003). Social networks, social integration, and social engagement determine cognitive decline in community-dwelling Spanish older adults. *The Journals of Gerontology Series B: Psychological Sciences and Social Sciences*, *58*, S93–S100.

Public Policies and the Next Steps in the Evolution of Women's Aging

Global Fact: *Between 2000 and 2050, the old-age dependency will double in more developed regions and triple in less developed regions. The potential socioeconomic impact on society that may result from an increasing old-age dependency ratio is an area of growing research and public debate.*

—*Global Aging (2001)*

Public policy relates to the care and support the aging population (Pampel, 1998; Rich & Baum, 1985). Currently, there are many quality-of-life concerns pertaining to the treatment of older adults in many different communities (Bowling, 2005; Hudson, 2010). Laws to protect the rights and independence of aging adults is an ethical issue to examine from a public policy perspective (eg, competency decision making; Moye & Marson, 2007). Across the life span, it is also important to better understand the cumulative impact of public policies on women and how it relates to their positive aging (eg, employment discrimination laws; Duncan & Loretto, 2004).

Ethical societies in the world must examine and continuously reexamine how they treat a growing aging population, ranging from aging-related public support programs to other social resources for older women. This examination is not a static process because the nature of an international aging population is evolving as they continue to live longer and their dynamic roles within family systems and other contexts (eg, the workplace) (Applebaum & Leek, 2008; Muramatsu & Akiyama, 2011). This dynamic aging process for women must be better understood from the constituents involved in order to best to design age- and gender-appropriate social policy education and interventions (eg, "aging in community" efforts) in many different cultures and countries across the world (Binstock, 2008; Chen, 2012; Zhang, Guo, & Zheng, 2012).

Women and Positive Aging.
DOI: http://dx.doi.org/10.1016/B978-0-12-420136-1.00015-3 **269**

The empowerment of women in many different cultures and countries across the world should be one of the initiatives underlying aging-related social policy reforms (eg, Nigeria; Nwagbara, Etuk, & Baghebo, 2012). The proceeding will present broad issues to consider under this topic.

CHANGING DEFINITION OF "QUALITY-OF-LIFE" STANDARDS FOR OLDER WOMEN ACROSS THE WORLD

Public policies directly impact the quality of life of those within a society, and everyone is a key "stakeholder" in the process of establishing standards of aging well (Everingham, Lui, Bartlett, Warburton, & Cuthill, 2010). For example, self-reported medication usage for older women is an important issue of education and health care system tracking that needs social policy and practice reforms for the health of many generations (in Australia; Dolja-Gore, Pit, Parkinson, Young, & Byles, 2013). Over time, different generations of women within different cultures have experienced changing standards of quality of life. The active involvement and input of older women for the development and/or implementation of societal public policy is a necessity to ensure accurate and effective quality-of-life outcomes.

EVOLVING DEFINITION OF "LATER ADULTHOOD" AS A PUBLIC POLICY CONCEPT

In a broad sense, public policy is best able to serve an aging population when it keep pace with the definitions of aging-related stages. When is the age at which a woman is old or is there really such a demarcation? If women are living longer than ever before (eg, "baby boomers"), the time periods at which a person enters middle adulthood and later adulthood is important to understand from a public policy perspective (eg, needs of the "golden age" cohort; Winter, Torges, Stewart, Henderson-King, & Henderson-King, 2006). The demographic "mapping" of when an aging woman's typical changes and associated developmental needs occur is important focus within and across cultures, because this understanding applies to the formulation and implementation of any societal policies. One important question to be addressed is whether aging-related public policies should be based upon a dynamic chronological definition (eg, older adults designated as being citizenry age 65 or older) or should it be based upon aging-related functional status (eg, chronological age versus functional age distinction). If public policy shifts its focus to be more "functional" in perspective related to the support of aging women, it is then imperative to have adequate assessment skill levels designed for specific skill-based contexts (eg, driving privileges).

QUOTES FROM FAMOUS POSITIVELY AGING WOMEN

"Aging is not lost youth but a new stage of opportunity and strength."

"It is easier to live through someone else than to complete yourself. The freedom to lead and plan your own life is frightening if you have never faced it before. It is frightening when a woman finally realizes that there is no answer to the question 'who am I' except the voice inside herself."
—*Betty Friedan, Feminist Activist and Author*

"You get to an age where you get tired of hiding behind whatever people think is correct."
—*Betty Wright, Musician*

SHIFTING SOCIAL IMAGE OF AN "OLDER WOMAN" IN DIFFERENT CULTURES

In addition to an evolving concept of later adulthood, there is also an analogous evolving concept related to what it means to be an "older woman" in many different parts the world. Increased longevity and general healthiness has created a new image of what it means to be a woman in later life. The continuation on different women's roles well past the traditional retirement age of 65 in the areas of work, family caregiving, and nonfilial social support redefines their social image as an active member of society. From a public policy perspective, it is important for public policies in the form of legislation and national, state, and local community programs to acknowledge and adapt to the reality of what it means to be an older woman in society.

Education is the key to this process to adapting public policies and community programs to better address the ongoing quality of life needs of older women in different societies (Manheimer, 2008). Education impacts how well an aging population adjusts to the many later-life changes encountered (Formosa, 2012). In any part of the world, "knowledge is power" for aging women. The focus of education and associated community initiatives to improve the lives of aging women can range from community-based exercise (Layne et al., 2008) to diversity education with very specific aging groups' cultural and functional needs highlighted (Sterns & Ansello, 2008; Yeo & McBride, 2008). To illustrate a critical issue for women across the life span, Beaulaurier, Seff and Newman (2008) suggested that community education is one important aspect of social policy reform needed to encourage older women's help-seeking motivation and behavior to seek help in response to experiencing intimate partner abuse. Education is needed for everyone in society, to better understand the complex processes involved in self and others' aging processes (Whitfield, Edwards, & Nelson, 2010) and how to best prepare a well-trained long-term care workforce with culturally diverse workers (eg, Browne & Braun, 2008).

TIPS FOR WOMEN'S EFFECTIVE SENIOR ACTIVISM

To be an effective political activist, aging women should

1. Be current on aging-related social topics requiring support.
2. Network with like-minded individuals/groups on issue of the political concern.
3. Voice your opinions through the social and public media.
4. Commit to "the cause" and see it to its fruition.

SPECIFIC ISSUES OF PUBLIC POLICY SUPPORTS

To support the positive aging of women in many different countries across the world, different societies must reexamine the growing aging trends regarding older adults' needs, motivations, preferences, and support resources (eg, off-label medication usage; Stephenson, Anderson, & Rochon, 2012) (Street, Burge, & Quadagno, 2009; Wolff, Kasper, & Shore, 2008). It is important to realize that any resources allocated to women as they age benefits all involved, not just simply older women but also those that they care for and depend upon. In general, all of the issues to be discussed in the proceeding impacts every member of society across the life span. The following will discuss specific areas of public as relates to the unique support needs of a growing global aging population of women.

Financial Protections and Resources

One of the two significant factors predicting life satisfaction for older adults is (i) financial security, older cohorts of women in many different societies are at a potential financial disadvantage because of disrupted workforce participation patterns due to caregiving responsibilities and (ii) other social restrictions on women's roles in the workplace and society (Marson & Sabatino, 2012). The concept of "feminization of poverty" (Minkler & Stone, 1985) relates to this idea of gender-related financial vulnerability for women. Disparities in wage gap regarding earnings between men and women over many generations also has been cited as contributing to aging women's relative financial insecurity.

In order to support the positive aging outcomes for women across the world, there needs to be greater attention paid to public policies related to financial protections and supportive programs to assist in the financial and personal independence of older adults (Callander, Schofield, & Shrestha, 2012). This situation may be further exacerbated by the realization that most women in many industrialized countries outlive their male counterparts and do not have shared resources for financial security in later life, although career and other family-related timing factors should be take into account (Jokinen-Gordon, 2012). Financial insecurity can undermine women's ability to afford health care for many different needs (mental and physical health, and substance use) (Domino et al., 2008).

Housing and Transportation

A significant issue for all communities to address is the degree to which aging adults' living environments are aging friendly and accessible to support viable "aging in place" situations (Lehning, 2011; Shenfil, 2009). The degree to which an aging woman can safely live and travel independently is a "universal" quality of life concern that public policies in countries across the world need to better address in planning for the growing international aging population (Fielding et al., 2011).

Housing is one of those specific environmental public policy topics that is showing recent trends in adapting to the needs and desires of aging residents (Matosevic, Knapp, Grand, & Fernandez, 2011) but much more needs to be done to ensure that housing design standards, community safety check programs, and independent living feasibility "check ins" by professional are needed and should be enforced through social policies (eg, Scarfo, 2011).

Understanding driving mobility capabilities and travel behavior "patterns" are equally crucial public policy issues related to supporting aging women needing to remain as independent as possible (Kulikov, 2011; Newbold, Scott, Spinney, Kanaroglou, & Páez, 2005). Education and support programs are of critical importance to both support quality of life needs and protect individuals as the ability to drive independently becomes increasingly a less viable option (Byles & Gallienne, 2012; Choi, Adams, & Kahana, 2013; Donorfio, Mohyde, Coughlin, & D'Ambrosio, 2008). In considering the creation of these community-based programs and social policies for diverse groups of aging adults, it is critical to acknowledge individual difference factors impacting their attitudes, activity of daily living (ADL) needs, and what would assist in their transition from driving to using public transportation (Choi, Mezuk, Lohman, Edwards, & Rebok, 2012). Part of the educational and social policy focus needs to be regarding consumer protection to ensure that ageism does not occur in response to service provisions (Bodner, Cohen-Fridel, & Yaretzky, 2011).

CHECK IT OUT!

Search the Internet to find different aging-related and gender-related public policies relevant to the well-being of a growing aging worldwide population of women. This search might address some unique issues related to aging women that are not being addressed through general aging policies. For example, public policies need to better acknowledge predominantly gender-specific eldercare programs and services, as well as protective legislation, especially significant to many aging women across the world who are faced with long-term primary caregiver role responsibilities over time. What role does culture have in the creation and implementation of public policies specifically targeting older women's issues in the world? What our diversity issues that would be important to understand and public policy legislation designed to assist and/or protect older women in society? As you are examining these factors, think about the following questions:

1. What are the cultural "messages" about older women and their later-life rights and responsibilities that impact public policies?
2. Are there apparent biases in public policies toward older women and, if yes, do they differ by culture?
3. In the coming decades, what are some current aging trends with aging women that will necessitate the creation of adaptive public policies to address future needs?

WORDS OF WISDOM

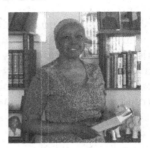

Sue is 86 years old, and is the Treasurer of AARP's Chicago Near South East Chapter in Chicago, Illinois. Sue has been treasurer for about a year but has been a member for longer. Before Sue retired she was a registered Nurse. She graduated from De Paul University with a bachelor's of science in nursing and worked for the Chicago Department of Health.

When Sue was asked what issues she thinks are associated with positive aging trends for women, Sue's response reflected some of her values. Sue believes that exercising, socializing, nutrition, and family are all things that should be a part of a women's life as they age. Sue goes for walk with one of her friends at least three days a week to stay active. Sue has a small group of close friends who all celebrate their birthdays together. They call themselves the "Four Seasons" because each of their birthdays is in a different season. Since Sue was diagnosed with type II diabetes, she follows a more nutritious diet and avoids taking diabetes medications. Sue stays in contact with her close family, her son and two grandchildren.

Sue has noticed that in Chicago the mayor has supported and influenced positive aging by opening senior centers where seniors can go to exercise and socialize. Senior centers have game rooms and also host speakers. Past speakers have been nutritionist and pharmacists who answer questions about healthy eating and medications.

Sue's word of advice to young women would be to get involved in different organizations, but do not just be a member. Be an active member. Ask questions and voice your ideas. Sue also believes that getting an education is very important. She advises younger women to go as far as they can in education. Sue states, "Education is the key to getting involved with public policies and make a change."

Health Care Coverage

A second significant factor that predicts life satisfaction among older adults is personal health status (Liao, Chang, & Sun, 2012). Public policies regarding proper health care for women across her life span into later life is a crucial issue in many countries across the world (Cole, 2007; Kuhlmann & Annandale, 2010). Past research suggests that women tend to underestimate their health needs and this may have a significant cumulative impact on their aging trajectory and associated quality of life. Community education for women, and those that care for them, is a necessary part of public policy initiatives in many different societies. As women typically live longer than male peers in many industrialized nations, the criticality of having quality health care education, outreach and assessment services, and support resources to address their personal mobility capabilities (eg, "user friendly" assessment tools; Rejeski, Ip, Marsh, & Barnard, 2010; Thorpe, Clay, Szanton, Allaire, &Whitfield, 2011), health screening (eg, pap smear screening; Adolfsson, Granevik, & Paulson, 2012) preventative fracture risk assessments (D'Souza et al., 2012), and healthy body weight maintenance (Gadalla, 2010) across woman's life span is increasingly a public policy concern on an international level.

Health and economic disparities, among other aging health determinants (eg, incarceration), have to be accounted for on both the national and international level in reforming social policies for women across their life spans (Miles, 2009; Williams, Stern, Mellow, Safer, & Greifinger, 2012; Zhenmei, Danan, & Hayward, 2008). The utilization of aging-friendly support policies and services needs in-depth analysis in both the short- and long-term to ensure that older women (and men) who need assistance actually utilize the program, services, and educational opportunities designed to satisfy their needs. Older adults' perceptions of available resources is critical for public policy makers to understand (Putnam, 2011; Singh, Sharma, Kumar, & Shinwari, 2012). Further, the need to better train and support the formal caregivers of older adults who may be immigrants from other countries and have their own adjustment needs is also an increasing issue for health care public policies (Redfoot & Houser, 2008). Mental health policies, outreach services, education, and support programs for aging women is even more of a public policy imperative because it can be unfortunately be a "hidden," stigmatized health issue in many different cultures (Akincigil et al., 2011; Bartels, 2011; Baskin et al., 2011).

Eldercare Resources and Caregiver Supports

Across many different cultures in the world, women are the traditional caregivers of family members (Lahaie, Earle, & Heymann, 2013). This social phenomenon of women as the expected "default" caregiver in many different cultures is important to acknowledge because being a caregiver impacts women's aging with physical, social, and mental health implications (Bertrand et al., 2012). The aim of supporting positive aging outcomes for women necessitates the need to have public policy-related resources in order to offset the financial, social, and physical demands related to balancing a woman's caregiving roles over time (Donorfio, Vetter, & Vracevic, 2010). The support and the involvement of family members is critical for both the aging woman who may be dealing with chronic health issues and is transitioning from self- to assisted care (Gallant, Spitze, & Grove, 2010).

Respite programs, community education for the entire family, and other community-based support would assist in optimizing woman's aging in terms of their physical and mental health. One important focus of such interventions would be to help in the care "transition" that is significant for all involved in the eldercare process (Arbaje, Boonyasai, & Dilworth-Anderson, 2011; Dilworth-Anderson, Hilliard, Williams, & Palmer, 2011; Gitlin &Wolff, 2011; Kietzrnan, Pincus, & Huynh, 2011; Reinhard & Lind, 2011; Stone & Bryant, 2011).

As aging women make this care transition, much more needs to be done through community education and legislative protection to protect women from self-neglect and/or abuse in its many forms from a culturally sensitive perspective (Dong, 2012; Dyer et al., 2008; Locher et al., 2008; Lowenstein, Eisikovits, Band-Winterstein, & Enosh, 2009). Many different regions of the world will experience an increased aging population through 2050 and beyond; this reality necessitates social policies and programs to encourage advanced care and "transition" planning for families, health care and long-term care institutions, and broader communities (Kwak, Allen, & Haley, 2011; Mor et al., 2011; Rockwell, 2010; Soonman, 2008).

Future Workplace Changes, Training, and Job Security

The aging population will meaningfully change the "landscape "of the workplace in many regions of the world (eg, health care career trends in nursing and dentistry; Spetz, 2005; Williams, 2005), and the associated needs of the older employees and their employers must be assessed and addressed through social policies (Bernard, 2008; Galinsky, 2007).

Concerns about aging discrimination, for example, as more middle-aged and older women continue in or reenter the workforce needs to be reevaluated under current protective legislation and associated workplace programs (eg, older worker training programs). From a public policy stance, there needs to be protection for adults working well past traditional retirement age due to financial, social, and/or motivational quality-of-life concerns (Börsch-Supan, 2003). The workplace can be a source of strong social support and cognitive stimulation for women that positively impacts how well they age. Public policies should be concerned with the growing aging workforce and that their rights be protected among qualified older women workers who might be simultaneously faced with eldercare duties (Katz, Lowenstein, Prilutzky, & Halperin, 2011). Otherwise, there might be the possibility of "triple jeopardy," in which women may be discriminated upon and prevented from employment because they may have differential educational training, are women, and are older (in Taiwan; Luo, 2010). An ethical society must have in place protective legislation for its most vulnerable and protection of employment rights, older women should be an increased concern in many different countries in the world (Slack & Jensen, 2008).

Retirement is becoming an extended and rather complex stage in an individual's life. There are more decision-making options related to this later life stage (Byles et al., 2013). The concept of "retirement," and any associated policies underlying the experience, has been linked to very specific time markers in history. Interestingly, policies toward retirement and retirement support systems can be found as early as thirteenth century, BC, in early Roman society when military soldiers retiring after 20 years of service were given a retirement pension. Many centuries later, German Chancellor Otto Von Bismarck enacted policies regarding retirement policies in response to the changing dynamics within his country at the time. His policies then became a preliminary retirement policy model for many different pension systems across Europe and in the United States in decades to follow. It is an ethical obligation for global societies to support and care for aging women (and men) who, for various reasons, become dependent and need assistance in retirement and other situations to maintain their quality of life (Gabriel & Bowling, 2004; Rich & Baum, 1985).

Historically, early retirement policies and programs were focused upon male workers because the role of workforce participant was traditionally relegated to men. The role of women in the workforce developed and expanded in the 1900s and the 2000s has seen further progress in women's career pursuits. Interestingly, nonwork roles for women have not necessarily dissipated but rather have become part of a "superwoman syndrome" in society (Shaevitz, 1984). One might argue that cohorts of women balancing multiple social roles and obligations will have a different trajectory than previous generations of women who may not have been expected to balance a full career and other role responsibilities equally.

The concept of "feminization of poverty" (Minkler & Stone, 1985; Stone & National Center for Health Services Research and Health Care Technology Assessment (U.S.), 1987) refers to the fact that older women may find themselves in the situation of not being able to afford to retire because of a disrupted workforce pattern and a lack of pension funds to rely upon in retirement. Although women are currently occupying more full-time careers in the work force than ever before, there is a wage gap that does created disparity in the accumulated lifelong earnings for aging women. This inequity in salary does create a potential need for aging women to remain in the workforce longer than desired or anticipated because of the need to maintain a certain level of financial security (Pampel, 1998).

As multiple generations of older adults live longer than ever before with chronic conditions, the likelihood of being a caregiver for an extended period of time has increased within a family system. At the same time, there are increasing numbers a multigenerational households creating patterns of dependency and financial support needs. Aging baby boomers currently are experiencing the phenomenon of supporting both older and younger generations in an unprecedented manner (ie, "sandwich generation;" Brody, 1985, 1990). Most middle-aged and older women encountering this situation may not find it feasible to retire as expected and, thus, instead focus on extended career succession efforts to remain in the workforce (ie, "women in the middle;" Brody, 1990).

The degree to which current public policies reflect the current aging workforce population requires constant updating and evaluation (Crystal, 1982). Circumstances surrounding cost of living, eldercare responsibilities, motivational needs, and other individual difference factors relate to the timing and extent of retirement for many people. Retirement is a complex process that needs to be continually reexamined in order to best meet the needs of its older workers.

SUMMARY

Effective public policies and associated social programs/legislation from these policies must respond to the evolving and dynamic nature of aging for women in many different cultures and circumstances. To best support and optimize a woman's aging, policies must continually assess anticipating needs. This assessment process requires an active involvement of older women's offering of input regarding adaptive public policies and associated support programs to best optimize their positive aging outcomes. With the coming decades, the dynamic and evolving role of older women today and in the future within communities and broader societies will continue to manifest itself in many different social processes and functions. To be effective, societies across the world must adapt to this changing role of aging women and achieve a balance of supporting autonomy while protecting the rights of this growing world population.

DISCUSSION QUESTIONS

1. What are some current age-related issues that public policy should be addressing for women across the world?
2. Are quality-of-life concerns being addressed by current public policies in many different countries? If not, what are some of the quality-of-life concerns that need to be addressed?
3. How can older women create differences in the development and implementation of public policies in their communities and countries?

4. In addition to needed public policies, what are some outdated programs and legislation that do not reflect the current status and needs of the aging female population?
5. How can community-based education positively affect public policies in communities and societies across the world for the benefit of older women?
6. What are the three different issues that you anticipate will need to be addressed by the growing numbers of aging women in the next three to four decades?
7. By 2050, underdeveloped countries will experience an even more dramatic increase in the numbers of older adults. What are some public policy concerns which should be discussed?
8. As aging is really human development over time, and impacts all women, how early should public policies focus on education and age-related services to promote positive aging outcomes for women across the life span? Please explain your answer.
9. How can aging women become more empowered to be involved in public policy matters on a local, national, and/or international platform?
10. If you were an advocate for older women's international rights, what specific issue would you pursue?

TEST YOUR KNOWLEDGE!

Take the following quiz about public policies in response to an aging population:

https://www.wisc-online.com/learn/career-clusters/health-science/ota2605/public-policy-and-aging

---

SUPPLEMENTAL BOOK READINGS

Over the past decades, there have been many books written on the topic of aging trends with women (among other aging groups) and the associated need for adaptive changes in social and public policies toward aging presently and in the future. Here are some *recommended additional readings*:

Barusch, A. S. (1994). *Older women in poverty: Private lives and public policies*. New York, NY: Springer Publishing Co.
This is a helpful resource for students, practitioners, policy makers, and aging adults wanting to better understand this

important ethic concern in public policies and community programs designed for women who may be faced with poverty across the life span. Topics of importance are the best way for countries across the world to address the needs of aging women including financial security and women's health care resources.

Li, Y. (2013). *Global aging issues and policies: Understanding the importance of comprehending and studying the aging process.* Springfield, IL: Charles C. Thomas Pub Ltd.
  The book emphasizes the need to acknowledge the global aging trends and the associated mutual exchange between the growing numbers of older adults worldwide and the societies in which they live. The aim of better understanding this demographic phenomena is to better address and plan for the needs of this subpopulation to enhance their quality of life in many different ways.

Koskiaho, B., Makinen, P., & Pattiniemi, M. (Editors). *Women, the elderly and social policy in Finland and Japan: The muse or the worker bee?* Denmark: Avebury.
  The book presents information of the aging experiences of women in two different countries, Finland and Japan. The interesting message from the book is that there is a critical need for all countries across the world to reevaluate the contributions of women to their communities and the growing needs of aging women within their communities. The authors strongly argue that governments should examine their public policies (eg, pension, work, and retirement) to ensure that they are effective in supporting this growing aging segment of the world population. Cross-culturally, women across the life span would benefit from the core "message" of this text—be proactive and question the cultural supports available for positive aging.

Special Committee on Aging United States Senate (2012). *Aging in America: Future challenges, promises, and potential.* Charleston, SC: CreateSpace Publishing.
  This report emphasizes the need to allocate more social and financial resources to programs supporting older adults of diverse backgrounds, needs, and circumstances. The report is a "call to action" for communities and policy makers to aid older adults in both meeting their needs and promoting their potential for growth and success in many different venues of social engagement.

Galasso, V. (2008). *The political future of social security in aging societies.* Cambridge, MA: MIT Press.

The author examines the issue of pension spending in a national economy with a simultaneously growing older population. The support ratio of younger workers to older workers is increasingly becoming imbalanced due to the "baby boom" demographic trend immediately followed by a historical time period of decreased births ("baby bust" generation).

Gutman, G., & Spencer, C. (Editors) (2010). *Aging, ageism and abuse: Moving from awareness to action.* Buffalo Grove, IL: Elsevier.

This book highlights the need for countries and local communities to assess and meet the needs of vulnerable groups of older adults who may not have their voices heard due to discrimination, poverty, or accessibility limitations. One such vulnerability is related to the crisis of elder abuse on a global level. Current social policies and programs that have been developed for the penal systems, support community services, and health care should be better monitored to avoid issues of ageism and abuse in the treatment of aging populations around the world.

Abbott, P., Carman, N., Carman, J., & Scarfo, B. (Editors) (2008). *Re-creating neighborhoods for successful aging.* Baltimore, MD: Health Professions Press.

The authors suggest that the design of living environments within communities and households should be "aging friendly," taking into account the physical, sensory, and other functional changes affecting the accomplishment of ADLs by an aging population. Suggestions are given regarding ways to create conducive living environments to support positive aging outcomes. Aging women would benefit from the information provided in this text as a catalyst for advocacy initiatives in their behalf to enhance community designs in regions across the world.

AGING VIDEOS

For learning purposes, the use of videos can be very beneficial for both instructors and readers. Here are recommended *supplemental videos*:

http://www.ucsd.tv/search-details.aspx?showID=23253&subject=health (Format: Website)

This is a great website that offers information and a video on the new "Age Wave" about the future of aging and associated public policy issues.

Can't Afford to Grow Old (Format: DVD)
This DVD addresses the important issue of the affordability of quality, long-term health care for most families and older adults. This is a worldwide issue because most countries are experiencing an influx of older adult patients within health care systems which are not equipped to deal with the complex chronic conditions of aging over a long-term care situation.

No Place Like Home: Long-Term Care For the Elderly (Format: DVD)
Alternatives to institutionalized care for aging clients are presented in case studies of different regions across the United States. Transportation to senior centers, in-home care options, and other alternatives to care should be considered and are illustrated within the film's segments.

House Calls (Format: DVD)
The video examines the growing social issue of aging adults wishing to remain independent as long as possible but the current health care system does not acknowledge nor support these quality of lie perceptions within this subpopulation. The demand for in-home care services will only grow—the question is whether the health care system will adapt to their needs.

ADDITIONAL INFORMATION LINKS

The following are some recommended *supplemental Internet links*:

Aging Society website: http://www.agingsociety.org/agingsociety/publications/public_policy/previous.html

AARP website: http://www.aarp.org/politics-society/advocacy/info-12-2010/make_aging_policy_ma.html

Heartland Institute website: http://heartland.org/policy-documents/past-present-and-future-aging

References

Adolfsson, A., Granevik, K., & Paulson, K. (2012). The reasons why women do not participate in the Pap smear screening and testing program in Sweden *Advances in Sexual Medicine* (2)3137http://dx.doi.org/10.4236/asm.2012.23006.

Akincigil, A., Olfson, M., Walkup, J. T., Siegel, M. J., Kalay, E., Amin, S., et al. (2011). Diagnosis and treatment of depression in older community-dwelling adults: 1992–2005. *Journal of the American Geriatrics Society, 59*(6), 1042–1051. http://dx.doi.org/10.1111/j.1532-5415.2011.03447.x.

Applebaum, R., & Leek, J. (2008). Bridging the academic/practice gap in gerontology and geriatrics: Mapping a route to mutual success. *Annual Review of Gerontology & Geriatrics, 28*, 131–147.

Arbaje, A. I., Boonyasai, R. T., & Dilworth-Anderson, P. (2011). The older person in transition: Implications for pathways of transitions of care. *Annual Review of Gerontology & Geriatrics, 31*, 15–30.

Bartels, S. J. (2011). Commentary: The forgotten older adult with serious mental illness: The final challenge in achieving the promise of Olmstead? *Journal of Aging & Social Policy, 23*(3), 244–257. http://dx.doi.org/10.1080/08959420.2011.579497.

Baskin, F., Marcus, L., Mays, W., Rawlings, R., Bruner-Canhoto, L., & O'Connor, D. (2011). Coalitions on mental health and aging: Lessons learned for policy and practice. *Journal of Aging & Social Policy, 23*(3), 323–332. http://dx.doi.org/10.1080/08959420.2011.579516.

Beaulaurier, R. L., Seff, L. R., & Newman, F. L. (2008). Barriers to help-seeking for older women who experience intimate partner violence: A descriptive model. *Journal of Women & Aging, 20*(3/4), 231–248.

Bernard, M. A. (2008). Workforce needs in the future: The institute of medicine 2008 report-retooling for an aging America. *Annual Review of Gerontology & Geriatrics, 28*, 13–17.

Bertrand, R. M., Saczynski, J. S., Mezzacappa, C., Hulse, M., Ensrud, K., & Fredman, L. (2012). Caregiving and cognitive function in older women: Evidence for the healthy caregiver hypothesis. *Journal of Aging & Health, 24*(1), 48–66. http://dx.doi.org/10.1177/0898264311421367.

Binstock, R. H. (2008). Social policy in gerontology and geriatrics education. *Annual Review of Gerontology & Geriatrics, 28*, 73–92.

Bodner, E., Cohen-Fridel, S., & Yaretzky, A. (2011). Sheltered housing or community dwelling: Quality of life and ageism among elderly people. *International Psychogeriatrics, 23*(8), 1197–1204. http://dx.doi.org/10.1017/S1041610211001025.

Börsch-Supan, A. (2003). Labor market effects of population aging. *Labour, 17*(s1), 5–44.

Bowling, A. (2005). *Ageing well: Quality of life in old age.* London, United Kingdom: McGraw-Hill Education.

Brody, E. M. (1985). Parent care as a normative family stress. *The Gerontologist, 25*, 19–29.

Brody, E. M. (1990). *Women in the middle: Their parent- care years.* New York, NY: Springer.

Browne, C. V., & Braun, K. L. (2008). Immigration and the direct long-term care workforce: Implications for education and policy. *Gerontology & Geriatrics Education, 29*(2), 172–188. http://dx.doi.org/10.1080/0270196080222327.

Byles, J., & Gallienne, L. (2012). Driving in older age: A longitudinal study of women in urban, regional, and remote areas and the impact of caregiving. *Journal of Women & Aging, 24*(2), 113–125. http://dx.doi.org/10.1080/08952841.2012.639661.

Byles, J., Tavener, M., Robinson, I., Parkinson, L., Smith, P., Stevenson, D., et al. (2013). Transforming retirement: New definitions of life after work. *Journal of Women & Aging, 25*(1), 24–44. http://dx.doi.org/10.1080/08952841.2012.717855.

Callander, E. J., Schofield, D. J., & Shrestha, R. N. (2012). Multiple disadvantages among older citizens: What a multidimensional measure of poverty can show. *Journal of Aging & Social Policy, 24*(4), 368–383. http://dx.doi.org/10.1080/08959420.2012.735177.

Chen, S. (2012). Historical and global perspectives on social policy and "aging in community". *Ageing International, 37*, 1–15. http://dx.doi.org/10.1007/s12126-011-9136-x.

Choi, M., Adams, K., & Kahana, E. (2013). Self-regulatory driving behaviors: Gender and transportation support effects. *Journal of Women & Aging, 25*(2), 104–118. http://dx.doi.org/10.1080/-08952841.2012.720212.

Choi, M., Mezuk, B., Lohman, M. C., Edwards, J. D., & Rebok, G. W. (2012). Gender and racial disparities in driving cessation among older adults. *Journal of Aging & Health, 24*(8), 1364–1379. http://dx.doi.org/10.1177/0898264312460574.

Cole, F. (2007). *US national debate topic, 2007–2008: Healthcare in Sub-Saharan Africa.* Bronx, NY: H. W. Wilson.

Crystal, S. (1982). *America's old age crisis: Public policy and the two worlds of aging.* New York, NY: Basic Books.

Dilworth-Anderson, P., Hilliard, T. S., Williams, S., & Palmer, M. H. (2011). A contextual conceptualization on transitions of care for older persons: Shaping the direction of care. *Annual Review of Gerontology & Geriatrics, 31*, 1–14.

Dolja-Gore, X., Pit, S. W., Parkinson, L., Young, A., & Byles, J. (2013). Accuracy of self-reported medicines use compared to pharmaceutical claims data amongst a national sample of older Australian women. *Open Journal of Epidemiology, 3*, 25–32. http://dx.doi.org/10.4236/ojepi.2013.31005.

Domino, M. E., Maxwell, J. J., Cody, M. M., Cheal, K. K., Busch, A. B., Van Stone, W. W., et al. (2008). The influence of integration on the expenditures and costs of mental health and substance use care: Results from the randomized PRISM-E study. *Ageing International, 32*(2), 108–127. http://dx.doi.org/10.1007/s12126-0089010-7.

Dong, X. (2012). Culture diversity and elder abuse: Implications for research, education, and policy. *Generations, 36*(3), 40–42.

Donorfio, L. K. M., Vetter, R., & Vracevic, M. (2010). Effects of three caregiver interventions: Support, educational literature, and creative movement. *Journal of Women & Aging, 22*(1), 61–75. http://dx.doi.org/10.1080/08952840903489094.

Donorfio, L. M., Mohyde, M., Coughlin, J., & D'Ambrosio, L. (2008). A qualitative exploration of self-regulation behaviors among older drivers. *Journal of Aging & Social Policy, 20*(3), 323–339.

D'Souza, M. S., Isac, C., Venkatesaperumal, R., Amirtharaj, A., Thanka, A., Balachandran, S., et al. (2012). Exploring fracture risk factors among Omani women: Implications for risk assessment. *Open Journal of Nursing, 2*, 365–371. http://dx.doi.org/10.4236/-ojn.2012.24054.

Duncan, C., & Loretto, W. (2004). Never the right age? Gender and age-based discrimination in employment. *Gender, Work & Organization, 11*(1), 95–115.

Dyer, C., Franzini, L., Watson, M., Sanchez, L., Prati, L., Mitchell, S., et al. (2008). Future research: A prospective longitudinal study of elder self-neglect. *Journal of the American Geriatrics Society, 56*, S261–S265. http://dx.doi.org/10.1111/j.15325415.2008.01978.x.

Everingham, J., Lui, C., Bartlett, H., Warburton, J., & Cuthill, M. (2010). Rhetoric to action: A study of stakeholder perceptions of aging well in two local communities. *Journal of Gerontological Social Work, 53*(8), 760–775. http://dx.doi.org/10.1080/01634372.2010.519974.

Fielding, R. A., Rejeski, W., Blair, S., Church, T., Espeland, M. A., Gill, T. M., et al. (2011). The lifestyle interventions and independence for elders study: Design and methods. *Journals of Gerontology Series A: Biological Sciences & Medical Sciences, 66A*(11), 1226–1237.

Formosa, M. (2012). Education and older adults at the university of the third age. *Educational Gerontology, 38*, 114–126. http://dx.doi.org/10.1080/03601277.2010.515910.

Gabriel, Z., & Bowling, A. (2004). Quality of life from the perspectives of older people. *Ageing and Society, 24*(05), 675–691.

Gadalla, T. M. (2010). Relative body weight and disability in older adults: Results from a national survey. *Journal of Aging & Health, 22*(4), 403–418. http://dx.doi.org/10.1177/08982643-10361367.

Galinsky, E. (2007). The changing landscape of work. *Generations, 31*(1), 16–22.

Gallant, M. P., Spitze, G., & Grove, J. G. (2010). Chronic illness self-care and the family lives of older adults: A synthetic review across four ethnic groups. *Journal of Cross-Cultural Gerontology, 25*(1), 21–43. http://dx.doi.org/10.1007/s10823-010-9112-z.

Gitlin, L. N., & Wolff, J. (2011). Family involvement in care transitions of older adults: What do we know and where do we go from here? *Annual Review of Gerontology & Geriatrics, 31*, 31–64.

Global Aging. (2001). The ageing of the world's population. Retrieved from: <http://www.globalaging.org/waa2/documents/theagingoftheworld.htm>.

Hudson, R. B. (Ed.). (2010). *The new politics of old age policy*. Baltimore, MD: Johns Hopkins University Press.

Jokinen-Gordon, H. (2012). Still penalized? Parity, age at first birth and women's income in later life. *Journal of Women & Aging, 24*(3), 227–241. http://dx.doi.org/10.1080/089528 41.2012.639671.

Katz, R., Lowenstein, A., Prilutzky, D., & Halperin, D. (2011). Employers' knowledge and attitudes regarding organizational policy toward workers caring for aging family members. *Journal of Aging & Social Policy, 23*(2), 159–181. http://dx.doi.org/10.1080/089594 20.2011.554120.

Kietzrnan, K. G., Pincus, H. A., & Huynh, P. T. (2011). Coming full circle: Planning for future pathways of transitions of care for older adults. *Annual Review of Gerontology & Geriatrics, 31,* 231–254.

Kuhlmann, E., & Annandale, E. (2010). *The Palgrave handbook of gender and healthcare.* New York, NY: Palgrave Macmillan.

Kulikov, E. (2011). The social and policy predictors of driving mobility among older adults. *Journal of Aging & Social Policy, 23*(1), 1–18. http://dx.doi.org/10.1080/08959420.2011.5 31991.

Kwak, J., Allen, J. Y., & Haley, W. E. (2011). Advance care planning and end-of-life decision making. *Annual Review of Gerontology & Geriatrics, 31,* 143–165.

Lahaie, C., Earle, A., & Heymann, J. (2013). An uneven burden: Social disparities in adult caregiving responsibilities, working conditions, and caregiver outcomes. *Research on Aging, 35*(3), 243–274. http://dx.doi.org/10.1177/0164027512446028.

Layne, J. E., Sampson, S. E., Mallio, C. J., Hibberd, P. L., Griffith, J. L., Das, S., et al. (2008). Successful dissemination of a community-based strength training program for older adults by peer and professional leaders: The people exercising program. *Journal of the American Geriatrics Society, 56*(12), 2323–2329. http://dx.doi.org/10.1111/j.1532-5415.2008.02010.x.

Lehning, A. J. (2011). City governments and aging in place: Community design, transportation and housing innovation adoption. *The Gerontologist, 52*(3), 345–356. http://dx.doi. org/10.1093/geront/gnr089.

Liao, P., Chang, H., & Sun, L. (2012). National health insurance program and life satisfaction of the elderly. *Aging & Mental Health, 16*(8), 983–992. http://dx.doi. org/10.1080/13607863.2012.-692765.

Locher, J. L., Ritchie, C. S., Robinson, C. O., Roth, D. L., West, D., & Burgio, K. L. (2008). A multidimensional approach to understanding under-eating in homebound older adults: The importance of social factors. *Gerontologist, 48*(2), 223–234.

Lowenstein, A., Eisikovits, Z., Band-Winterstein, T., & Enosh, G. (2009). Is elder abuse and neglect a social phenomenon? Data from the first national prevalence survey in Israel. *Journal of Elder Abuse & Neglect, 21*(3), 253–277. http://dx.doi.org/10.1080/08946560902997629.

Luo, L. (2010). Employment among older workers and inequality of gender and education: Evidence from a Taiwanese national survey. *International Journal of Aging & Human Development, 70*(2), 145–162. http://dx.doi.org/10.2190/AG.70.2.c.

Manheimer, R. J. (2008). Lifelong learning in aging societies: Emerging paradigms. *Annual Review of Gerontology & Geriatrics, 28,* 111–127.

Marson, D. C., & Sabatino, C. P. (2012). Financial capacity in an aging society. *Generations, 36*(2), 6–11.

Matosevic, T., Knapp, M., Grand, J. L., & Fernandez, J. (2011). Changes over time: The motivations of independent sector care home managers and owners in England between 1994 and 2003. *Ageing and Society, 31,* 1389–1405. http://dx.doi.org/10.1017/ S0144686X10001480.

Miles, T. P. (2009). Health care reform and health disparities. *Annual Review of Gerontology & Geriatrics, 29*(275–289), R13.

Minkler, M., & Stone, R. (1985). The feminization of poverty and older women. *The Gerontologist, 25*(4), 351–357. http://dx.doi.org/10.1093/geront/25.4.351.

Mor, V., Gruneir, A., Feng, Z., Grabowski, D. C., Intrator, O., & Zinn, J. (2011). The effect of state policies on nursing home resident outcomes. *Journal of Applied Gerontology, 59,* 3–9.

Moye, J., & Marson, D. C. (2007). Assessment of decision-making capacity in older adults: An emerging area of practice and research. *The Journals of Gerontology Series B: Psychological Sciences and Social Sciences, 62*(1), P3–P11.

Muramatsu, N., & Akiyama, H. (2011). Japan: Super-aging society preparing for the future. *The Gerontologist, 51*(4), 425–432. http://dx.doi.org/10.1093/geront/gnr067.

Newbold, K. B., Scott, D. M., Spinney, J. E., Kanaroglou, P., & Páez, A. (2005). Travel behavior within Canada's older population: A cohort analysis. *Journal of Transport Geography, 13*(4), 340–351.

Nwagbara, E. N., Etuk, G. R., & Baghebo, M. (2012). The social phenomenon of women empowerment in Nigeria: A theoretical approach. *Sociology Mind, 2*(4), 388–393. http://dx.doi.org/10.4236/sm.2012.24051.

Pampel, F. C. (1998). *Aging, social inequality, and public policy.* Thousand Oaks, CA: Sage.

Putnam, M. (2011). Perceptions of difference between aging and disability service systems consumers: Implications for policy initiatives to rebalance long-term care. *Journal of Gerontological Social Work, 54*(3), 325–342.

Redfoot, D. L., & Houser, A. N. (2008). The international migration of nurses in long-term care. *Journal of Aging & Social Policy, 20*(2), 259–275.

Reinhard, S. C., & Lind, K. D. (2011). Public policy implications for pathways through transitions: The rise of the transitional care concept. *Annual Review of Gerontology & Geriatrics, 31,* 209–229.

Rejeski, W., Ip, E. H., Marsh, A. P., & Barnard, R. T. (2010). Development and validation of a video-animated tool for assessing mobility. *Journals of Gerontology Series A: Biological Sciences & Medical Sciences, 65A*(6), 664–671.

Rich, B. M., & Baum, M. (1985). *The aging: A guide to public policy.* Pittsburg, PA: University of Pittsburgh Press.

Rockwell, J. (2010). Deconstructing housework: Cuts to home support services and the implications for hospital discharge planning. *Journal of Women & Aging, 22*(1), 47–60. http://dx.doi.org/10.1080/08952840903489052.

Scarfo, B. (2011). Building a more sustainable future for senior living. *Educational Gerontology, 37*(6), 466–487. http://dx.doi.org/10.1080/03601277.2011.570198.

Shaevitz, M. H. (1984). *The superwoman syndrome.* New York, NY: Warner Books.612

Shenfil, S. (2009). Pathways to positive aging: A program to build an aging-friendly community. *Generations, 33*(2), 82–84.

Singh, L. P., Sharma, A., Kumar, M., & Shinwari, S. (2012). Public health care in Afghanistan: An investigation in suboptimal utilization of facilities. *Health, 4*(10), 794–801. http://dx.doi.org/10.4236/health.2012.410123.

Slack, T., & Jensen, L. (2008). Employment hardship among older workers: Does residential and gender inequality extend into older age? *Journals of Gerontology Series B: Psychological Sciences & Social Sciences, 63B*(1), S15–S24.

Soonman, K. (2008). Future of long-term care financing for the elderly in Korea. *Journal of Aging & Social Policy, 20*(1), 119–136.

Spetz, J. (2005). The aging of the nurse workforce: Recent trends and future challenges. *Annual Review of Gerontology & Geriatrics, 25*(65–87), R10–R11.

Stephenson, A., Anderson, G. M., & Rochon, P. (2012). Off-label prescribing in older people: The need for increased awareness and caution. *Drugs & Aging, 29*(6), 435–436.

Sterns, A. A., & Ansello, E. F. (2008). Education about special aging populations: Intellectually disabled, incarcerated, and non-English speaking. In H. L. Sterns & M. A. Bernard (Eds.), *Annual review of gerontology and geriatrics, gerontological and geriatric education* (Vol. 28, pp. 185–216). New York, NY: Springer.http://dx.doi.org/10.1891/0198-879428185.

Stone, R., & National Center for Health Services Research and Health Care Technology Assessment, (1987). *The feminization of poverty and older women.* Rockville, MD: US Department of Health and Human Services, Public Health Service, National Center for Health Services Research and Health Care Technology Assessment.

Stone, R. I., & Bryant, N. S. (2011). Educating direct care workers on transitions of care. *Annual Review of Gerontology & Geriatrics, 31*, 167–188.

Street, D., Burge, S., & Quadagno, J. (2009). The effect of licensure type on the policies, practices, and resident composition of Florida assisted living facilities. *Gerontologist, 49*(2), 211–223. http://dx.doi.org/10.1093/geront/gnp022.

Thorpe, R. J., Clay, O. J., Szanton, S. L., Allaire, J. C., & Whitfield, K. E. (2011). Correlates of mobility limitation in African Americans. *Journals of Gerontology Series A: Biological Sciences & Medical Sciences, 66A*(11), 1258–1263.

Whitfield, K. E., Edwards, C. L., & Nelson, T. L. (2010). Methodological considerations for the examination of complex systems in aging. *Annual Review of Gerontology & Geriatrics, 30*, 35–56.

Williams, B. A., Stern, M. F., Mellow, J., Safer, M., & Greifinger, R. B. (2012). Aging in correctional custody: Setting a policy agenda for older prisoner health care. *American Journal of Public Health, 102*(8), 1475–1481. http://dx.doi.org/10.2105/JPH.2012.300704.

Williams, J. N. (2005). The aging dental workforce: Implications for the 21st century. *Annual Review of Gerontology & Geriatrics, 25*(89–97), R12.

Winter, D. G., Torges, C. M., Stewart, A. J., Henderson-King, D., & Henderson-King, E. (2006). Pathways toward the third age: Studying a cohort from the "golden age". *Annual Review of Gerontology & Geriatrics, 26*(103–129), R10–R11.

Wolff, J. L., Kasper, J. D., & Shore, A. D. (2008). Long-term care preferences among older adults: A moving target? *Journal of Aging & Social Policy, 20*(2), 182–200.

Yeo, G., & McBride, M. (2008). Cultural diversity in gerontology and geriatrics education. In H. L. Sterns & M. A. Bernard (Eds.), *Annual review of gerontology and geriatrics, gerontological and geriatric education* (Vol. 28, pp. 93–109). New York, NY: Springer.http://dx.doi.org/10.1891/0198879428185.

Zhang, N. J., Guo, M., & Zheng, X. (2012). China: Awakening giant developing solutions to population aging. *The Gerontologist, 52*(5), 589–596. http://dx.doi.org/10.1093/geront/gns105.

Zhenmei, Z., Danan, G., & Hayward, M. D. (2008). Early life influences on cognitive impairment among oldest old Chinese. *Journals of Gerontology Series B: Psychological Sciences & Social Sciences, 63B*(1), S25–S33.

Aging Knowledge and Attitude Surveys

Palmore's Facts on Aging Quiz
—Harris, D. K., Changas, P. S., & Palmore, E. B. (1996).
Palmore's first facts on aging quiz in a multiple-choice format.
Educational Gerontology, 22, 575–589.

Instructions: Please select one option for each question.

1. The proportion of people over 65 who are senile (have impaired memory, disorientation, or dementia) is:
   A. about 1 in 100.
   B. about 1 in 10.
   C. about 1 in 2.
   D. the majority.

2. The senses that tend to weaken in old age are:
   A. sight and hearing.
   B. taste and smell.
   C. sight, hearing, and touch.
   D. all five senses.

3. The majority of old couples:
   A. have little or no interest in sex.
   B. are not able to have sexual relations.
   C. continue to enjoy sexual relations.
   D. think sex is only for the young.

4. Lung vital capacity in old age:
   A. tends to decline.
   B. stays about the same among nonsmokers.
   C. tends to increase among healthy old people.
   D. is unrelated to age.

5. Happiness among old people is:
   A. rare.
   B. less common than among younger people.
   C. about as common as among younger people.
   D. more common than among younger people.

6. Physical strength:
   A. tends to decline with age.
   B. tends to remain the same among healthy old people.
   C. tends to increase among healthy old people.
   D. is unrelated to age.

7. The percentage of people over 65 in long-stay institutions (such as nursing homes, mental hospitals, and homes for the aged) is about:
   A. 5%.
   B. 10%.
   C. 25%.
   D. 50%.

8. The accident rate per driver over age 65 is:
   A. higher than for those under 65.
   B. about the same as for those under 65.
   C. lower than for those under 65.
   D. unknown.

9. Most workers over 65:
   A. work less effectively than younger workers.
   B. work as effectively as younger workers.
   C. work more effectively than younger workers.
   D. are preferred by most employers.

10. The proportion of people over 65 who are able to do their normal activities is about:
    A. one-tenth.
    B. one-quarter.
    C. one-half.
    D. three-fourths.

11. Adaptability to change among people over 65 is:
    A. rare.
    B. present among about half.
    C. present among most.
    D. more common than among younger people.

12. As for old people learning new things:
    A. most are unable to learn at any speed.
    B. most are able to learn, but at a slower speed.
    C. most are able to learn as fast as younger people.
    D. learning speed is unrelated to age.

13. Depression is more frequent among:
    A. people over 65.
    B. adults under 65.
    C. young people.
    D. children.

14. Old people tend to react:
    A. slower than younger people.
    B. at about the same speed as younger people.
    C. faster than younger people.
    D. slower or faster than younger people, depending on the type of test.

15. Old people tend to be:
    A. more alike than younger people.
    B. the same as younger people in terms of alikeness.
    C. less alike than younger people.
    D. more alike in some respects and less alike in others.

16. Most old people say:
    A. they are seldom bored.
    B. they are sometimes bored.
    C. they are often bored.
    D. life is monotonous.

17. The proportion of old people who are socially isolated is:
    A. almost all.
    B. about half.
    C. less than a fourth.
    D. almost none.

18. The accident rate among workers over 65 tends to be:
    A. higher than among younger workers.
    B. about the same as among younger workers.
    C. lower than among younger workers.
    D. unknown because there are so few workers over 65.

19. The proportion of the U.S. population now age 65 or over is:
    A. 3%.
    B. 13%.
    C. 23%.
    D. 33%.

20. Medical practitioners tend to give older patients:
    A. lower priority than younger patients.
    B. the same priority as younger patients.
    C. higher priority than younger patients.
    D. higher priority if they have Medicaid.

21. The poverty rate (as defined by the federal government) among old people is:
 A. higher than among children under age 18.
 B. higher than among all persons under 65.
 C. about the same as among persons under 65.
 D. lower than among persons under 65.

22. Most old people are:
 A. employed.
 B. employed or would like to be employed.
 C. employed, do housework or volunteer work, or would like to do some kind of work.
 D. not interested in any work.

23. Religiosity tends to:
 A. increase in old age.
 B. decrease in old age.
 C. be greater in the older generation than in the younger generations.
 D. be unrelated to age.

24. Most old people:
 A. are seldom angry.
 B. are often angry.
 C. are often grouchy.
 D. often lose their tempers.

Correct Answers:

1. B	6. A	11. C	16. A	21. D
2. D	7. A	12. B	17. C	22. C
3. C	8. C	13. B	18. C	23. C
4. A	9. B	14. A	19. B	24. A
5. C	10. D	15. D	20. A	

Aging Perceptions Questionnaire (APQ)
—Barker, M., O'Hanlon, A., McGee, H. M., Hickey, A., & Conroy, R. M. (2007). Cross-sectional validation of the Aging Perceptions Questionnaire: A multidimensional instrument for assessing self-perceptions of aging. BMC Geriatrics, 7(9), published online. doi:10.1186/1471-2318-7-9.

Instructions: These questions assess your views and experiences of getting older. Since everyone is getting older, these questions can be answered by anyone of any age. There are no right or wrong answers—just your experiences and views. Even if the statement relates to something you do not often think about in relation to yourself, please try to give an indication of your views by answering every question.

A. VIEWS ABOUT AGING

We are interested in *your own personal views and experiences* about getting older. Please indicate your views on the following statements (strongly disagree, disagree, neither agree nor disagree, agree, or strongly agree). Circle the response that best describes your view for each statement.

	Strongly disagree	Disagree	Neither agree nor disagree	Agree	Strongly agree
1. I am conscious of getting older all of the time	□₁	□₂	□₃	□₄	□₅
2. I am always aware of my age	□₁	□₂	□₃	□₄	□₅
3. I always classify myself as old	□₁	□₂	□₃	□₄	□₅
4. I am always aware of the fact that I am getting older	□₁	□₂	□₃	□₄	□₅
5. I feel my age in everything that I do	□₁	□₂	□₃	□₄	□₅
6. As I get older I get wiser	□₁	□₂	□₃	□₄	□₅
7. As I get older I continue to grow as a person	□₁	□₂	□₃	□₄	□₅
8. As I get older I appreciate things more	□₁	□₂	□₃	□₄	□₅
9. I get depressed when I think about how ageing might affect the things that I can do	□₁	□₂	□₃	□₄	□₅
10. The quality of my social life in later years depends on me	□₁	□₂	□₃	□₄	□₅
11. The quality of my relationships with others in later life depends on me	□₁	□₂	□₃	□₄	□₅
12. Whether I continue living life to the full depends on me	□₁	□₂	□₃	□₄	□₅
13. I get depressed when I think about the effects that getting older might have on my social life	□₁	□₂	□₃	□₄	□₅
14. As I get older there is much I can do to maintain my independence	□₁	□₂	□₃	□₄	□₅
15. Whether getting older has positive sides to it depends on me	□₁	□₂	□₃	□₄	□₅

16. Getting older restricts the things that I can do	$\Box_1$	$\Box_2$	$\Box_3$	$\Box_4$	$\Box_5$
17. Getting older makes me less independent	$\Box_1$	$\Box_2$	$\Box_3$	$\Box_4$	$\Box_5$
18. Getting older makes everything a lot harder for me	$\Box_1$	$\Box_2$	$\Box_3$	$\Box_4$	$\Box_5$
19. As I get older I can take part in fewer activities	$\Box_1$	$\Box_2$	$\Box_3$	$\Box_4$	$\Box_5$
20. As I get older I do not cope as well with problems that arise	$\Box_1$	$\Box_2$	$\Box_3$	$\Box_4$	$\Box_5$
21. Slowing down with age is not something I can control	$\Box_1$	$\Box_2$	$\Box_3$	$\Box_4$	$\Box_5$
22. How mobile I am in later life is not up to me	$\Box_1$	$\Box_2$	$\Box_3$	$\Box_4$	$\Box_5$
23. I have no control over whether I lose vitality or zest for life as I age	$\Box_1$	$\Box_2$	$\Box_3$	$\Box_4$	$\Box_5$
24. I have no control over the effects that getting older has on my social life	$\Box_1$	$\Box_2$	$\Box_3$	$\Box_4$	$\Box_5$
25. I get depressed when I think about getting older	$\Box_1$	$\Box_2$	$\Box_3$	$\Box_4$	$\Box_5$
26. I worry about the effects that getting older may have on my relationships with others	$\Box_1$	$\Box_2$	$\Box_3$	$\Box_4$	$\Box_5$
27. I go through cycles in which my experience of aging gets better and worse	$\Box_1$	$\Box_2$	$\Box_3$	$\Box_4$	$\Box_5$
28. My awareness of getting older comes and goes in cycles	$\Box_1$	$\Box_2$	$\Box_3$	$\Box_4$	$\Box_5$
29. I feel angry when I think about getting older	$\Box_1$	$\Box_2$	$\Box_3$	$\Box_4$	$\Box_5$
30. I go through phases of feeling old	$\Box_1$	$\Box_2$	$\Box_3$	$\Box_4$	$\Box_5$
31. My awareness of getting older changes a great deal from day to day	$\Box_1$	$\Box_2$	$\Box_3$	$\Box_4$	$\Box_5$
32. I go through phases of viewing myself as being old	$\Box_1$	$\Box_2$	$\Box_3$	$\Box_4$	$\Box_5$

B. EXPERIENCE OF HEALTH-RELATED CHANGES

The next list describes some health-related changes you may have experienced. Can you tell me whether you have experienced these changes in the last 10 years and whether you believe that the changes experienced are specifically related to getting older or not.

		HAVE you experienced this change?		"In terms of the changes you HAVE experienced: Do you think this change is ONLY related to, or due to the fact that, you are getting older"?	
		Yes	No	Yes	No
Id1	Weight problems	$\square_1$	$\square_0$	$\square_1$	$\square_0$
Id2	Sleep problems	$\square_1$	$\square_0$	$\square_1$	$\square_0$
Id3	Back problems or slipped disc	$\square_1$	$\square_0$	$\square_1$	$\square_0$
Id4	Painful joints	$\square_1$	$\square_0$	$\square_1$	$\square_0$
Id5	Not being mobile	$\square_1$	$\square_0$	$\square_1$	$\square_0$
Id6	Loss of balance	$\square_1$	$\square_0$	$\square_1$	$\square_0$
Id7	Loss of strength	$\square_1$	$\square_0$	$\square_1$	$\square_0$
Id8	Slowing down	$\square_1$	$\square_0$	$\square_1$	$\square_0$
Id9	Cramps	$\square_1$	$\square_0$	$\square_1$	$\square_0$
Id10	Bone or joint conditions	$\square_1$	$\square_0$	$\square_1$	$\square_0$
Id11	Cardiac or heart problems	$\square_1$	$\square_0$	$\square_1$	$\square_0$
Id12	Ear or hearing problems	$\square_1$	$\square_0$	$\square_1$	$\square_0$
Id13	Vision and eyesight changes	$\square_1$	$\square_0$	$\square_1$	$\square_0$
Id14	Respiratory problems	$\square_1$	$\square_0$	$\square_1$	$\square_0$
Id15	Foot problems	$\square_1$	$\square_0$	$\square_1$	$\square_0$
Id16	Depression	$\square_1$	$\square_0$	$\square_1$	$\square_0$
Id17	Anxiety	$\square_1$	$\square_0$	$\square_1$	$\square_0$

Scoring:
A. Views about getting older
 Timeline acute/chronic: Mean of items 1, 2, 3, 4, and 5
 Timeline cyclical: Mean of items 27, 28, 30, 31, and 32
 Emotional representations: Mean of items 9, 13, 25, 26, and 29
 Control positive: Mean of items 10, 11, 12, 14, 15
 Control negative: Mean of items 21, 22, 23, and 24 (items are reverse-scored)
 Consequences positive: Mean of items 6, 7, and 8
 Consequences negative: Mean of items 16, 17, 18, 19, and 20
B. Experience of health-related changes
 Number of health-related changes experienced=sum of Id1a, Id2a, Id3a, Id4a, Id5a, Id6a, Id7a, Id8a, Id9a, Id10a, Id11a, Id12a, Id13a, Id14a, Id15a, Id16a, Id17a
 Number of health-related changes attributed to aging=sum of Id1b, Id2b, Id3b, Id4b, Id5b, Id6b, Id7b, Id8b, Id9b, Id10b, Id11b, Id12b, Id13b, Id14b, Id15b, Id16b, Id17b
 Identity score: (number of changes attributed to aging/number of health-related changes experienced) × 100

Can You Spot Age Discrimination in the Workplace? (AARP Quiz)
 —*Carole Fleck (June 2014) AARP. http://www.aarp.org/work/on-the-job/info-2014/workplace-age-discrimination-quiz.html.*

1. The Age Discrimination in Employment Act (ADEA) of 1967 protects workers 40 and older from personnel decisions based on age, including hiring, firing, layoffs, promotions or demotions.
 A.____True **B.**____ False

2. The deadline to file an age discrimination claim is generally within 180 days from the date the suspected discrimination took place.
 A.____True **B.**____ False

3. A bill called the *Protecting Older Workers Against Discrimination Act*, introduced in Congress in 2012, would:
 A.____Amend the Age Discrimination in Employment Act
 B.____Clarify standards for discrimination claims
 C.____Strengthen age discrimination laws
 D.____All of the above

4. If you see employers do this, it is illegal:
 A.____Mention in job ads that they want to hire energetic young workers
 B.____Force workers to retire at a certain age
 C.____Fire older workers for performance issues
 D.____Both A and B

5. What are some warning signs that you could be facing age discrimination at work?
   A.____Years of solid performance reviews suddenly turn negative.
   B.____You're given new demands or quotas that seem harsh and unreasonable.
   C.____Younger employees are given on-the-job training courses that you and other older workers are not offered.
   D.____All of the above

6. Which federal agency investigates age discrimination claims?
   A.____Consumer Financial Protection Bureau
   B.____Federal Communications Commission
   C.____Federal Bureau of Investigation
   D.____Equal Employment Opportunity Commission

7. How many age discrimination claims were filed in 2013?
   A.____4702
   B.____8410
   C.____15,050
   D.____21,396

8. If you're considering filing an age discrimination claim, you should:
   A.____Talk with a lawyer who specializes in employment issues.
   B.____Keep a record of documents, situations, comments or anything else that suggests age discrimination.
   C.____Have a lawyer review the documents your employer asked you to sign before you leave your job.
   D.____All of the above

Scoring: 1. A, 2. A, 3. D, 4. D, 5. D, 6. D, 7. D, 8. D.

EXPERIENCED WORKFORCE QUIZ

Learn Why Older Workers Are a Valuable Asset (AARP)
   —*AARP (June 2013). http://www.aarp.org/work/on-the-job/info-06-2013/experienced-workforce-quiz.html?intcmp*=AE-WOR-RELBOX.

1. By 2016, what portion of the total workforce will be age 50 or older?
   A.____One-fifth
   B.____One-third
   C.____One-half
   D.____Three-fifths

2. Why is it important to attract and retain experienced employees?
   A.____There's a need to fill critical skills shortages so companies can retain their competitive edge.
   B.____Unemployment rate needs to be lower.
   C.____Experienced workers have a better work ethic than younger workers.
   D.____None of the above

3. Which of the following is not considered to be one of the fastest-growing careers by 2018?
   A.____Home health aide
   B.____Computer software engineer
   C.____Skin care expert
   D.____Lawyer

4. Approximately how many people ages 44–70 are interested in starting their own business?
   A.____1 in 4
   B.____2 in 3
   C.____1 in 3
   D.____1 in 2

5. Which of the following would most workers *not* consider a key feature of their ideal job?
   A.____The chance to use their skills and talents
   B.____A friendly work environment
   C.____Feeling respected by coworkers
   D.____On-site cafeteria

6. In 2010, one of the most common jobs for someone age 55-plus was as a registered nurse. Approximately how many people were employed as RNs?
   A.____1 million
   B.____636,000
   C.____763,000
   D.____559,000

7. What percentage of Americans are interested in teaching as a second career?
   A.____25%
   B.____46%
   C.____37%
   D.____31%

8. By 2020, approximately how many Americans are likely to be teleworkers?
   A.____50 million
   B.____60 million
   C.____70 million
   D.____40 million

9. What do employers value in experienced workers?
   A.____Reliability and trustworthiness
   B.____Stability and consistency
   C.____Expertise
   D.____All of the above

10. AARP has an awards program that recognizes organizations that value an experienced workforce. What is the name of that awards program?
    A.____Best employers for workers over 50
    B.____Best employers for older workers
    C.____Best places to work when you are over 50
    D.____Top companies for workers over 50

Scoring: 1. B, 2. A, 3. D, 4. A, 5. D, 6. B, 7. D, 8. B, 9. D, 10. A.

List of National and International Support Resources by Topic

NATIONAL AND INTERNATIONAL WOMEN'S ORGANIZATIONS

Mentoring Women's Network Foundation

Address: 202 East Market Street, Indianapolis, IN 46204
Telephone: 317-240-4482
Website: www.mentoringwomensnetwork.com
Description: The mentoring women's network is focused on developing women through mentoring relationships so that women can reach their full potential professionally. To participate as a mentor or mentee one must join as a member. The services include networking events (local and virtual), leadership skills, development training, and access to up to four mentors per year. The website offers very helpful forums for communicating through "chat" as well as photos, videos, and posted opportunities for members to communicate.

Women's Business Development Center

Address: 8 S. Michigan Ave., 4th Floor, Chicago, IL 60603
Telephone: 312-853-3477
Email: wbdc@wbdc.org
Website: www.wbdc.org
Description: Women's Business Development Center offers guidance and courses to women starting a new business or women who are currently in business. The website offers assistive information regarding international business development opportunities and business-related contacts. There is also an opportunity for certification under the Women's Business

Enterprise (WBE) certification program, which is offered in Midwestern states of Illinois, Iowa, Kansas, Minnesota, Missouri, Nebraska, North Dakota, South Dakota, and Wisconsin.

There are helpful resources and tools and ways to connect with women for lifespan business opportunities.

The Lilac Tree

Address: 1123 Emerson St., Suite 215, Evanston, IL 60201
Telephone: 847-328-0313
Email: info@thelilactree.org
Website: www.lilactree.org
Description: The Lilac Tree offers resources for divorcing women. The organization includes individual information sessions, support groups, workshops, and seminars. The website offers the opportunity for women contemplating or undergoing divorce to better understand the normative experiences of other women. Divorce University is offered as an educational experience for women across the life span. This is a difficult decision that impacts both the aging woman and her family system, and this website and organization helps women realize that they are not alone.

Advancing Women

Website: www.advancingwomen.com
Description: Advancing Women is a recruiting website that connects companies with jobs seeking women in the fields of engineering, manufacturing, construction, technology, biotech, medical, financial, government, and the defense/security industry. There is a variety of information presented to help women of diverse backgrounds connect with employers and clients for the purpose of career mentoring. Research as well as very practical advice is offered to assist women in becoming successful business entrepreneurs. This is especially relevant as many women are delaying retirement and are faced with the task of establishing a new second, third, or "more" career in later life.

Wing to Wing Women's Mentoring Project

Website: www.wing2wingproject.com
Description: Wing to Wing offers mentor relationship opportunities for women to achieve personal and professional growth. The website presents information about how women can get involved to be a volunteer mentor, and help women of different regions of the world psychologically and emotionally grow across life stages. Women can share personal stories of

learning and wisdom. This forum of sharing and communicating life experiences can be a wonderful resource for aging women as they deal with many different concerns about elder caregiving, adjustment to personal aging, and all the different role-related adjustments of women as they age.

Women's Resource Center

Address: 113 W. Wayne Ave., P.O. Box 596, Wayne, PA 19087
Telephone: 610-687-6391
Email: info@womensrc.org
Website: www.womenresourcecenter.net
Description: The Women's Resource Center website offers helpful information for girls and women living in the Philadelphia, Delaware, Chester, Montgomery, and Bucks County locations regarding resources, events, and support services. The aim of the organization is to support the positive development of women over life span, building self-esteem, social skills, and effective life skills for positive adaptation over time. Although an aging woman may not be in this specific regional location, the ideas presented through the organization's website may still be useful in terms of starting community program initiatives for women in their unique region of the world.

Office of Women's Policy and Initiatives

Address: John A. Wilson Building, 1350 Pennsylvania Ave., NW, Suite 327, Washington, DC 20004
Telephone: 202-724-7690
Email: women@dc.gov
Website: www.owpi.dc.gov
Description: The website offers resources for domestic violence, financial literacy; wellness and health; workforce development and preparedness; and resources for women. This is a critical social and ethical issue for many different communities across the world. This website offers important public policy information about events, research, and legislation, tackling issues impacting the quality of life of women of all ages and backgrounds in the United States and across the world.

Older Women's League

Address: 1627 Eye Street, NW, Suite 600 Washington, DC 20006
Telephone: 202-450-8986
Email: info@owl-national.org
Website: http://www.owl-national.org/

Description: The mission of the Older Women's League (OWL) is to empower and give a voice to older women age 40 and older. The website offers information regarding various media-related resources and ways to connect with other women age 40 and above interested in the many different opportunities for older women's self-growth and development in careers (eg, encore careers), education, volunteerism, and other activities in society. The website encourages older women to be active, involved participants in politics, public policy, and personal initiatives.

Red Hat Society

Address: 431 S. Acacia Avenue Fullerton, CA 92831
Telephone: 866-386-2850 (US), 714-738-0001 (International)
Website: http://www.redhatsociety.com/
Description: The Red Hat Society is an interesting organization for aging women who wish to maintain and acquire a wonderful social network of women within communities. The aim of the organization is to break down social barriers, eradicate negative stereotypes, and promote positive images of older women in society. The Red Hat Society promotes a very positive message about celebrating the power and beauty of aging women.

Supportive Older Women's Network

Address: 4100 Main Street, Suite 403 Philadelphia, PA 19127
Telephone: 215-487-3000; *Fax*: 215-487-3111
Email: info@sown.org
Website: http://www.sown.org/
Description: The mission of Supportive Older Women's Network (SOWN) is to strengthen the quality of life in older women's lives through various networking opportunities. Through the different networking activities and information presented on the website, older women are encouraged to share and learn from personal insights/stories, problem-solving strategies, coping skills, and ideas in how to gain personal control over their lives when aging creates so many personal changes and alterations in daily life activities.

Strong Women

Address: Friedman School of Nutrition Science and Policy, Tufts University, 150 Harrison Ave., Boston, MA 02111
Telephone: N/A
Email: strongwomen@tufts.edu
Website: www.strongwomen.com

Description: Strong Women is a national community-based training program established by Dr. Miriam E. Nelson and colleagues' research on bone density in older adults. The program focuses on two curricula: Strong Woman Strength training, which focuses on building muscle mass for middle to older age women and Strong Women-Healthy Heart, which focuses on nutrition and fitness as women age. Local programs and upcoming workshops can be found by searching on the website.

Canadian Network of Women's Shelters and Transition Houses

Telephone: 613-680-5119
Email: info@endvaw.ca
Website: www.endvaw.ca
Description: The Canadian Network of Women's Shelters and Transition Houses is an online service directing women to shelters and transition homes in their area. These homes and shelters are for the purpose of supporting women and their families who are involved in abusive and violent relationships.

Women for Women International, Global Headquarters

Address: 2000 M Street, NW, Suite 200 Washington, DC 20036
Telephone: 202-737-7705
Fax: 202-737-7709
Email: general@womenforwomen.org
Website: http://www.womenforwomen.org/
Description: As an international resource Women for Women aids those in war stricken countries to gain education and to learn skills relevant to providing income for themselves and their family members. The program also educates women on health management and human rights. These women in turn go on to educate others in their communities to advocate for change in war stricken countries. A list of the current countries is hosted on the website provided.

Women's Institute for a Secure Retirement

Address: 1140 19th St. NW, Suite 550 Washington, DC 20036
Telephone: 202-393-5452
Fax: 202-393-5890
Email: info@wiserwomen.org
Website: www.wiserwomen.org

Description: The Women's Institute for Secure Retirement (WISER) organization and associated website is focused upon assisting women in achieving and maintaining financial security into later life through informational workshops, helpful research resources, and networking opportunities within communities and with experienced financial mentors. Complex topics are presented, ranging from the impact of divorce women's financial status to the issues of planning for retirement, and associated pension planning.

Office of Women's Health, US Department of Health and Human Services

Address: Department of Health and Human Services, 200 Independence Ave. SW Room 712 E, Washington, DC 20201
Telephone: 202-690-7650 or Help line 800-994-9662
Website: www.womenshealth.gov
Description: This program is focused on supporting women's health throughout the United States. The website provides research-based facts on current health topics for women. The helpline assists with directing inquiries to regionally based women's health programs. The main goal of the office of women's health is to improve policies, education, and model programs focused on women's health.

GENERAL AGING INFORMATION RESOURCES

National Institute on Aging

Address: 31 Center Dr., MSC 2292, Bethesda, MD 20892
Telephone: 800-222-2225
Email: niaic@nia.nih.gov
Website: www.nia.nih.gov
Description: The National Institute in Aging (NIH) website offers research-based information on topics in women's aging such as menopause and sexuality in later life. The website hosts a variety of topics in aging such as loss of spouse, skin care, Alzheimer's disease, and even advice for communicating with the doctor.

American Association of Retired Persons

Website: http://www.aarp.org
Description: The American Association of Retired Persons (AARP) the membership organization for adults aged 50 and older who are interested

in receiving information regarding consumer protection, eldercare, and/ or financial planning into later life. For aging women, all of these topics would be very important for their continued positive adjustment on financial, social, and psychological bases. From a public policy perspective, AARP offers representation as a "voice" in politics for many different legislative issues that are vital to older woman.

American Society on Aging

Address: 575 Market St., Suite 2100 San Francisco, CA 94105-2869
Telephone: 415-974-9600, 800-537-9728
Fax: 415-974-0300
Website: http://www.asaging.org
Description: The American Society on Aging (ASA) is a comprehensive website offering opportunities for aging women in terms of educational and business resources and information toward the diverse experiences of different groups and their related issues as they age. National conferences, web seminars, publications, and other helpful information (eg, MindAlert) will empower aging women to seek and utilize information and resources to age more positively and help those in their communities. There is important dual focus for older women, which is providing both information and training for older adults and those that care for them (eg, healthcare workers). This information can also be utilized as professional development for women as they decide to transition into professional careers within the aging field.

Alliance for Aging Research

Address: 1700 K St., NW, Suite 740 Washington, DC 20006
Telephone: 202-293-2856
Fax: 202-955-8394
Email: info@agingresearch.org
Website: http://www.agingresearch.org
Description: The Alliance for Aging Research focuses on public policy and health information to improve the quality of health and lives of aging adults. Information regarding public policy initiatives, healthcare-related information, and associated advocacy organizations is presented on the organization's website to help inform the aging population about resources and guidelines. Beyond general aging issues, older women would benefit from information pertaining to gender-specific issues of health- and role-related responsibilities, which could impact personal issues of adaptation (eg, caring for a significant other with Alzheimer's disease).

Association for Gerontology in Higher Education

Address: 1220 L Street, NW, Suite 901 Washington, DC 20005-4018
Telephone: 202-289-9806
Fax: 202-289-9824
Email: aghe@aghe.org
Website: http://www.aghe.org/
Description: The Association for Gerontology in Higher Education (AGHE) as a professional membership organization has the primary aim of educating both professionals, students, faculty, and the general public regarding many different aging-related phenomenon and trends from national and international perspectives. Annual meetings, publications, and website resources that offer excellent educational opportunities, and social networking venues for older women to better understand their personal aging trajectories and how they can better apply it to their personal lives and or professional practices.

Gerontological Society of America

Address: 1220 L Street NW, Suite 901 Washington, DC 20005
Telephone: 202-842-1275
Website: http://www.geron.org/
Description: The Gerontological Society of America (GSA) is an organization that has been concerned over many decades with a positive promotion of aging issues through training, information dissemination, and networking amongst professionals in the field. The website offers information that would be helpful to both women interested in starting or changing their career into the aging field, as well as investigating personal information related to aging. Although it is a national conference, it encompasses research and professional networking for many different countries across the world.

HelpAge International

Website: http://www.helpage.org/home
Description: HelpAge International as an organization has the overarching aim of protecting and expanding the rights of older adults across the world. Issues of healthcare, age-friendly environments, economic security, living conditions, and safety concerns are just a sample of the initiatives promoted through this advocacy organization. Certainly aging issues but also gender by aging biases and stereotypes that need to be rectified in societies that this organization would assist with through 100 affiliates in 65 countries.

Leadership Council of Aging Organizations

Telephone: 202-434-2470
Email: LCAO@aarp.org
Website: http://www.lcao.org/
Description: The Leadership Council of Aging Organizations is an interesting advocacy coalition that may not directly invite an aging population as membership, but does have very significant functioning as a united membership of national nonprofit aging service organizations. Knowledge of such coalitions can certainly benefit older women as they seek out local and national resources regarding elder advocacy organizations, which may be able to help with their aging-related needs and concerns. The power of such organizational coalitions is that they can be the "voice" for aging women's issues and can be the impetus for public policy change on a local, state, and/or national level.

National Association of Area Agencies on Aging

Address: 1730 Rhode Island Ave, NW, Suite 1200 Washington, DC 20036
Telephone: 202-872-0888
Fax: 202-872-0057
Website: http://www.n4a.org
Description: The National Association of Area Agencies on Aging (n4a) is a user-friendly website, which allows people to input their location to find qualified and reliable eldercare services, managed care locations, and preferred providers of healthcare. This is a valuable resource for aging women concerned with locating reputable healthcare resources to support their positive aging health outcomes as well as help those that they care for.

National Council on the Aging

Address: 1901 L Street, NW, 4th Floor Washington, DC 20036
Telephone: 202-479-1200
Website: http://www.ncoa.org
Description: The National Council on the Aging (NCA) is an informational organization website providing information for older adults, elder advocates, eldercare givers, and practitioners working with aging populations. The website is user-friendly and offers helpful information regarding the quality of life of aging women, financial security (eg, information on reverse mortgages), positive aging in place (eg, falls prevention), food security (eg, community food programs), and opportunities for socializing with other older adults in the community (eg, local senior centers).

QUALITY OF LIFE IN AGING RESOURCES

Health in Aging Foundation

Address: 40 Fulton St., 18th floor, New York, NY
Telephone: 800-563-4916
Email: info@healthinaging.org
Website: www.healthinaging.org
Description: The Health in Aging Foundation website was created by the American Geriatrics Society for the purpose offering health advice and resources to older persons and those who are caring for older, aging individuals. Geriatric healthcare professionals can be located through the website as well as information about medications and other health-related topics in aging older adults.

United Nations, Ageing Social Policy and Development Division

Website: http://www.un.org/esa/socdev/ageing/
Description: This is a great website which offers a truly international perspective regarding advocacy and public policy initiatives to protect the rights of older persons across locations of the world. The stated mission of the organization is to implement initiatives which follow and satisfy the Madrid International Plan of Action on Ageing to create quality-of-life standards for all aging individuals. The website offers useful information regarding issues of poverty, family, disability, employment, community education, social integration, social protection, among other issues relevant to an aging society.

ELDER ABUSE AND NEGLECT PROTECTION RESOURCES

Clearinghouse on Abuse and Neglect of Older Adults

Address: College of Human Resources, University of Delaware, Newark, DE 19716
Telephone: 302-831-3525
Fax: 302-831-6081
Website: http://www.cane.udel.edu/
Description: This website is a wonderful clearinghouse of information related to all issues of elderly abuse and neglect. Information ranges from peer-reviewed articles, hearing transcripts, videos, agency reports, books, and other resources that can assist an aging woman in better

understanding her rights and responsibilities as both an elder caregiver and recipient.

Hosted by the University of Delaware Center for Community Research and Service, this website offers helpful web links, a large bibliography of informational resources, and a link to the National Center on Elder Abuse.

National Adult Protective Services Association

Address: 1900 13th Street Suite 303 Boulder, CO 80302
Telephone: 720-565-0906
Fax: 720-565-0438
Website: http://www.napsa-now.org/
Description: This is an extremely useful website for practical information and professional services related to the protection and the safety of older adults within communities across the world. Older adults can be some of the most vulnerable individuals in the community and protection of their rights is increasingly an ethical issue in society (eg, knowledge about protective services regarding physical, mental, and/or financial abuse at the hands of caregiver). Aging women would benefit from this knowledge about the many different resources in the community as well as nationwide that can protect them from harm or abuse.

National Association of States United for Aging and Disabilities (NASUAD)

Address: 1225 I Street, N.W., Suite 725 Washington, DC 20005
Telephone: 202-898-2578
Email: NCEA@nasua.org
Website: http://www.nasuad.org
Description: Formerly the National Association of State Units on Aging (NASUA), this organization advocates for both individuals with disabilities and aging adults. This organization encompasses 56 state and regional agencies focused on support services in the community and home. Older women would benefit the information presented in various publications, as well as information regarding public policy and state-related technical assistance that can be offered as resources for support in their lives and for those for whom they may be caring.

National Center on Elder Abuse

Address: 1225 I Street, N.W., Suite 725 Washington, DC 20005
Telephone: 202-898-2578
Email: NCEA@nasua.org
Website: http://www.ncea.aoa.gov

Description: Associate with administration on aging national center on elder abuse (CEA) presents useful information about what is elder abuse and how to stop or prevent it from occurring. This is a major ethical concern because there may be many "hidden" victims of elder abuse who do not feel that they can come forward and report it. For aging women, the knowledge about this potential threat to their quality of life can help them have a "voice" and be empowered to both avoid such situations and/or help others in such circumstances.

National Clearinghouse on Abuse in Later Life

Address: 1245 E. Washington Ave., Suite 150, Madison, WI 53703
Telephone: 608-255-0539
Fax: 608-255-3560
Email: ncall@wcadv.org
Website: http://www.ncall.us/
Description: This website offers a bill information for both the older adult being cared for as well as those that the older adult may be caring for and not adequately knowledgeable about resources and community support to engage in such activities. Women across her life span are typically the caregivers of others and is very important for them to understand all the different sources of information regarding legal options and various community awareness events and opportunities. Equally important is this information for women to avoid being victims of the many different forms of abuse, which are explained on this website.

Institute on Aging

Address: 2700 Geary Boulevard. San Francisco, CA 94118
Telephone: 415-447-1989, X513
Email: elderabuseprevention@ioaging.org
Website: http://www.ioaging.org
Description: The Institute on Aging website offers many different forums for support services for both care recipient and caregivers into later life. The website contains a drop-down menu with relevant topics in a blog as well as informational resources regarding services for elders and caregivers, adults with disabilities, elder protection, and general education/ training for older adults. The website deals with many different important quality-of-life issues such as suicide invention, grief support, and general crisis counseling. This website is wonderful resource for older women who may not have the social supports available to assist them in working through the many different stressors in later life.

Wisconsin Coalition Against Domestic Violence

Address: 307 South Paterson, Suite #1 Madison, WI 53703
Telephone: 608-255-0539
Fax: 608-255-3560
Email: wcadv@inxpress.net
Website: http://www.endabusewi.org/
Description: Domestic violence is one form of violence that can certainly be related to later life elder abuse for women. The website offers many different descriptions of ways to advocate and educate others. Within the community to help protect and support the many different survivors of domestic abuse within the state of Wisconsin. More importantly, the issues and education presented relates to any state and any country in the world. The website promotes the idea of educating service providers, legislators, law enforcement, and the general community in understanding and identifying signs of domestic violence in order to help victims and prevent future violence from occurring.

ALZHEIMER'S DISEASE SUPPORT SERVICES AND EDUCATION

Alzheimer's Foundation of America

Address: 322 Eighth Ave., 7th fl., New York, NY 10001
Telephone: 1-866-232-8484 (Toll-Free)
Website: http://www.alzfdn.org
Description: As the number of people living longer is increasing over the next four or more decades, the issue of better understanding and addressing issues related to Alzheimer's disease is an ethical and social imperative in many different countries across the world. The website offers a national toll-free helpline as well as important caregiving resources member support organizations and national events, which can benefit women either experiencing Alzheimer's firsthand or caring for others undergoing Alzheimer's disease. Knowledge is key to help support quality of life of women involved in such a family circumstance.

Alzheimer's Organization

Address: National office 225 N. Michigan Ave., Floor 17 Chicago, IL 60601-7633
Telephone: 312-335-8700
Fax: 866-699-1246
Website: http://www.alz.org

Description: This website by the national Alzheimer's Association organization has a wealth of information related to on-going research for both professionals and laypeople experiencing directly or indirectly exposure to Alzheimer's disease through care activities. The Alzheimer's Association website offers a comprehensive body of content ranging from local support resources to online learning and everything in between related to knowledge and caregiving tools to best support a growing segment of the national and international population living with Alzheimer's disease. Aging women, as has been said before, are by default caregivers of aging family members and thus need to consult informational websites such as this one help to better understand these age-related changes and associated caregiving support resources for their own positive aging outcomes as well as those that they care for.

DIVERSITY IN HEALTH EDUCATION RESOURCES

National Aging Pacific Center on Aging

Address: 1511 Third Avenue, #914 Seattle, WA 98101
Telephone: 800-336-2722
Fax: 206-624-1023
Website: http://www.napca.org
Description: The diversity of the aging experience is a critical social factor to acknowledge from the constituents within the aging population. This website does a great job of offering information from the many different perspectives of the aging experience: from the older adult to the family caregiver, to the service provider, to the public policy makers/legislators involved in elder advocacy issues. This organization is focused upon the quality of life in positive aging outcomes of both Asian-Americans and Pacific Islanders. In a broader sense, it might be argued that this website is wonderful "model" of how different aging subgroups may experience aging in a very culturally based qualitatively different way and thus need specific focus through both education and service provisions. Older women within the specific racial and ethnic communities would especially benefit from the information and resources provided on this website.

National Caucus and Center on Black Aging

Address: 1220 L Street NW, Suite 800, Washington, DC 20005
Telephone: 202-637-8400
Fax: 202-347-0895
Website: http://www.ncba-aged.org

Description: This website provides helpful information about diversity of aging experiences in many different ways for African-Americans age 50 and older. The variety of cultural and social factors affecting people's aging experiences is vital to understand as it relates to their positive aging outcomes in the United States and across the world. For aging African-American women, this website offers health links to informational resources, as well as social support services that can help them age well, as well as help those in their family and broader community. The National Caucus and Center on Black Aging (NCBA) organization has the purpose of empowering and promoting the well-being of a growing segment of aging adults in the African-American community and nation. Older women within the African-American community would benefit greatly from the information provided for their own positive aging.

National Hispanic Council on Aging

Address: The Walker Building, 734 15th Street NW Suite 1050, Washington, DC 20005
Telephone: 202-347-9733
Fax: 202-347-9735
Website: http://www.nhcoa.org
Description: The National Hispanic Council on Aging (NHCOA) website offers information and resources focused on promoting the quality of life of Hispanic older adults. The website presents helpful healthcare and advocacy information for both benefit of the older adults, their families, and the larger Hispanic community. News about public policies and community events for older adults and caregivers in the Hispanic community would benefit older women who are directly or indirectly dealing with aging issues.

National Indian Council on Aging

Address: 10501 Montgomery Blvd. N.E., Suite 210, Albuquerque, NM 87111
Telephone: 505-292-2001
Fax: 505-292-1922
Website: http://www.nicoa.org
Description: This website by the National Indian Council on Aging (NICOA) presents information for both aging adults and their caregivers, as well as policy makers, for the purposes of supporting and advocating for both American Indians and Alaska native elders. The economic well-being and social services/healthcare support of this population is emphasized through the organization's mission statement and

the resource presented. Aging women within these communities would significantly benefit from the information presented to enhance their "voice" in society.

Asociación Nacional Pro Personas Mayores

Address: National Association for Hispanic Elderly 234 East Colorado Boulevard, Suite 300 Pasadena, CA 91101
Telephone: 626-564-1988
Website: http://www.anppm.org/
Description: The website of the National Association for Hispanic elderly presents links to access a wide variety of services, community projects, and resources in the hopes of improving the quality of life for Hispanic individuals across many communities in the world. Services range from training for older workers to affordable housing opportunities. Different community projects range from Medicare outreach to emergency preparedness education. Resources range from health prevention to art and cultural events in local regions. This information would be very useful to aging Hispanic women, as well as others in their lives, who would benefit from such physical and mental health-related initiatives within communities.

American Foundation for the Blind (Aging Population)

Address: 2 Penn Plaza, Suite 1102 New York, NY 10121
Website: http://www.afb.org/seniorsitehome.asp
Description: The American Federation for the Blind (AFB) website offers supportive information and resources focused on issues of eye health into later life for aging women and those they may care for into later life. Information regarding conditions of glaucoma, cataracts, macular degeneration, and diabetic retinopathy is presented in understandable terms for older adults needing guidance in this life-changing aging issue. Practical issues of vision changes and its impact on everyday activities of conducting ADLs, IADLs, working, driving, and other daily activities. Personal stories, events, and other support resources are offered through this website that can help women both identify with aging vision as well as learn how to better cope with such changes.

Centers for Disease Control and Prevention

Address: Healthy Aging Program, 4770 Buford Highway, N.E., Mailstop F-78, Atlanta, GA 30341-3717
Telephone: 800-CDC-INFO or 800-232-4636
Website: http://www.cdc.gov/aging/

Description: The Centers for Disease Control (CDC) website presents great information on general aging topics related to promoting independence and well-being of an aging population. Aging women would benefit from accessing the materials presented in *Healthy Aging Program* and *The Healthy Brain* initiatives. Both research and practical advice is given to help older women optimize their aging outcomes in a comprehensive manner. Among other information, links within the website highlight aging-related topics of emergency preparedness, various health information links (eg, fall prevention), care planning, and early disease detection advice.

World Health Organization (WHO)/Ageing (Kobe Centre)

Address: Avenue Appia 20 1211, Geneva 27, Switzerland
Telephone: +41 22 791 21 11
Fax: +41 22 791 31 11
Website: http://www.who.int/kobe_centre/ageing/en/
Description: Through the research efforts of the WHO's Kobe Centre, reports and information is presented on "age-friendly cities," international aging trends and needs, and global health events for promoting positive aging across the world. Women from many different countries would benefit from the international information about support resources and public policies designed to assist with positive aging outcomes in many countries.

CAREGIVING SUPPORT ORGANIZATIONS

Family Caregiver Alliance

Address: 785 Market St., Suite 750, San Francisco, CA 94103
Telephone: 800-445-8106
Website: http://www.caregiver.org
Description: This website produced by the Family Caregiver Alliance (FCA) does a fantastic job presenting topics of interest for caregivers from every stage (planning, on-going, and post) and type of care (daily, in-home, and/or long-distance). Information regarding educational opportunities, caregiving support networks, and public policy information/initiatives is displayed on the website. The range of information will assist any woman planning, currently engaged, or transitioning to role closure in caregiving responsibilities (self-care, other's care).

Caregiver Action Network

Address: 1130 Connecticut Ave NW, Suite 300 Washington, DC 20036
Telephone: 202-454-3970

Email: info@caregiveraction.org

Website: http://www.caregiveraction.org

Description: The Caregiver Action Network (CAN) website is a very user-friendly resource tool for women who are seeking help in different life circumstances of being a caregiver. Not only focused on aging, this website presents different care topics that can certainly impact an aging woman's life (eg, adult aging children caring for aging parents with Alzheimer's disease). Helpful caregiving information, caregiving coping resources, and peer support resources are offered as links. This is a proactive resource which gives a "voice" to caregivers in many different ways, from the "Caregiver Voices" link to suggesting opportunities to become an advocate in the community.

HOUSING AND TRANSPORTATION ORGANIZATIONS

National Resource Center on Supportive Housing and Home Modification

Address: University of Southern California Andrus Gerontology Center, Los Angeles, CA 90089-0191

Telephone: 213-740-1364

Website: http://www.homemods.org/index.shtml

Description: This website represents a project of the National Resource Center on Supportive Housing and Home Modification, in affiliation with the Fall Prevention Center of Excellence, funded by the Archstone Foundation. The focus of the website is to offer training and information promoting initiatives toward "aging in place" and independent living for adults across the life span. The specific aim is to educate both laypeople and practitioners on home modification services and offers updated resource tools such as a National Directory of Home Modification and Repair Resources. Online courses are offered to help train individuals wanting to be proactive in personal home modifications to professionals working with aging clients faced with "aging in place" adjustment issues. This is a universal design topic that any aging woman would benefit from researching for personal aging or for other reasons (eg, care of an aging parent).

Rebuilding Together (Aging in Place)

Address: National Headquarters 1899 L Street NW, Suite 1000 Washington, DC 20036

Telephone: 1-800-473-4229

Website: http://rebuildingtogether.org/resource/age-in-place-checklist/

Description: Sponsored by *Rebuilding Together*, this website represents an initiative to help older adults live in their homes for extended periods of time (ie, "aging in place") with the avoidance of falls and optimization of functioning ability in the accomplishment of ADLs. The website represents on-going advocacy efforts initiatives in coordination with Area Agencies on Aging, AARP, American Occupational Therapy Association, National Association of Home Builders, National Council on Aging, and other related housing and aging organizations. A helpful checklist is offered, which can be a great tool for older women wishing to remain in their homes longer.

Rural Transit Assistance Program

Address: 122 C Street NW, Suite 520 Washington, DC 20001
Telephone: 202-772-2039
Fax: 202-772-3101
Website: http://www.nationalrtap.org/
Description: The website by the National Rural Transit Assistance Program (RTAP) Resource Library is a great resource for older women residing in rural areas of the United States who need to understand transportation resources in their community. Links on the website present rural transit-related materials, including training modules (webinars, "2 the Point" Training), reports, technical briefs, and articles that you can view, order, or download. Tribal transit is one of the resources offered. Access to transportation is a key aspect of positive aging outcomes for women and/or those who receive their care.

HOME-BASED AND FORMAL CARE SETTING ORGANIZATIONS

Assisted Living Federation of America

Address: 1650 King Street, Suite 602, Alexandria, VA 22314
Telephone: 703-894-1805
Fax: 703-894-1831
Website: http://www.alfa.org
Description: This Assisted Living Federation of America (ALFA) website is a wonderful informational resource regarding senior living communities. Advocacy issues covering residents' rights of autonomy in decision making, quality in care and overall dignity in treatment. ALFA's programs offer helpful professional development resources through educational opportunities, research reports, and networking opportunities to achieve professional excellence in senior living care. Aging women would benefit

from such as informational resource to assist in personal and/or family planning for present care needs and/or future eldercare.

Leading Age

Address: 2519 Connecticut Avenue NW, Washington, DC 20008
Telephone: 202-783-2242
Email: info@leadingage.org
Website: http://www.leadingage.org
Description: LeadingAge's website is a great resource for aging individuals and their families who need information on eldercare planning services, caregiving resources, and a directory of not-for-profit aging services across different aging needs, preferences, and situations. In addition to these informational resources, learning opportunities are provided through both online training courses and downloadable resource publications. Aging women would directly benefit from the information given regarding support services to achieve their own positive aging over time, as well as how to better care for others in their lives.

National Adult Day Services Association

Address: 1421 E. Broad Street, Suite 425 Fuquay Varina, NC 27526
Telephone: 877-745-1440
Fax: 919-825-3945
Email: info@NADSA.org
Website: http://www.nadsa.org
Description: The National Adult Day Services Association's (NADSA) website suggests questions to ask when deciding an adult day service center. From a practitioners' perspective, information regarding consumer-related factors in considering the quality of care services, public policy initiatives, and networking with experienced adult day services colleagues. Whether a layperson or a professional within the industry, the information and learning opportunities presented would benefit older women considering issues related to adult day services.

National Association for Home Care and Hospice

Address: 228 Seventh Street, SE, Washington, DC 20003
Telephone: 202-547-7424
Fax: 202-547-3540
Website: http://www.nahc.org
Description: The National Association for Home Care & Hospice's (NAHC) website advocates for the many different professionals who provide quality in-home care to older adults and other clients who are

chronically ill and/or disabled. Information is provided regarding ways to attain and maintain a high standard of care. Whether a professional within the industry or a family caregiver seeking care resources, the information presented would benefit older women considering issues related to in-home care services.

National Association of State Long-Term Care Ombudsman Programs

Address: 1414 Wayfield Lane, Mount Juliet, TN 37122
Telephone: 615-533-4856
Website: http://www.nasop.org
Description: The National Association of State Long-Term Care Ombudsman Programs' (NASOP) website presents important information regarding the mission of the Long-Term Care Ombudsman Program (ie, to seek resolution of problems and advocate for the rights of residents of long-term care facilities with the goal of enhancing the quality of life and care of residents). The website has interesting informational resource links related to this advocacy effort, from reports, position papers, services, and public policy information. Older women would learn much from the advocacy information presented, both for personal purposes and use as an impetus within the community.

National Consumer Voice for Quality Long-Term Care

Address: 1001 Connecticut Avenue, NW, Suite 425 Washington, DC 20036
Telephone: 202-332-2275
Fax: 866-230-9789
Email: info@theconsumervoice.org
Website: http://www.theconsumervoice.org/
Description: The Consumer Voice's website communicates the need to ensure consumers' rights in receiving ethical, quality long-term care services, and supports. The organization through its website provides supportive information and tools for many different key "stakeholders" in the eldercare process, from consumers, families, caregivers, advocates, and ombudsmen. Training individuals to be better long-term care consumers, training practitioners to be better able to achieve their goals of supplying quality care to aging clients, and empowering older adults and their families to be better advocates of quality care are just some of the efforts presented on the website. Whether a layperson or a professional within the industry, the information and learning opportunities presented would benefit older women considering issues related to long-term care services.

DIET AND NUTRITION ORGANIZATIONS

Meals on Wheels Association of America

Address: 413 N. Lee Street, Alexandria, VA 22314
Telephone: 888-998-6325
Fax: 703-548-5274
Website: http://www.mowaa.org
Description: The Meals on Wheels' website offers great background information regarding the mission of the organization to meet the physical and social needs of residents "aging in place" in communities. The role of a person as either a volunteer or a recipient of services is equally emphasized as a "quality of life" outcome for all involved in the community. This website would be helpful to aging women looking for either volunteer opportunities in their community or for services to address elder care issues of the self or others.

National Association of Nutrition and Aging Services Programs

Address: 1612 K Street, NW, Suite 400 Washington, DC 20006
Telephone: 202-682-6899
Fax: 202-223-2099
Email: pcarlson@nanasp.org
Website: http://www.nanasp.org
Description: National Association of Nutrition and Aging Services Programs' (NANASP) website offers information pertaining to local, state, and national public policies in maintaining a quality standard of nutrition and other services for a growing aging population. The information presents an aging network of organizations (eg, Elder Justice Coalition) and their associated advocacy efforts on many different levels within society. This information regarding agencies and organizations addressing the quality of care needs is important for all aging women, and should inspire further advocacy efforts with communities.

WORK, RETIREMENT, AND VOLUNTEERISM ORGANIZATIONS

International Social Security Association

Website: http://www.issa.int
Description: The International Social Security Association's (ISSA) website displays great informational links regarding excellence in social security systems from a global perspective. Expert advice and other helpful

resources educate both laypeople and experts faced with this growing societal, financial issue. Aging women would benefit from reviewing the international information on this important topic, which impacts later quality of life for all members of society.

OECD Pensions

Website: http://www.oecd.org/insurance/privatepensions/

Description: This website by OECD Pensions presents illuminating information regarding critical topics of population aging and its final implications, pension changes and reforms; private pensions, retirement savings, and retirement strategies in both OECD and non-OECD countries. The organization advocates an international perspective in understanding pension trends and what is needed regarding international public policy initiatives to best support this growing international aging population. Aging women facing the affordability of retirement would benefit from the information presented on this website.

International Social Security Programs

Website: http://www.ssa.gov/policy/docs/progdesc/

Description: This website presents an in-depth description of the programs under the Social Security Act and explains how these programs operate in response to an aging populations. Information about different programs is organized into different categories that are easy to search (ie, assistance programs, health insurance, social insurance, and services for specific group constituencies, such as aging veterans). Annual publications are offered as links which explain eligibility provisions and the maximum levels of assistance for aging individuals and/or couples receiving supplementary payments. This information would help educate and empower aging women who need to better understand their financial status as they prepare to retire or adjust to retirement.

Service Corp of Retired Executives

Address: Washington, DC Chapter (Different Locations by State), 409 3rd Street, SW Suite 100A, Washington, DC 20024

Telephone: 202-619-1000

Website: https://www.score.org/

Description: The Service Corp of Retired Executives (SCORE) website is a great informational website about how retired older adults can give back to their communities and offer their vast areas of expertise to help others in their world. The organizations conveys an empowering message that older adults' wisdom is to be societally valued and utilized. This is a great social message to aging women who are looking for ways to be more active in their communities, benefitting their own positive aging and those of others that they come in contact with through their mentoring efforts.

Senior Corps—Corporation for National and Community Service

Address: 1201 New York Avenue, NW Washington, DC 20525
Telephone: 202-606-5000
Fax: 800-833-3722
Email: info@cns.gov
Website: http://www.nationalservice.gov/programs/senior-corps
Description: Senior Corps' website is a great resource for both laypeople aged 55 years or older and practitioners working with this growing segment of the world population. The website gives information and resources to assist people in becoming companions, coaches, and/or mentors to older adults in need through community projects and organizations. Volunteers find information about how to best serve the community while also enriching their own lives and aging outcomes. Volunteer programs include the "Foster Grandparents" program which older volunteers help young children learn how to read and the "Senior Companions" program which offers respite time and support for formal or informal caregivers as well as help for the care recipients. Older women would benefit from the greatly benefits from the opportunities to be active community volunteers in their lives.

Urban Institute: Older Workers

Address: 2100 M Street NW, Washington, DC 20037
Telephone: 202-833-7200
Website: http://www.urban.org/research-area/older-workers
Description: This website by the Urban Institute offers up-to-date research and information related to changing workforce trends in response to an aging population. This information would be helpful for aging women across the world who are dealing with different issues related to staying or re-entering the workforce in later life.

Urban Institute: Retirement Policy

Address: 2100 M Street NW, Washington, DC 20037
Telephone: 202-833-7200
Website: http://www.urban.org/retirees/index.cfm

Description: This website by the Urban Institute offers up-to-date research and information related to public policies on retirement trends in response to an aging population. This information would be very assistive for aging women who are preparing to make the transition or are currently in retirement and who need to optimize the retirement experience of aging.

Index

Note: Page numbers followed by "*b*" refer to boxes.

A

ACTIVE (Advanced Cognitive Training for Independent and Vital Elderly), 110
Active social participation, 254
Active Start, 131
Activity of daily living (ADL), 273–275
Activity theory, 13, 75, 186, 254
Adaptation to aging
  definition, 27
  tips for women, 32*b*
Aerobic exercise, 123–124
Age Discrimination and Employment Act, 1967, 223
"Age friendly" for women, 143–144
Age of Champions documentary, 127*b*
Aging
  anxiety, 88–89
  assisted living and, 191
  changing living situations with, 150–151
  in a community setting, 32, 192
  double standard of, 241
  female "baby boomers", 59–60
  knowledge and attitude surveys, 289
  in place, 190–191, 258–259
  quality-of-life factors, 152–156
    aging women's financial resources/opportunities, 153
    mobility status, 153
    physical and mental health, 152–153
    social support for older women, 153–154
    societal attitudes toward aging women, 154–155
  research, 3–4
Aging self-acceptance, 51
  cultural roles and, 51–52
  education and mental health interventions, 54–56
  optimizing, 63
  personal adjustments to, 54–56
  physical, 52–53

  positive psychosocial adjustment and, 58–60
  predictor of, 62–63
  realistic aging and sense of self, 60–63
  societal feedback and its impact on, 53–54
  tips for, 55*b*
  words of wisdom, 55*b*–56*b*
Aging women's mental health
  outcomes, factors determining, 10–12
    social belongingness, 11
    technology, 11
  quality of life and, 7–8
  role of culture in, 12
Aging women's resources and mental health, 5
  famous quotes, 5*b*
  impact of caregiver role, 4–5
  "mind-body" connection, 8–10
  tips for positive mental health, 6*b*
  websites regarding cultural ideas, 7*b*
Alzheimer's disease support services and education
  Alzheimer's Association, 313–314
  Alzheimer's Foundation of America, 313
"Appropriate" aging reactions and coping mechanisms for aging women, 145

B

Bandura's concept of enactive mastery, 58
Beauty, concept of, 93
Beauty culture, 88–89
"Better aged" societies, 143–144
Body image, older women's adaptive reactions to, 87–89
  adaptive protection against a negative body image, 88
Botulinum toxin type A ("Botox") injections, 93
Brain drain, 221, 258–259

Brief Aging Perceptions Questionnaire, 61–62
Brief Resilient Coping Scale, 4

C

Career work life expectancy, strategies to improve, 225–226
 continual skill updating, 228
 employability enhancing practice, 224–225
 long-term career succession planning, 228
 skill assessments, need for, 228–229
Caregiver role, in aging woman's positive, 4–5, 30, 150
 feeling of a "role reversal" in caring for aging parents, 172
Caregiving support organizations
 Caregiver Action Network (CAN), 317–318
 Family Caregiver Alliance (FCA), 317
CHAMPS (Community Health Activities Model Programming for Seniors), 131
Civic engagement of aging women, 251–252
 benefits of, 252–260
 active social participation, 254
 extended social support resources, 253–254
 having a "voice" in politics and community activities, 255
 intergenerational learning and mentoring, 252–253
 mentoring from experienced older adults, 255–260
 positive "role models" of aging, 255
 tips for, 258b
 words of wisdom, 259b
Civic Engagement Scale, 256b–258b
Cognitive decline, 106
Cognitive functioning, 110
Contact hypothesis, 244
Continuity theory, 75–76
Convoy, 187
Cosmetic surgery, 91–92
Culture, role in aging women's positive mental health, 12, 146, 154–155, 260
 cultural roles and aging self-acceptance, 51–52
 degree of women's aging acceptance, 59–60
"Culture" of youth, 91–93

D

Daily physical activity for older women
 amount of, 129b
 moderate-intensity activities, 129
 vigorous activities, 129
 barriers to working out, 128–130
 "beginning" vs "maintaining" an exercise regime, 125
 behavioral intentions, 131
 being active, benefit of, 121–123
 body, influence on, 124
 brain, influence on, 123–124
 factors supporting, 125–128
 motivation, 127
 sense of community, 125–127
 famous quotes, 123b
 promotion of regular exercise, 130–131
 recommendations/interventions, 130–132
 tips for, 130b
 utilization of assistive devices during, 128
 walking, 131–132
 words of wisdom, 126b
 workplace interventions, 131
Defy aging, 53–54
Diet and nutrition organizations
 Meals on Wheels Association of America, 322
 National Association of Nutrition and Aging Services Programs' (NANASP), 322
Disengagement theory, 186
Diversity, 143–144
 "aging paradigm" and, 148–149
 famous quotes, 148b
 quality-of-life perceptions and, 146–148
 words of wisdom, 155b
Double jeopardy bias, 4, 9, 149–150
Double standard of aging, 241
Downward social comparison, 89–90

E

Ecology of women's positive aging, 31–33
Educational achievement and health and longevity, 106–107
Education for women, 151–152
Effective self-regulation, 73
"Ego integrity" psychosocial stage, 58
Elder abuse and neglect protection resources
 Clearinghouse on Abuse and Neglect of Older Adults, 310–311
 Institute on Aging, 312

National Adult Protective Services Association, 311
National Association of States United for Aging and Disabilities (NASUAD), 311
National Center on Elder Abuse, 311–312
National Clearinghouse on Abuse in Later Life, 312
Wisconsin Coalition Against Domestic Violence, 313
Emotional reaction of getting older, 54–56
Empowerment of older women, 260
Erikson's theory, 58
Ethnicity, and developmental experiences, 148–149
Experienced workforce quiz, 297–299

F
Family relationships and health and longevity, 105
Female "baby boomers," aging, 59–60, 259–260
Feminization of poverty, 4, 57, 278
Fit, being, 145, 156

G
Gendered ageism, 93
Gender identity and positive aging, 151
Gender role, 169–170
General aging information resources
Alliance for Aging Research, 307
American Association of Retired Persons (AARP), 306–307
American Society on Aging (ASA), 307
Association for Gerontology in Higher Education (AGHE), 308
Gerontological Society of America (GSA), 308
HelpAge International, 308
Leadership Council of Aging Organizations, 309
National Association of Area Agencies on Aging (n4a), 309
National Council on the Aging (NCA), 309
National Institute in Aging (NIH), 306
Generational experiences of woman's aging, 149
Generativity, 221
Gerontophobia, 88–89
Gerotranscendance, 38–39
Grandparents, 11–12

H
Halo effect of attractiveness, 90–91
Happy Neuron, 74
Harmonious aging, 4–5, 144
balance between mental health and functional status, 4–5
Health and longevity
benefits of never smoking, or quitting smoking, 108–109
educational achievement and, 106–107
family relationships and, 105
income level and, 102–104
interventions for, 109–111
physical activity, role of, 107–108
relationship between marital status and longevity, 105
social support interventions, 104–106, 110
socioeconomic status, role of, 102–103
Health education resources
American Foundation for the Blind (Aging Population), 316
Asociación Nacional Pro Personas Mayores, 316
Centers for Disease Control and Prevention, 316–317
National Aging Pacific Center on Aging, 314
National Caucus and Center on Black Aging, 314–315
National Hispanic Council on Aging (NHCOA), 315
National Indian Council on Aging, 315–316
World Health Organization (WHO)/ Ageing (Kobe Centre), 317
Health-related risks, 34–35
Healthy aging, 102–103
Healthy People 2020, 104*b*
Home-based and formal care setting organizations
Assisted Living Federation of America, 319–320
Leading Age, 320
National Adult Day Services Association's (NADSA), 320
National Association for Home Care & Hospice's (NAHC), 320–321
National Association of State Long-Term Care Ombudsman Programs' (NASOP), 321
National Consumer Voice for Quality Long-Term Care, 321

Housing and transportation organizations
National Resource Center on Supportive
Housing and Home Modification,
318
Rebuilding Together (Aging in Place),
318–319
Rural Transit Assistance Program, 319
Hypoactive Sexual Desire Disorder
(HSDD), 207

I

Implicit Association Test (IAT), 92, 243–244
Income, 102–104
Individual differences in the aging
experience for women, 146
Intergenerational learning and mentoring,
252–253
Internalized self-identity, 148–149

J

Job centrality, 220–221
Job involvement, 220–221

K

"Know thyself" in context of personal
aging, 60–62

L

Later-life role transitions of women, 6–7,
56–57
health-related risks and, 34–35
sleeping behavior, 6
social-economic status, perceived, 6
social roles, 6
work and retirement, 35
Learned helplessness, 37
Lookism, 91

M

Maslow's hierarchy of needs model, 58–59
Mature worker
advantages of a, 222–223
stereotypes of, 223–225
tips for, 222*b*
McCoy Female Sexuality Questionnaire,
205
Mental aerobics, 71, 170–172
famous quotes, 73*b*
idea of continual cognitive engagement,
73
interventions with older women, 74
later-life health correlation with, 75–77

older women and, 71–72
as a preventative or rehabilitative factor
for aging women, 74–75
tips for, 74*b*
Mental exercise interventions and positive
aging, 72. *See also* Mental aerobics
Mentoring, 252–253, 255–260
Mind-body connection in aging women's
mental health, 8–10, 33, 71–72

N

National and international women's
organizations
Advancing Women, 302
Canadian Network of Women's Shelters
and Transition Houses, 305
The Lilac Tree, 302
Mentoring Women's Network
Foundation, 301
Office of Women's Health, US
Department of Health and Human
Services, 306
Office of Women's Policy and Initiatives,
303
Older Women's League, 303–304
Red Hat Society, 304
Strong Women, 304–305
Supportive Older Women's Network
(SOWN), 304
Wing to Wing Women's Mentoring
Project, 302–303
Women for Women International, Global
Headquarters, 305
Women's Business Development Center,
301–302
Women's Institute for a Secure
Retirement, 305–306
Women's Resource Center, 303
Nonnormative events, 146, 152
Normative biological events, 146
Normative historical events, 146

O

Older woman
role within a culture, 7–8
social power, empowerment, and coping
of, 7–8
resiliency responses, 8
Older Women's Activity Questionnaire,
122
On-the-job protection of aging worker, 225
"Other focused" orientation, 31–32

P

Physical activity, 107–108, 144–145. *See also* Daily physical activity for older women
  aerobics, 153
Physical aging, women's adaptive reactions to, 87
  body image, 87–89
  famous quotes, 89*b*
  "halo effect of attractiveness", 90–91
  psychological mechanisms and cognitive biases, 89–91
  role of "rosy retrospection", 90
  tips for, 90*b*
Physical aging self-acceptance, 52–53
Positive aging attitudes and adaptation, 3–4, 51, 101–102, 143–146, 186
  aging self-acceptance. *See* Aging self-acceptance
  to biological changes, 39–40
  ecology of, 31–33
  famous quotes, 30*b*, 52*b*, 104*b*, 226*b*, 241*b*, 271*b*
  gender issues, 155–156
  lifespan factors predicting, 144
  "mind-body" connection for aging women, 8–10
  personal control, 37–38
  positive cultural attitudes and influences, 37–38
  psychological resilience, 37
  social roles influences, 30
  societal "messages" of, 13–15
  with spirituality, 38–39
  stereotypes impacting, 237–241
  subjective perceptions, 10
  tips for promoting, 239*b*
  value of education and, 39–40
  at workplace, 222
Positive psychosocial adjustment and self-actualization, 58–60
Positive "role models" of aging, 255
Positivity Scale, 9
"Programmed theories" of aging, 175–176
Pro-older adults, 243–244
Psychological resilience, 37
Public policies for aging population, 269
  early retirement policy and programs, 278
  evolving definition of "later adulthood", 270–271
  "quality-of-life" standards, 270

social image of an "older woman" in different cultures, 271–272
  specific issues of supports, 272–279
  eldercare resources and caregiver supports, 276–277
  financial protections and resources, 273
  future workplace changes, training, and job security, 277–279
  health care coverage, 275–276
  housing and transportation, 273–275
  words of wisdom, 275*b*

Q

Quality of life in aging resources
  Health in Aging Foundation, 310
  United Nations, Ageing Social Policy and Development Division, 310

R

Race, and developmental experiences, 148–149
Realistic aging and sense of self, 60–63
Realistic aging processes, 3
Red Hat Society, 188
Regular exercisers, 125–127
Reproductive capacity, 93
Residential relocation, 185–186
Resiliency responses to aging, 8
  definition, 27
  generativity activities in a society, 33–35
  health-related stress level and functional status, 9
  as a learning process, 7–8
  personal growth, 33–35
  personal patterns of, 35
  quality-of-life outcomes and, 32
  social roles and, 4–5
  in Westernized cultures, 6
Retirement
  early, policy and programs, 278
  issues related to, 219–220. *See also* Work
Role conflict, 169–170
Role theory, 169–170
Rosy retrospection, 90

S

Selective optimization with compensation, 6
Self-efficacy scores, 128
Self-esteem in later adulthood, 51, 59
  social comparison of, 89–90
  working-related, 227

"Self-focused" orientation, 31–32
Self-fulfilling prophecy, 37
Self-regulation theory, 73
Sexual Aversion Disorder (SAD), 207
Sexuality and aging women, 56, 201–203
   barriers, 203–205
   biology of women's later-life sexual
      desire, 205–208
   famous quotes, 204b
   gender identity in later life, 151
   positive supports for, 208–210
   predictors of sexual desire, 210
   sexual arousal, 207–208
   sexual drive and desire, 207
   tips for sexual health, 209b
   treatment options for sexual dysfunction,
      208–210
      "biopsychosocial" approach to
         improve, 209–210
      sexual "homework" exercises, 208
   words of wisdom, 206b
"Similar to me" bias, 148–149
Smoking, 108–109
Social belongingness, 59
Social capital, 11
Social engagement, 75, 186
Social image of an "older woman" in
   different cultures, 271–272
Social optimization, 170
Social reciprocity of care, 58
Social relationships in aging adults,
   186–188
Social support. See also Public policies for
   aging population
   associated with widowhood, 57
   extended social support resources,
      253–254
   importance of, 185–186
      physical and mental/cognitive health,
         189–192
   quality and function of, 188–189
   quality of life and, 104–106, 110
   role of genetics, 188–189
   tips for aging women's, 189b
   words of wisdom, 190b–191b
Societal "messages" of women's positive
   aging, 13–15
Societal status for older women, 149–150
   of paid employment, 173–174
Socioeconomic status, 102–103
Socioemotional selectivity, 187
Socioemotional selectivity theory, 187

Spirituality, 38–39
Stereotypes of aging women
   associated with poor health outcomes,
      242
   harmfulness of, 241–243
   impacting positive aging, 237–241
   implicit age stereotypes, 240
   interventions for combating, 243–244
   negative stereotypes, 238
   pitying stereotype, 240
   "trumped" gender stereotypes, 240
   words of wisdom, 238b–239b
Stimulating cognitive exercises, benefits of,
   74–75
Successful aging, 101–102
Superwoman syndrome, 6, 172

T
Tant culture, 56–57
Theory of planned behavior, 131
Triple jeopardy, 9, 91, 277–278

U
Usual aging, 101–102

W
Wear and Tear theory, 175–176
"Women in the middle," idea of, 175–176
Women's effective senior activism, 272b
Women's roles in societies
   concept of a social optimization with
      compensation strategy with social
      roles, 170
   different role responsibilities of women,
      171
   expansion and change of, 170–172
   famous quotes, 170b, 176b
   multiple, 172–175
      elder caregiving role, 172–173
      volunteer and other social activities,
         174–175
      work and retirement roles, 173–174
   quality of women's aging and, 176–177
   social engagement activities, 174–175
   tips for balancing, 171b
   within-role task expansion, 175–177
Womentoring, 255–256
Work
   advantages of a mature worker, 222–223
   career work life expectancy, strategies to
      improve, 225–226

on-the-job protection, 223
positively aging at workplace, 222
psychological function of, 220–222
relationship between job satisfaction and
    age, 221
tips for aging women workers, 222b
white-collar jobs, 227–228
Work, retirement, and volunteerism
    organizations
International Social Security
    Association's (ISSA), 322–323

International Social Security Programs,
    323
OECD Pensions, 323
Senior Corps—Corporation for National
    and Community Service, 324
Service Corp of Retired Executives
    (SCORE), 323–324
Urban Institute: Older Workers, 324
Urban Institute: Retirement Policy,
    324–325

Printed in the United States
By Bookmasters